Thoracoscopy for Pulmonologists

Thoracoscopy for Pulmonologists

A Didactic Approach

Philippe Astoul • GianFranco Tassi

Jean-Marie Tschopp

Editors

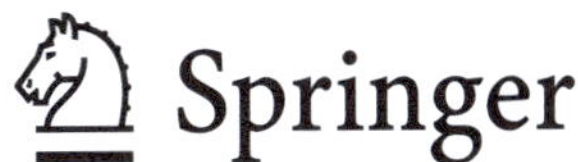
Springer

Editors
Philippe Astoul
Division of Thoracic Oncology, Pleural
Diseases, and Interventional Pulmonology
Hôpital NORD
Marseille
France

Jean-Marie Tschopp
Département de Médecine Interne
Centre valaisan de pneumologie
CHCVs
Montana
Switzerland

GianFranco Tassi
Divisione di Pneumologia
Spedali Civili di Brescia
Brescia
Italy

ISBN 978-3-662-50592-2   ISBN 978-3-642-38351-9   (eBook)
DOI 10.1007/978-3-642-38351-9
Springer Heidelberg New York Dordrecht London

Foreword

Carlo Forlanini, in Pavia, in 1882, had the brilliant idea to create, by simple air insufflation in the pleural space, an artificial pneumothorax for the treatment of tuberculous cavities in an attempt to 'put the lung to rest'. Unfortunately, in a significant number of cases, pleural adhesions would not allow complete lung collapse, limiting the impact of the procedure. This limitation was eventually addressed by Hans Jacobeus who in 1910 performed the first thoracoscopy using a cystoscope in Stockholm. This simple but ingenious procedure pioneered the field of minimally invasive surgery and laparoscopy.

Therefore pleuroscopy, before being recognized primarily as a diagnostic tool, served a therapeutic purpose by allowing lysis of pleural adhesions via electrocautery, hereby allowing for complete collapse of the lung then regarded as an effective treatment for tuberculosis in the pre-streptomycin era. The instruments used at the time had of course a number of limitations. One important issue was the poor visibility of the pleural space. The operator was often tempted to increase the intensity and the light bulb would frequently burn out, requiring the operator to hold temporarily the procedure in order to replace the defective equipment. This was clearly not an ideal scenario.

Later on, endoscopic photography, then cinema, was developed in the 1940s by P. Holinger in Chicago and Hashimoto in 1952. In France, Fourestier-Gladu-Vulmiere introduced his endoscope equipped with a camera, which was quite successful, and was quickly adopted for a host of procedures including thoracoscopy.

A number of individuals should also be mentioned for their valuable contributions to the field of thoracoscopy, including Sattler in Austria, Brandt in Berlin and Swierenga in the Netherlands. The equipment used for thoracoscopy gradually improved, with many contributions from the companies Storz and Wolf, and the technique rapidly spread throughout the world.

Surgeons eventually adopted the technique in the 1970s and 1980s and expanded its indications, ushering the era of video-assisted thoracoscopic surgery (VATS), whereas pulmonologists continued to develop 'medical thoracoscopy' introducing novel techniques such as flexible-rigid thoracoscopy and mini-thoracoscopy.

The current book edited by Philippe Astoul, GianFranco Tassi and Jean-Marie Tschopp is proof that the field continues to advance. These experts in medical thoracoscopy are internationally recognized for their clinical competence, educational qualities and efforts and contributions to the medical literature. As a result, the authors of this book have come from many geographic backgrounds, attesting of the remarkable international network of experts developed throughout their careers. The Art of Teaching demonstrated in this book is unparalleled, whether the concepts taught are simple ('so simple to do') or complex. The potential for knowledge acquisition offered through this book is in my view exceptional.

I congratulate the editors for the remarkable achievement and wish with all my heart that this book will meet the success it deserves.

Marseille, France   Christian Boutin

Preface

Over the last two decades, the increased incidence of pleural-related disease has added a significant workload for pulmonologists. It is now accepted that thoracoscopy is an integral component and best practice in the workup of pleural pathology. Indeed, thoracoscopy has become the cornerstone investigation for the pleura and allows accurate diagnosis, staging and, in many cases, therapeutic options. There is great worldwide interest from pulmonologists in this procedure, and this can be easily appreciated at the many courses dedicated to the technique. Indeed, these courses are frequently oversubscribed, and there are often long waiting lists to obtain training. We therefore believe that a new 'practical thoracoscopy book' (the first was published in 1991) is long overdue.

Advances in medical technologies have frequently resulted in new and potentially less invasive techniques. In the setting of diagnostic and therapeutic chest procedures, a distinction must be made between thoracoscopy done by pulmonologists, which may be video assisted, and surgical thoracoscopy or video-assisted thoracoscopic surgery (VATS). In all cases where a chest tube is required, it should take a pulmonologist only a few additional minutes to introduce an endoscope via the same incision, to inspect the pleura, to locate any adhesions, to obtain pleural samples and to verify that the chest tube is well positioned. In patients with primary pleural cancer, thoracoscopy has consistently been demonstrated as the only procedure capable of obtaining a diagnosis at an early stage of the disease. In other diseases associated with a pleural effusion, direct vision biopsy has a diagnostic rate of more than 95 % of patients.

This dedicated book discusses the considerable progress made with this technique. These advances are due to improvements in the endoscopic telescopes with extremely high optical quality despite their very small diameter, high-quality instruments – including video camera, forceps, endoscopic scalpel and stapler. All of these tools enable the physician or surgeon to carry out interventional thoracoscopy. The progress in anaesthetic care has allowed physicians to perform thoracoscopy in a range of setting from local anaesthesia in an outpatient facility to general anaesthesia in theatre. This book will provide the reader with a clear, concise and practical guide to the technique. This will allow the operator to perform a full exploration of the pleural cavity but at the same time utilizing a technique which is much less invasive and incapacitating than thoracotomy. The technique is associated with few complications – especially when the procedure is performed according to appropriate recommendations.

It is clear that this book is the result of a long collaboration by all members of the 'thoracoscopy' family spread throughout the world and especially in Europe. We thank all these pulmonologists for their enthusiasm, commitment, creativity and open-mindedness which has mirrored the spirit of Christian Boutin, who is generally accepted as the father of modern thoracoscopy.

Finally, we would like to thank Richard Wolf GmbH (Knittlingen – Germany) for its continued support over the years. They have readily listened to physicians and this has allowed ongoing improvement of the instruments used for this technique.

Marseille, France
Brescia, Italy
Montana, Switzerland

Philippe Astoul
GianFranco Tassi
Jean-Marie Tschopp

Contents

Part VI Future in the Field of Thoracoscopy

Contributors

Philippe Astoul Division of Thoracic Oncology, Pleural Diseases, and Interventional Pulmonology, Hôpital NORD, Marseille, France

Andrew Bentley Department of Respiratory and Intensive Care Medicine, North West Lung Center, Manchester Academic Health Science Centre, University Hospital of South Manchester, Manchester, UK

David P. Breen Department of Respiratory Medicine, Galway University Hospitals, Galway, Ireland

Martin H. Brutsche Division of Pneumology, Kantonsspital St. Gallen, St. Gallen, Switzerland

Miltiadis G. Chrysanthidis Department of Pulmonology, Sismanoglio Hospital, Athens, Greece

Cyrus Daneshvar Department of Respiratory Medicine, Galway University Hospitals, Galway, Ireland

Robert J.O. Davies Department of Respiratory Medicine, Oxford Pleural Unit, Oxford Centre for Respiratory Medicine, Oxford Radcliffe Hospital, Churchill Hospital Site, Oxford, UK

Antoine Delage Department of Pulmonology, Thoracic Oncology, and Intensive Care, Hôpital Pasteur, Nice, France

Christophe Dooms Pulmonology Department, University Hospital Gasthuisberg, Leuven, Belgium

Wolfgang Frank Department of Pulmonary Diseases, Lungenklinik, AmseeWaren, Müritz, Germany

Marios Froudarakis Department of Pulmonology, University Hospital of Alexandroupolis, Alexandroupolis, Greece

Seamus Grundy NIHR Translational Research Facility, University Hospital of South Manchester, Manchester, UK

Jeroen Hendriks Department of Surgery, University Hospital Antwerp, Edegem, Belgium

Felix Herth Department of Pneumology and Critical Care Medicine, Thoraxklinik/University of Heidelberg, Heidelberg, Germany

Atsuko Ishida Division of Respiratory and Infectious Diseases, Department of Internal Medicine, St Marianna University School of Medicine, Kawasaki, Japan

Julius Janssen Department of Pulmonary Diseases, Canisius Wilhelmina Hospital, Nijmegen, The Netherlands

Patrick Lauwers Department of Thoracic and Vascular Surgery, Antwerp University Hospital, Antwerp, Belgium

Gian Pietro Marchetti Division of Pneumology, Spedali Civili di Brescia, Brescia, Italy

Charles-Hugo Marquette Department of Pulmonology, Thoracic Oncology, and Intensive Care, Hôpital Pasteur, Nice, France

Teruomi Miyazawa Division of Respiratory and Infectious Diseases, Department of Internal Medicine, St Marianna University School of Medicine, Kawasaki, Japan

Daniella Negrini Department of Experimental and Clinical Biomedical Sciences, University of Insubria, Varese, Italy

Marc Noppen Interventional Endoscopy Clinic, University Hospital UZ Brussel, Brussels, Belgium

Bernard Paelinck Department of Cardiology, Antwerp University Hospital, Antwerp, Belgium

Francisco Rodríguez-Panadero Unidad Médico-Quirúrgica de Enfermeda des Respiratorias, Hospital Universitario Virgen del Rocío, Sevilla, Spain

Beatriz Romero Romero Unidad Médico-Quirúrgica de Enfermeda des Respiratorias Hospital Universitario Virgen del Rocío, Sevilla, Spain

Saiyad A. Sarkar Pulmonary and Critical Care Department, Franklin Square Hospital Center, Baltimore, MD, USA

Nicolas Schönfeld Department of Pulmonology, Lungenklinik Heckeshorn, HELIOS Klinikum Emil von Behring, Berlin, Germany

GianFranco Tassi Division of Pneumology, Spedali Civili di Brescia, Brescia, Italy

Pascal Thomas Division of Thoracic Surgery, Hôpital NORD, Marseille, France

Delphine Trousse Division of Thoracic Surgery, Hôpital NORD, Marseille, France

Jean-Marie Tschopp Département de Médecine Interne Centre valaisan de pneumologie, CHCVs, Montana, Switzerland

Johan Vansteenkiste Respiratory Oncology Unit (Pulmonology) and Leuven Lung Cancer Group, University Hospital Gasthuisberg, Leuven, Belgium

Paul Van Schil Department of Thoracic and Vascular Surgery, Antwerp University Hospital, Antwerp, Belgium

Part I

The Pleura and Thoracoscopy Technique

Introduction to the Pleura and Thoracoscopy Technique

1

Philippe Astoul, GianFranco Tassi,
and Jean-Marie Tschopp

One hundred years ago, Jacobeus published the first paper describing the technique of thoracoscopy. The procedure became well known and played an important role as a first treatment for tuberculosis before the advent of chemotherapy. It is important to look to the past to better understand the new developments of this technique. In the 1950s, medical thoracoscopy was neglected in Great Britain and the United States of America, simply because it was considered out of date. However in some chest centers of continental Europe, especially in Berlin (Germany) and Marseille (France), pulmonologists went on using this technique and developed tools allowing not only a better view of the thoracic cavity but combining also the videothoracoscopy with new tools such as ultrasounds of the pleura. In the same way, the technique of sedation and local anesthesia and the great improvements in the equipment available have made this technique simple, provided physicians desiring to perform thoracoscopy receive good training and have access to the experience developed over the years.

P. Astoul (✉)
Division of Thoracic Oncology, Pleural Diseases,
and Interventional Pulmonology, Hôpital NORD,
Marseille, France
e-mail: pastoul@ap-hm.fr

G. Tassi
Division of Pneumology, Spedali Civili di Brescia,
Brescia, Italy
e-mail: gf.tassi@tin.it

J.-M. Tschopp
Département de Médecine Interne
Centre valaisan de pneumologie,
CHCVs, Montana 3963, Switzerland
e-mail: jean-marie.tschopp@hopitalvs.ch

P. Astoul et al. (eds.), *Thoracoscopy for Pulmonologists*,
DOI 10.1007/978-3-642-38351-9_1, © Springer-Verlag Berlin Heidelberg 2014

Thoracoscopy: An Old Technique for a Modern Work-Up of the Pleural Cavity

Gian Pietro Marchetti and GianFranco Tassi

2.1 Introduction

Internal exploration of a living (human) body – endoscopy, from the Greek *endo* (inside) and *skopein* (to observe with care) – was always the aspiration of physicians. However, until the beginning of the nineteenth century, it was simply not possible to perform – through a lack of scientific knowledge and unavailability of appropriate instruments.

2.2 Precursors

The first endoscopists were probably the gynaecologists of antiquity, if we accept the fact that the speculum was the first endoscopic instrument. Hippocrates referred to a "speculum" used to examine the rectum, and in the Roman period, similar instruments were developed to a high degree of sophistication. Excavations at Pompeii and Herculaneum produced a large number of particularly well-made instruments, and Avicenna makes mention of them in his writings.

But recent history in this field began in the early nineteenth century with Philipp Bozzini, a gynaecologist from Frankfurt. He carried out internal examinations using a concave mirror with light from a wax candle inside a tin tube covered with leather, creating an instrument which in 1806 was named "*Lichtleiter*" (light conductor) (Bozzini 1806).

The term "endoscopy" was first coined by the French urologist Desormeaux (Desormeaux 1865). He was a leading pioneer in this field and designed a cystoscope which used an intense white light which was produced by a mixture of alcohol and turpentine. This method provided clinically acceptable results. In 1868, Adolf Kussmaul, a German physician, attempted to view the stomach by means of a straight rigid metal tube, illuminated by the Desormeaux method. Later, in Berlin the urologist Maximilian Nitze used an incandescent platinum wire on the tip of the instrument for illumination. In 1877 he presented his cystoscope for the first time. It was the true forerunner of all modern instruments.

With regard to thoracic endoscopy, the "Father" of rigid bronchoscopy, Gustav Killian, should be remembered. He was a German laryngologist at the University of Freiburg, and in 1897 he succeeded in extracting a foreign body from the right bronchus under local anaesthesia (Killian 1898).

The first physician to observe the pleural cavity in vivo was the Irish endoscopist *Richard Francis Cruise* in 1866. He designed a binocular cystoscope illuminated by a camphor-based mixture. Working with Samuel Gordon, an internist from Dublin, he introduced the instrument through a pleuracutaneous fistula and examined the pleural cavity of a child suffering from

G.P. Marchetti (✉) • G. Tassi
Division of Pneumology, Spedali Civili di Brescia,
Brescia, Italy
e-mail: marchetti.giampietro@libero.it; gf.tassi@tin.it

P. Astoul et al. (eds.), *Thoracoscopy for Pulmonologists*,
DOI 10.1007/978-3-642-38351-9_2, © Springer-Verlag Berlin Heidelberg 2014

chronic empyema (Gordon 1866). This is the first recorded observation of the pleural cavity; however, this was not followed by any further practical utilisation of the technique.

2.3 The Pioneer: H.C. Jacobaeus

Although the clinical application of thoracoscopy was to be used on a worldwide scale for the lysis of pleural adhesions caused by tuberculosis, its original purpose was diagnostic, and it was only later that it became an almost exclusively therapeutic technique.

Both approaches were initiated by the person who is unanimously recognised as the "Father of Thoracoscopy", the Swedish internist Hans Christian Jacobaeus. At the age of 31, he published a report on 4 October 1910 in the German-language journal *Münchener Medizinische Wochenschrift*, entitled "Über die Möglichkeit die Zystoskopie bei Untersuchung seröser Höhlungen anzuwenden" ("On the possibility of performing cystoscopy in the examination of serous cavities") (Jacobaeus 1910).

The article is divided into three parts: the introduction, which deals with materials and methods; then the longer second part (100 lines) dedicated to laparoscopy; and then the final part (47 lines) on thoracoscopy. This is not only the first publication on thoracoscopy but also the first on human laparoscopy, accompanied by a drawing with two small stylised figures to demonstrate the trocar he used. He used a trocar, created with the assistance of Dr Ahlstrom, in which a 14 Nitze (4.6 mm) rigid cystoscope of adapted exactly. This system used a one-way automatic valve which prevented air escaping from either the abdominal cavity or the thorax. The total diameter was 17 F (5.6 mm) and the 90° lateral-vision optic was 22 cm long with an Osram lamp at the tip. The report described only two cases of thoracoscopy and no figures or endoscopic pictures were provided. It is possible that technical problems prevented a complete examination of the cavity; however, it is clear from the article that the author's intention was solely diagnostic, and there was nothing to suggest its future therapeutic evolution, apart

perhaps from the Forlanini method used in the treatment of tuberculosis.

In an edition of the same journal in September 1911, Jacobaeus published a larger clinical series (Jacobaeus 1911), including 45 laparoscopies and 27 thoracoscopies (10 acute pleural effusion, 5 chronic pleural effusions, 3 empyemas, and 9 pneumothoraces). For the first time in the literature, a normal pleural cavity anatomy is described. The author also discussed some orientation points, as well as the course of the intercostal muscles, the intercostal vessels and nerves, the diaphragm with its "shiny" tendinous centre surrounded by normal muscle, and the cardiac pulsation which was better visible from the left, and he also discussed the problems with exploring the mediastinal pleura. Some pathological modifications are also described, such as the change in colour of atelectatic lungs. Jacobaeus was a strong advocate for the method (Fig. 2.1) and published articles in German, French, and Swedish. In January 1912 he travelled to Hamburg, where the influential surgeon Ludolph Brauer was working, who was organising the Seventh International Congress on Tuberculosis which was due to take place in Rome on 12 April 1912. (The meeting was to become famous for the official international recognition of the Forlanini method.) Brauer became very interested in laparo-thorocoscopy and published, a few months later, a 170-page article (Brauer 1912) entitled *"Über Laparoskopie und Thorakoskopie von HC Jacobaeus"* (On the laparoscopy and thoracoscopy from HC Jacobaeus). In Hamburg, Jacobaeus achieved reliable and revolutionary results in the treatment of pulmonary tuberculosis by pneumothorax. In addition he also provided a wealth of knowledge on the safety of the procedure even after the introduction of large quantities of air (up to 2 l). He also described the difficulties encountered in treating tuberculosis by therapeutic pneumothorax if pleural adhesions were present. In The Lancet, dated 23 August 1913, there is a report from the 17th International Congress of Medicine which was held in London. It contains a few lines documenting that Dr HC Jacobaeus gave an admirable presentation describing the practical utility of

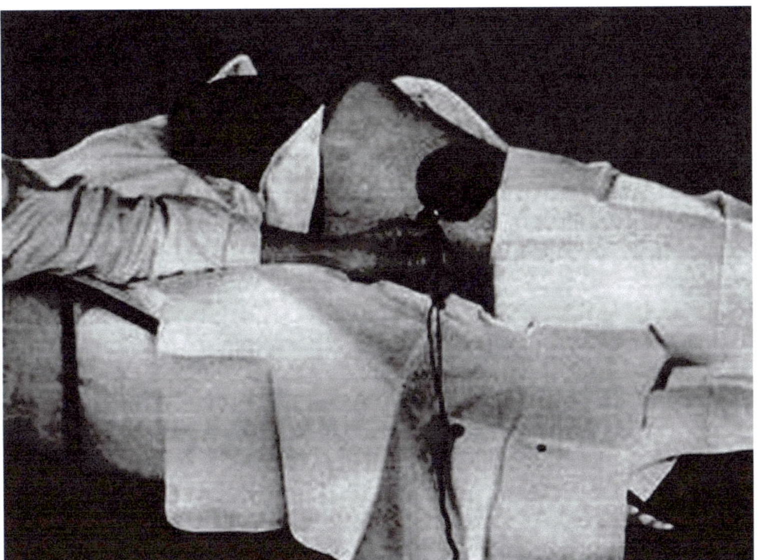

Fig. 2.1 Thoracoscopy in 1912: Jacobaeus

laparo-thorocoscopy in the diagnosis of 200 patients without complication. Jacobaeus also presented some coloured drawings which illustrated the principal endoscopic alterations in the cases he had examined.

1913 is also remembered in the field of thoracoscopy because in that year at the hospital of St. Göran in Stockholm, Jacobaeus sectioned *"with the thoracoscope as a guide, fragments of pulmonary pleura in a case of pleural tumour"*, thereby making the first attempt to perform lysis of pleural adhesions, and continued *"with an even smaller trocar, I introduced an instrument similar to larynx scissors, and cut a small piece from the pulmonary area. There was no discomfort for the patient either during or after the operation"*. On 21 May 1914, he performed a thoracoscopy under local anaesthesia for the management of a case of cavitary pulmonary tuberculosis. This procedure used separate entry portals for the optic and the cautery, in the fifth and third intercostal space, respectively. He saw a false adherence which joined the parenchyma to the diaphragm and a true one located on the right upper lobe, the size of a little finger. He cauterised it, causing the instant collapse of the lung. The patient returned to his room on foot, and there were no immediate consequences. On 23 May a new insufflation of air was carried out:

300 cc with a pressure of +7 cm H2O; this was considerably lower than that used prior to the intervention. The outcome was positive, with the cessation of expectoration within a few days. An examination a month later showed that the lung remained collapsed, the cavity was compressed, and the patient was well.

In subsequent years (Fig. 2.2) his described clinical techniques including thoracoscopic lysis of adhesions which were preventing pneumothorax (later to be known as the "Jacobaeus operation") became more numerous. They were published in international journals such as the British Medical Journal and the American Review of Tuberculosis, where the first 78 cases treated with 55 positive results were reported.

Two other articles go into more detail: one in English which was published in 1923 in the Archives of Radiology and Electrotherapy, from the Proceedings of the Royal Society of Medicine, and a more extensive review published in German entitled *"Die Thorakoskopie und ihre praktische Bedeutung"* (Thoracoscopy and its practical meaning) (Jacobaeus 1925). This comprehensive paper details all of Jacobaeus' clinical work and includes five drawings of the main endoscopic features encountered, of which three of the images were primarily concerned with tuberculosis pleural effusions. The paper also included a

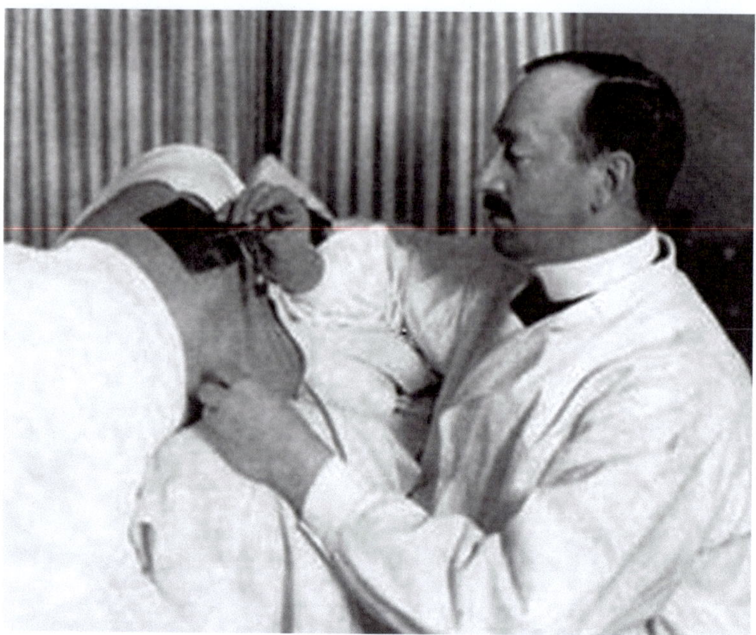

Fig. 2.2 Thoracoscopy in 1920: Jacobaeus

photograph which demonstrated the exact position of the hands and the correct positioning of the trocar during the operation. More attention is paid to tuberculosis than to tumours, which comprises 30–40 cases; these are endoscopically distinguishable from tuberculosis by being characterised by lesions with nodules-masses and/or pleural thickening. In the cases with tumours, there is a clear prevalence of metastatic pleurisy, but Jacobaeus also described five cases with the non-specific term "endothelioma". In his conclusions he stresses that thoracoscopy, preceded by careful examination of x-rays and preparatory pneumothorax, is fundamental in order to achieve accurate diagnosis of the nature and cause of any type of pleural tumour.

Jacobaeus also worked closely with the thoracic surgeon at his hospital, Einar Key, which enabled an appropriate and complete management of intrathoracic pathologies. In 1922 an article was published in Surgery, Gynecology and Obstetrics entitled "The practical importance of thoracoscopy in surgery of the chest" which gives an account of five cases of thoracoscopy prior to therapeutic thoracotomy. In these cases Jacobaeus first induces a pneumothorax and examines the pleural cavity, identifying the endothoracic tumour and providing useful information for the subsequent thoracotomy.

Jacobaeus was willing to collaborate with anyone who was interested in the field of research he had created and was in turn respected and recognised without envy as the initiator of thoracoscopy. For example, together with Unverricht, he improved the technical characteristics of the thoracoscope to make it more reliable and effective and always cited the contribution of others in his work.

2.4 Diffusion of the Method

The path opened by Jacobaeus was rapidly followed by others, and the application of the method spread to various countries.

In France, notable physicians were Dumarest, author of an important paper on artificial pneumothorax (Dumarest et al. 1954), and Douady and Meyer, whose manual on pleuroscopy and sectioning of adhesions was widely circulated (Douady and Meyer 1942).

In Germany the initiator of thoracoscopy was Unverricht, who introduced it in 1915 and collaborated with Jacobaeus in the creation of the

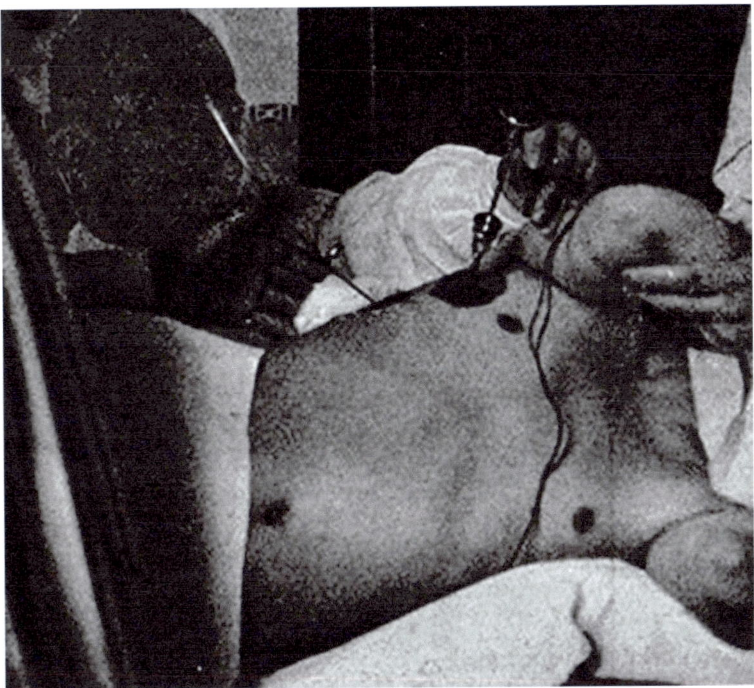

Fig. 2.3 Thoracoscopy in 1925: Unverricht

instrument that was most commonly used at that time. His personal experience comprised of approximately 2,500 interventions (Fig. 2.3), and he published a short article on the method (Unverricht 1923) which was illustrated with explanatory watercolours. Other important German physicians in this field included Diehl and Kremer who published a complete monograph on the subject (Diehl and Kremer 1929).

In 1923 in Scandinavia, Holmböe designed special haemostatic forceps with a mechanical action to prevent haemorrhage, and Güllbring worked extensively on improving the illumination of the optic and also invented an adjustable operating bed which was widely used in Europe. He extended the treatment of lysis of adhesions even in cases with apparent complete pneumothorax.

Singer and Davidson became known in the United States mainly for the introduction of complex combined instruments in the attempt to replace the old thoracoscope, which, despite their efforts, remained the instrument of preference (Fig. 2.4). However, the most significant American contribution came from Matson (Fig. 2.5), who performed 350 interventions over a 15-year period

and adopted an effective strategy to avoid endopleural haemorrhage, using the recently introduced electrocautery scalpel with excellent results (Matson 1936).

In Switzerland the most important contribution came from G Maurer, a thoracic surgeon in Davos, who, concerned by the problem of frequent haemorrhage, developed a technique to isolate the point of attachment of adhesions.

Chandler was undoubtedly the best-known thoracoscopist in Britain of that period, and he is noted for the introduction of his eponymous combined thoracoscope. This instrument had an optical deviation of 30° which permitted the rapid passage from coagulation to sectioning of the adhesions without changing cautery. It was used principally in Britain and was described in a 1930 article in the Lancet, which was an important contribution regarding thoracoscopy in a journal with such a wide distribution (Chandler 1930).

In Spain in 1924, Xalabarder invented a simple new technique of transillumination of adhesions by placing the cautery behind them and bringing it quickly to a high temperature, thereby generating an intense red-white light. The Portuguese Lopo de Carvalho, a noted scholar of pulmonary

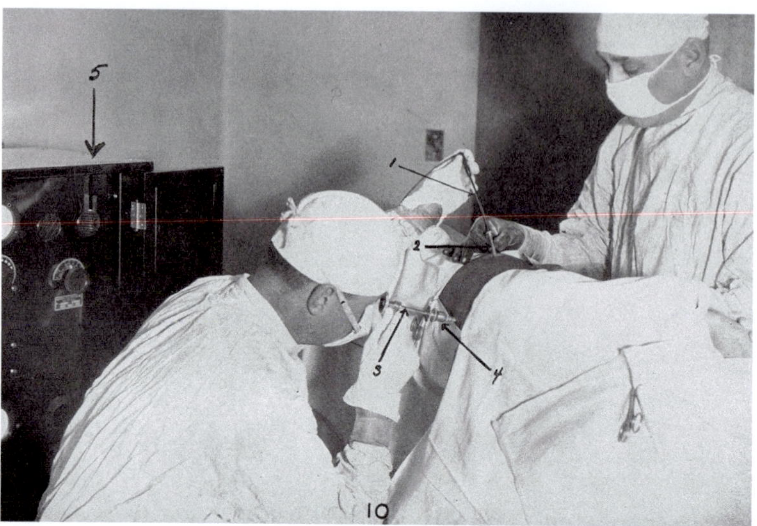

Fig. 2.4 Thoracoscopy in 1929: Matson

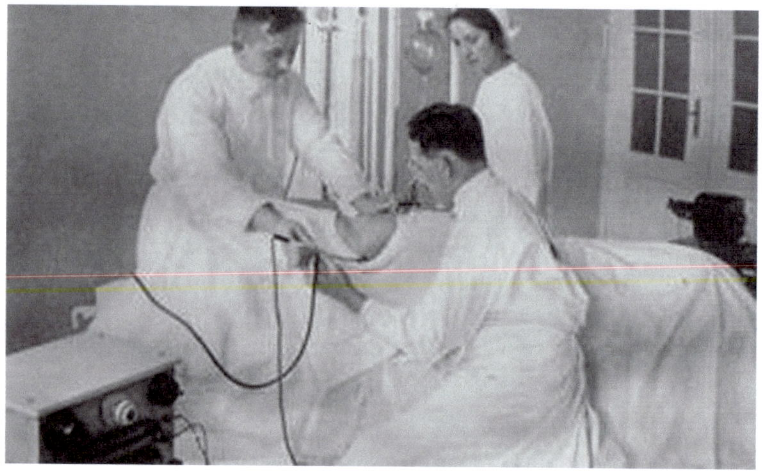

Fig. 2.5 Thoracoscopy in 1926: unknown

angiography, was among the first to use thoracoscopy in the treatment of tuberculosis.

The Canadian thoracic surgeon Norman Bethune (1890–1939) designed a number of new instruments which were integrated with existing ones. He patented lights to transilluminate adhesions and invented staples to position adherences before sectioning, and his name is connected to the first nebulisation of talc in the pleural cavity (Bethune 1935).

In Italy, Stolkind was the first to use the thoracoscope; and in 1914 he wrote, referring to the experience of Jacobaeus, that " *la toracoscopia rappresenta uno degli importanti mezzi ausiliari di diagnosi dei tumori del cavo pleurico, dei noduli tubercolari e del punto di lacerazione del polmone nel pneumotorace"* (thoracoscopy represents one of the important auxiliary methods of diagnosis of tumours of the pleural cavity, of tubercular nodules and the point of laceration of the lung in pneumothorax) (Stolkind 1914). But the brightest star was Felice Cova, who was called the "Paganini of the thoracoscope" because of his consummate skill and dexterity with the instrument and who published a magnificent book entitled the *Atlas Thoracoscopicon,* which includes many excellent didactic illustrations (Cova 1928).

A large number of books on the subject of thoracoscopy were published in that period – in

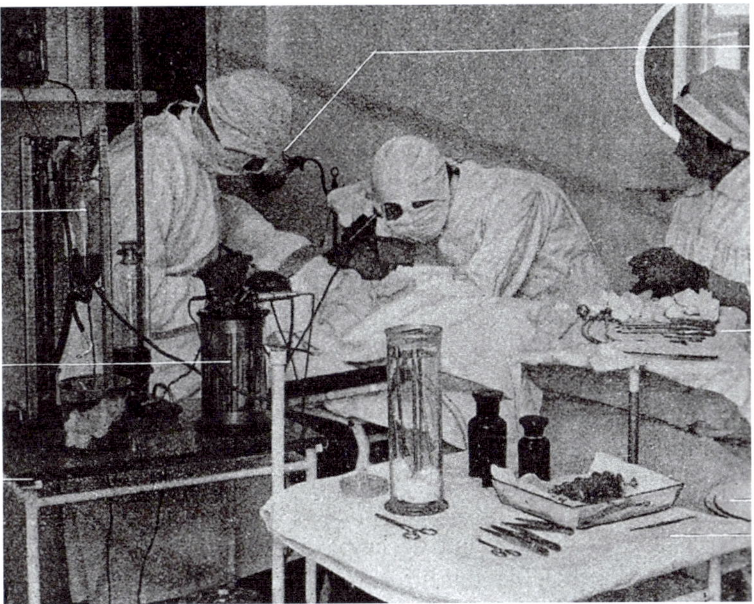

Fig. 2.6 Thoracoscopy in the 1930s: unknown

various countries and languages. These were copiously illustrated and by and large complete works. Some of the most significant texts are those by Unverricht (Unverricht 1923), Cova (Cova 1927), and Dihel and Kramer (Diehl and Kremer 1929). But perhaps the most complete is that by Mistal, a Swiss physician entitled "*Endoscopie et pleurolyse*" with a preface by Jacobaeus. It is a comprehensive monograph of 400 pages in 11 chapters with numerous drawings and photographs including 557 bibliographical references (Mistal 1935).

There is no doubt that thoracoscopy was the principal method used for the lysis of adhesions (Fig. 2.6) (Jacobaeus operation) as it now had become reliable and recognised both experimentally and in practice. Dedicated endoscopic rooms were developed, nursing staff were appropriately trained, and thorax models were created and widely distributed in order to teach the Jacobaeus operation.

However, there was no improvement to biopsy forceps (staging of endothoracic cancer was still being carried out with open thorax). There was still no talk of pleurodesis, pneumothorax prior to the examination of the pleural cavity was seen as a dangerous manoeuvre, and even biopsy was considered unsafe because of the risk of haemorrhage.

But diagnostic thoracoscopy, for indications other than tuberculosis and without performing therapeutic pneumothorax, had begun.

At first only anecdotal evidence suggested the verification of occasional cases of metastatic tumours or mesothelioma or cases of spontaneous pneumothorax. For example, the French physicians Sergent and Kourilsky published in the "*Travaux originaux*" section of *Presse Medicale* an article entitled "*Contribution a l' étude de l'endothéliome pleural – Image radiologique e pleuroscopique*" (Contribution to the study of pleural endothelioma – radiological and pleuroscopic image). It discusses the case of a 62-year-old patient with a history of repeated thoracentesis, parietal thoracic swelling, and radiological verification of pleural nodules. Pleuroscopy was carried out for diagnosis with only a macroscopic exam performed and without tissue biopsy (Sergent and Kourilsky 1939). This initial contribution was followed by a paper from Fourestier and Duret who maintained, again in the *Presse Medicale,* that pleural biopsy is essential for the diagnosis of endothelioma, citing three clinical cases they had observed (Fourestier and Duret 1943). They stressed the importance of distinguishing between true primary pleural tumours (endotheliomas), which are extremely rare, and pulmonary tumours which develop later and are more common. In reality the two pathologies, although prognostically very different, *"sont parfaitement susceptibles de revêtir la même morphologie"* (are perfectly capable of assuming the same morphology).

The pleuroscopic approach with these three patients followed a long course which comprised of preparatory thoracentesis and complex differential diagnoses. Only when these are in place can the biopsy be performed. This was defined as *"la clef du problème"* (the key to the problem). The case of the third patient is notable in that he was a 40-year-old man who in the course of 1 year, from 14 February 1942 to 14 February 1943, underwent 159 thoracentesis – one every 2 days – during which a total of 310 l of pleural liquid was drawn off.

In the field of diagnostic thoracoscopy, mention should be made to an article published by Fabri and Parmeggiani reporting their observations on exudative pleuritis (Fabri and Parmeggiani 1942). It deals with ten cases of acute pleuritis, nine of which were shown to be related to tuberculosis and in which the diagnosis was exclusively macroscopic. In the single non-tubercular case, a hyperaemic visceral pleura is described on which yellowish nodules and plaques are present. This had a gelatinous aspect and was apparently neoplastic in nature. According to the authors the advantage of thoracoscopy lay in highlighting in vivo circulatory modifications *within* the pleural cavity, something clearly impossible in a post-mortem examination. It is interesting to note that in their conclusions they state that "questo *intervento deve essere attuato tempestivamente, sia a versamento formato sia anche davanti a modiche quantità di liquido, onde evitare la formazione di dannose aderenze"* (this intervention should be performed rapidly, both with large and small effusions, in order to avoid damaging adherences).

J.M.C. Branco described his experience in diagnostic thoracoscopy which included its use in the examination of thoracic trauma caused by a penetrative wound (Branco 1946). First, he assessed the extent of the wounds in five patients and then successfully coagulated the injured vessel, arterial or venous depending on the case. Finally, he washed the pleural cavity with saline solution and subsequent aspiration of the fluid. He suggested that in cases where thoracotomy is unavoidable, thoracoscopy may be useful in identifying the best point of access to the thorax.

It is also worth noting the report by Coulaud and Deschamps described the serendipitous pleuroscopic discovery of an asymptomatic pulmonary perforation (Coulaud and Deschamps 1947). The patient underwent four successive thoracoscopies in order to assess the evolution of the fistula, which, after injection of 10 g of crisalbine around the edges, healed in about 2 months.

The use of thoracoscopy in pneumothorax is primarily accredited to Anton Sattler, who dedicated a large part of his professional life to the study of this condition and its management. His most important work on the subject was the article "Zur Behandlung des Spontanpneumothorax mit besonderer Berücksichtigung der Thorakoskopie" (On the treatment of spontaneous pneumothorax with special attention to thoracoscopy) (Sattler 1937). Sattler considered the pleura to be the mirror of the most diverse pathological processes and was a strong advocate of the diagnostic importance of thoracoscopy and of the need to induce pneumothorax before carrying out the examination.

2.5 Pleurodesis

The first contribution on pleurodesis is from the French physicians Quénu and Longuet, who published a systematic review where they discussed the various methods up to that point to keep the lung distended once the thoracic cavity was open (Quenu and Longuet 1896). At the time, single lung intubation did not exist, and parenchymal collapse after thoracotomy was viewed with extreme trepidation. Trials with Saurbach's negative pressure chamber only began at the beginning of the twentieth century.

The list of techniques to achieve pleurodesis is long and diverse: including simple irritants such as iodoform gauze, hot needles, needle puncture, and thermoelectrical irritation; chemical irritants such as zinc chloride and potassium hydroxide; and agglutinants such as sealing wax, glue, and mistletoe – often more injurious than efficacious. In some cases it became a real surgical intervention which involved scarification of the serous membranes or the introduction of binding substances in order to suture the lung to the thoracic wall. All these attempts were ineffective. Samuel Robinson, a famous American thoracic surgeon stated *"If one lobe can be anchored so that remains in position during resection of the others lobe or lobes, the chief obstacle to successful lobectomy will be removed"* (Mumford and Robinson 1914). This anchorage was considered necessary for a two-stage lobectomy, and in particular for bronchiectasis, which at the time was a frequent and disabling disease. It would therefore have been necessary to firstly carry out a pleurodesis before performing the lobectomy.

This objective was achieved by the Canadian thoracic surgeon Norman Bethune who published an article in the Journal of Thoracic Surgery entitled *"Pleural poudrage - A new technique for the deliberate production of pleural adhesions as a preliminary to lobectomy"* (Bethune 1935). The article describes the process of pleurodesis on animals and demonstrated its efficacy in producing adhesions – poor after a week, but adequate after a month. Bethune used the method in four patients with bronchiectasis where "pleural poudrage" was carried out 1 or 2 months prior to the lobectomy – the procedure was successful in all cases. He used instruments he had designed himself, such as the two-way insufflator: an entrance for insufflation and an exit which emptied the cavity of the smallest amount of air in order to maintain a constant endopleural pressure.

This technique remained largely neglected for many years. However, the technique gained a renaissance when effective adhesions for neoplastic pleuritis were being sought. It was only then that the modernity and foresight of this pioneering work was appreciated.

2.6 Post-World War Decline

In the 1950s enormous changes in the management of tuberculosis was realised, mainly from the positive impact of the introduction of antibiotics. However, this also had a negative impact on thoracoscopy. The "Jacobaeus operation" (Fig. 2.7) was gradually abandoned, as was lobar collapse therapy in general.

Paradoxically, it was the operation's diffusion in the previous years, with emphasis on the lysis of adhesions, which meant that for many people it had become almost a synonym for thoracoscopy. Evidently the small number of works dedicated to its diagnostic application was not sufficient to create a solid foundation for the technique.

During that period, pleural needle biopsy (DeFrancis et al. 1955) was introduced. It was easier to perform than thoracoscopy and was seen as a potential replacement for thoracoscopy to obtain pleural biopsies. It achieved a moderate level of acceptance, in particular in English-speaking countries, where thoracoscopy had not been in widespread use, became almost completely forgotten to the point that until recent times the alternative to non-diagnostic needle biopsy was thoracotomy.

In some parts of Europe, however, thoracoscopy continued to be practised, principally for diagnostic purposes. However, there was also a widening of the areas of application of the technique, for example, with the introduction of pulmonary biopsy. During the 1960s there was a slow revival of the technique, demonstrated by the publication of large clinical studies dealing with hundreds of patients: 130 cases by Bergquist and Nordenstam (1966); 488, Sattler (1968); and 1,130 subjects in the Brandt paper (Brandt and Mai 1971).

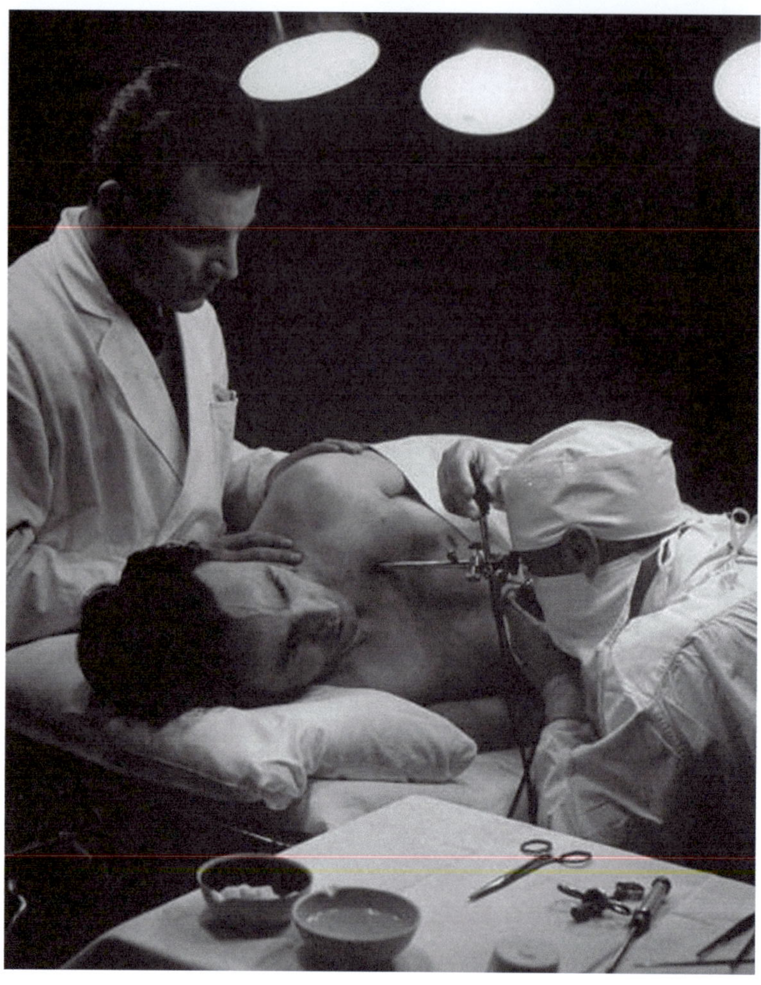

Fig. 2.7 Thoracoscopy in the 1950s: unknown

2.7 Renaissance

The real renaissance began in the 1970s, when there was a tangible increase in the utilisation of pleural endoscopy. Publications on the subject increased greatly (over 100 papers between 1970 and 1980), and at the same time there were significant technical improvements such as the use of cold light and better-quality optics.

In Europe the important role of pulmonologists was recognised, and many became reference centres in their various countries due to their long clinical experience and scientific research: Alcozer in Italy, Boutin in France, Brandt and Loddenkemper in Germany, Sattler in Austria, and Swierenga and Viskum in Scandinavia.

In 1980 Boutin organised the first "International Symposium on Thoracoscopy" in Marseille, which was attended by 140 physicians from 16 countries (Boutin et al. 1981). He initiated an educational programme entitled "Course on Thoracoscopy" which in subsequent years has become an international point of reference in the training of numerous professionals throughout the world. Christian Boutin deserves recognition not only for having improved the quality and increased the diffusion of thoracoscopy (his is still the most commonly used thoracoscope) but also for having placed it in a larger context. It is now applied in all aspects of pleural disease, such as staging in mesothelioma or giving indications for effective pleurodesis without complications.

There are a number of publications dealing exclusively with thoracoscopy during the last four decades. Swierenga published the first photographic atlas of thoracoscopy which had wide distribution in Europe (Swierenga 1978), and in 1983 the *"Atlas der diagnostischen Thorakoskopie"* was published by Brandt and colleagues and this was later translated into English (Brandt et al. 1985). *"La toracoscopia diagnostica"* by Alcozer and Dorigoni appeared in 1984 with numerous illustrations in colour (Alcozer and Dorigoni 1984). It was the result of a long personal experience and was the first publication in Italian on the subject of thoracoscopy since Cova, cited above.

A volume entitled "Toracoscopia" was published in Spain by Quetglas, Velasquez, and Pujol with contributions from various Spanish pulmonologists and thoracic surgeons (Quetglas et al. 1985).

In 1991 Boutin and collaborators published "Practical Thoracoscopy" (Boutin et al. 1991). It is an exceptional synthesis of technical knowledge and application of a method. It has now become an integral text of endoscopy for pulmonologists.

2.8 Surgical Thoracoscopy

The 1990s was another major phase in the history of the technique: the development of a thoracoscopic technique that was exclusively surgical.

Similar to the early stages of endoscopy, where cystoscopy led the way for other applications, it was laparoscopic surgery which provided the impetus to surgeons around the world to rediscover thoracoscopy.

In the early 1990s laparoscopic cholecystectomy was developed with considerable success and subsequently numerous applications. Immediately after, publications began to appear describing experiences of thoracic surgeons in thoracoscopy: pulmonary biopsy, treatment of the pneumothorax with resection of pustules and blebs, removal of pulmonary nodules, interventions on the mediastinum, and even lobectomy and pneumonectomy.

The evolution and diffusion of the method has been extremely fast and is directly linked to technological progress, in particular video technology and the design of dedicated surgical instruments.

The use of video support has meant the coining of new terminology, such as *videothoracoscopy, surgical videothoracoscopy, and video assisted thoracic surgery or VATS.*

At the same time there has been a virtual explosion of literature on the subject. Publications were not slow to appear: Gossot *"Surgical thoracoscopy"* (Gossot et al. 1994), Krasna *"Atlas of thoracoscopic surgery"* (Krasna and Mack 1994), and Inderbitzi *"Surgical thoracoscopy"* (Inderbitzi 1995). These are just a few of the earlier volumes published.

Surgery appeared to follow its own path and continued to strengthen its indications. In addition internists have attempted to improve the performance and reduce the degree of invasiveness. Attempts are being made to reduce the size of optics (minithoracoscopy) (Inculet and Malthaner 1998; Tassi and Marchetti 2003) and semiflexible instruments similar to those used in bronchoscopy (Colt and Lee 2005).

However, these newer techniques are perhaps too recent to qualify as being "history" rather than just "news" of events which are currently evolving.

References

Alcozer G, Dorigoni A (1984) La toracoscopia diagnostica. Nardini, Firenze

Bergquist S, Nordenstam H (1966) Thoracoscopy and pleural biopsy in the diagnosis of pleurisy. Scand J Respir Dis 47:64–74

Bethune N (1935) Pleural poudrage: a new technique for deliberate production of pleural adhesions as a preliminary to lobectomy. J Thorac Surg 4:251–261

Boutin C, Viallat JR, Cargnino P et al (1981) La Thoracoscopie en 1980. Revue générale. Poumon Coeur 37:11–19

Boutin C, Viallat JR, Aelony Y (1991) Diagnostic thoracoscopy for pleural effusions. In: Boutin C, Viallat JR, Aelony Y (eds) Practical thoracoscopy. Springer, Berlin, pp 51–64

Bozzini P (1806) Lichtleiter, eine Erfindung zur Anschauung innerer Teile und Krankheiten nebst der Abbildung. J Pract Arzn Wund 24:107–124

Branco JMC (1946) Thoracoscopy as a method of exploration in penetrating injuries of the chest. Dis Chest 12:330–335

Brandt HJ, Mai J (1971) Differential diagnose des Pleuraergusses durch Thorakoskopie. Pneumologie 145:192–203

Brandt HJ, Loddenkemper R, Mai J (1985) Atlas of diagnostic thoracoscopy. Indications – technique. Thieme, New York

Brauer L (1912) Über Laparo- und Thorakoskopie von HC Jacobaeus, Privatdozent Stockholm. Beitr Klin Tuberk 25:I–II

Chandler F (1930) A new thoracoscope. Lancet I: 232–233

Colt HG, Lee P (2005) Rigid and semirigid pleuroscopy: the future is bright. Respirology 10:418–425

Coulaud E, Deschamps P (1947) Découverte pleuroscopique d'une importante perforation pulmonaire asymptomatique. Guérison rapide spontanée. Rev Tuberc 11:825–827

Cova F (1927) Toracoscopia. Operazione di Jacobaeus. Sperling & Kupfer, Milano

Cova F (1928) Atlas thoracoscopicon. Sperling & Kupfer, Milano

DeFrancis N, Klosk E, Albano E (1955) Needle biopsy of the parietal pleura. A preliminary report. N Engl J Med 252:948–949

Desormeaux A (1865) De l'endoscopie et de ses applications au diagnostic et au traitement des affections de l'urèthre et de la vessie. Baillière, Paris

Diehl K, Kremer W (1929) Die Tuberkulose und ihre Grenzgebiete in Einzeldarstellungen. Volume 7. Thoraskopie und Thorakokaustik. Springer, Berlin

Douady D, Meyer A (1942) Manuel de pleuroscopie et de section de brides dans le pneumothorax thérapeutique. Legrand et Bertrand, Paris

Dumarest J, Galy P, Germain J (1954) La pratique du pneumothorax thérapeutique. Masson, Paris

Fabri G, Parmeggiani D (1942) Osservazioni toracoscopiche nelle pleuriti essudative. Policlinico Sez Prat 49:1347–1359

Fourestier M, Duret M (1943) Nécessité de la biopsie pleurale pour le diagnostic de l'endo- théliome de la plèvre. Presse Med 32:467–468

Gordon S (1866) Clinical reports of rare cases, occurring in the Whitworth and Hardwicke Hospitals: most extensive pleuritic effusion rapidly becoming purulent, paracentesis, introduction of a drainage tube, recovery, examination of interior of pleura by the endoscope. Dublin Q J Med Sci 41:83–90

Gossot D, Kleinmann P, Levi JE (1994) Surgical thoracoscopy. Springer, Paris

Inculet RI, Malthaner RA (1998) Minithoracoscopy for pleural effusions. Can Respir J 5:253–254

Inderbitzi R (1995) Surgical thoracoscopy. Springer, Berlin

Jacobaeus HC (1910) Über die Möglichkeit, die Zystoskopie bei Untersuchung seröser Höhlungen anzuwenden. Münch Med Wochenschr 40:2090–2092

Jacobaeus HC (1911) Kurze Übersicht ber meine Erfahrungen der Laparo-Thorakoskopie. Münch Med Woch 58:1612

Jacobaeus HC (1925) Die Thorakoskopie und ihre praktische Bedeutung. Ergeb Gesamten Med 7:112–166

Killian G (1898) Über directe Bronchoskopie. Münch Med Woch 27:844–877

Krasna MJ, Mack MJ (1994) Atlas of thoracoscopic surgery. Quality Medical Publishing, St Louis

Matson RC (1936) The role of thoracoscopy in the diagnosis and management of lung tumors. Surg Gynecol Obstet 63:617–624

Mistal O (1935) Endoscopie et pleurolyse. Masson, Paris

Mumford JG, Robinson S (1914) The surgical aspects of bronchiectasis. Ann Surg 60:29–35

Quenu E, Longuet L (1896) Note sur quelques recherches experimentales concernant la chirurgie thoracique. C R Soc Biol Paris 4:1007–1008

Quetglas FS, Velasquez AS, Pujol JL (1985) La toracoscopia. Jarpyo, Madrid

Sattler A (1937) Zur Behandlung der Spontapnumothorax mit besonderer Berücksichtigung der Thorakoskopie. Beitr Klin Tuberk 89:395–408

Sattler A (1968) Die Bedeutung der endoskopischen Untersuchung des Pleuraraums fur die Diagnostik und Therapie. Méd Hyg 26:630–638

Sergent E, Kourilsky R (1939) Contribution à l'étude de l'endothéliome pleural.Images radiologiques et pleuroscopiques. Presse Med 14:257–259

Stolkind E (1914) Contributo alla diagnosi delle malattie polmonari colla pleuroscopia. Gazz Osp Clin 76:801–803

Swierenga A (1978) Atlas of thoracoscopy. Boehringer, Ingelheim/Rhein

Tassi G, Marchetti G (2003) Minithoracoscopy: a less invasive approach to thoracoscopy. Chest 124:1975–1977

Unverricht W (1923) Technik und Methode der Thorakoskopie. Vogel, Leipzig

Macroscopic Approach to the Pleural Cavity

3

Delphine Trousse and Pascal Thomas

3.1 General Information

In humans, the thoracic organs are protected within a bony wall, muscles, and membranes. Thus, to ensure its best protection and function, the lung is surrounded by chest ribs, thick muscles of the chest wall, and the pleura. The outer surface of the lung and the inner surface of the thoracic cage are covered by a thin elastic serous membrane which is called the pleura. The pleura and the pleural cavity are essential for the efficient function of the lung as are the pericardium and the pericardial cavity for the heart.

The pleura is formed by two serosal membranes: the visceral pleura and the parietal pleura. The first one is called the visceral pleura and covers the whole lung surface. The second membrane, called the parietal pleura, covers the inner surface of the chest wall and the mediastinum (Fig. 3.1). The parietal pleura is divided into three different parts. The first part is represented by the costal pleura and covers the inner part of the chest ribs. The second component covers the diaphragm, and the last one is represented by the pleura surrounding the mediastinum. At this level the reflection covers the different constituents of the pulmonary hilum including the main pulmonary artery, the pulmonary veins, and the main

bronchus. Inferiorly the reflection extends down to the diaphragm. The overall shape of this reflection looks like a racket. The handle of this racket forms the ligament joining the lung to the diaphragm and is called the pulmonary ligament (Brizon and Castaing 1989) (Fig. 3.2).

Dissection of this ligament is usually one of the first surgical steps in thoracic surgical procedures and allows for a complete release and mobilization of the lung for further intervention. This pulmonary ligament contains several lymph nodes important in lung cancer staging. Indeed this area is an important part of the radical lymphadenectomy associated with pulmonary resection and is currently designated as station 9 in the international lymph node classification (Mountain 1997) (Fig. 3.3).

The space delineated by the two serosal layers of the pleura is commonly called the pleural space or pleural cavity. Both pleural surfaces have two layers: a superficial mesothelial cell layer facing the pleural space and an underlying connective tissue layer (Lee and Olak 1994).

The pleural space is a thin negative pressure cavity with a small amount of fluid. The amount of fluid is strictly regulated by processes of filtration and absorption. Indeed the lung has to change volume continuously during respiration. One of the primary roles of the pleural fluid is to transmit the transpleural forces occurring during the respiratory cycle and to ensure adequate coupling between the lung and the chest wall during normal breathing. The pleural cavity plays a major role in decreasing friction during respiration (Wang 1998).

D. Trousse (✉) • P. Thomas
Division of Thoracic Surgery, Hôpital NORD,
Marseille, France
e-mail: delphine.trousse@ap-hm.fr;
pascalAlexandre.thomas@ap-hm.fr

P. Astoul et al. (eds.), *Thoracoscopy for Pulmonologists*,
DOI 10.1007/978-3-642-38351-9_3, © Springer-Verlag Berlin Heidelberg 2014

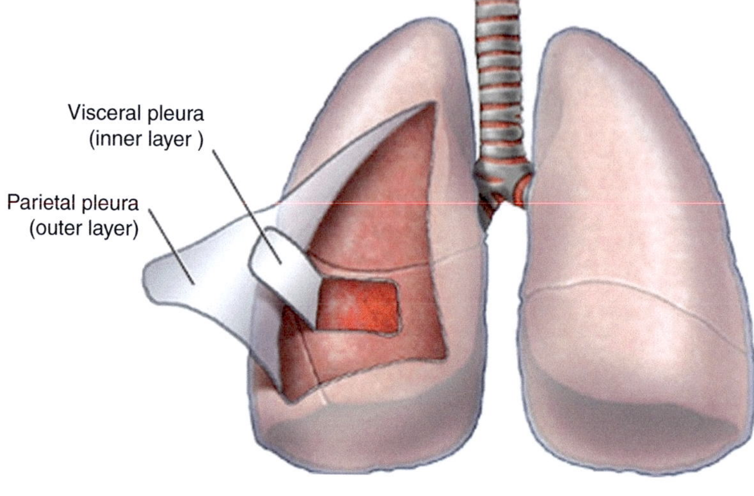

Fig. 3.1 The two layers of the pleura

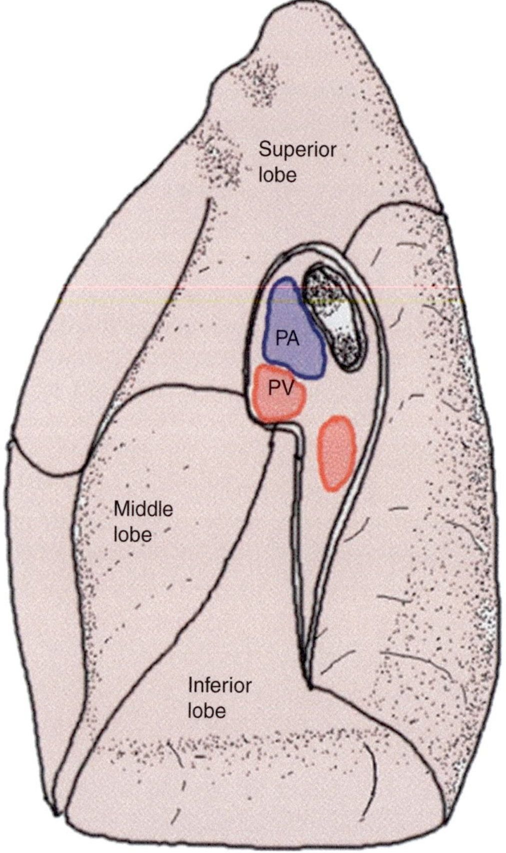

Fig. 3.2 The transition between the two layers at the level of the pulmonary hilum

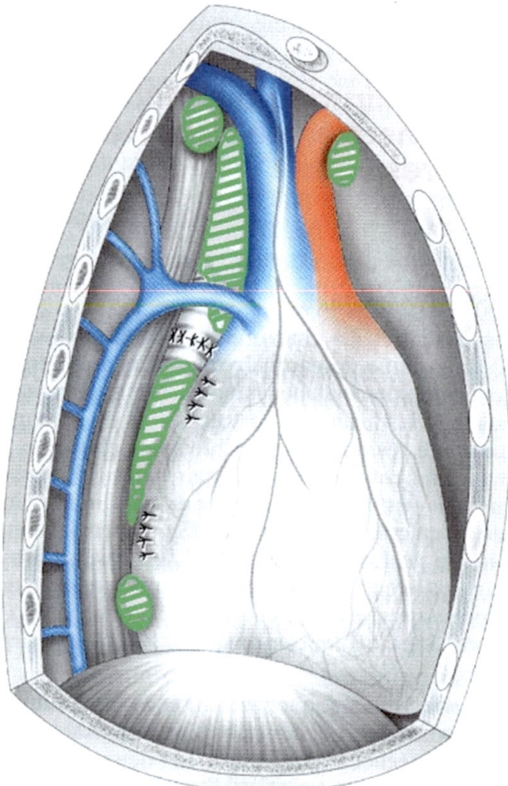

Fig. 3.3 Lymph node stations as approached by thoracoscopic

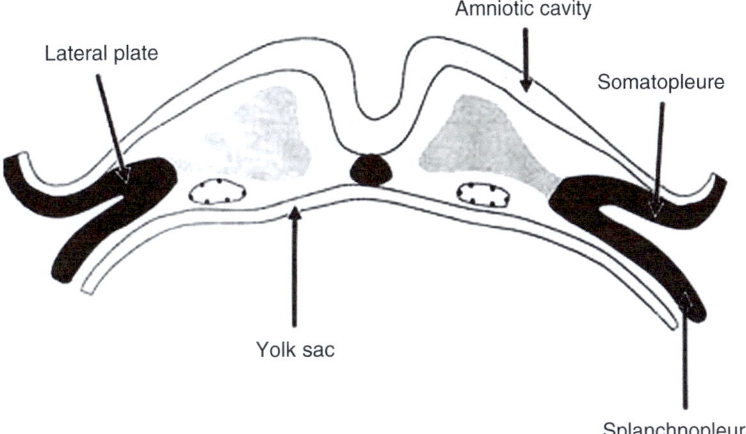

Fig. 3.4 The somatic mesoderm and the splanchnic mesoderm form the lateral plate

3.2   Embryology

The pleural cavity is created between the fourth and the seventh week of embryologic development and at that stage is lined by the splanchnopleure and the somatopleure. These embryonic components of the visceral and parietal pleura develop different anatomic characteristics with respect to vascular, lymphatic, and nervous supply (Lee and Olak 1994; Wang 1998).

During the third week of gestation, there is differentiation of the embryonic mesoderm into three different parts; these are called the paraxial mesoderm, the intermediate mesoderm, and the lateral plates. The lateral plate is formed by two different layers: the first one is the somatic mesoderm or somatopleure and the second one is represented by the splanchnic mesoderm which is also referred to as the splanchnopleure. The somatopleure is the original membrane for the parietal pleura while the splanchnopleure will become the visceral layer of the pleura (Fig. 3.4).

There is creation of the intraembryonic cavity by ventral migration of the somatopleure towards the midline. The intraembryonic coelom is the primitive cavity that will form the three major body cavities: pericardium, pleura, and peritoneum (Fig. 3.5). The pleural cavity is

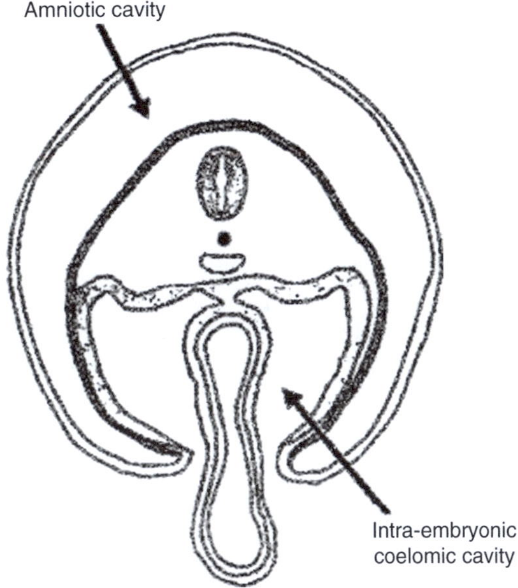

Fig. 3.5 The creation of the intraembryonic coelom

later separated by the diaphragm from the peritoneal cavity inferiorly. Superiorly the pleuropericardial fold divides into the heart and the lung buds at the end of the fifth week of gestation. There is midline fusion of the pleuropericardial folds and separation of the pleural cavity from the pericardial sac. The pleural cavity continues to expand until the end of the third month (Fig. 3.6).

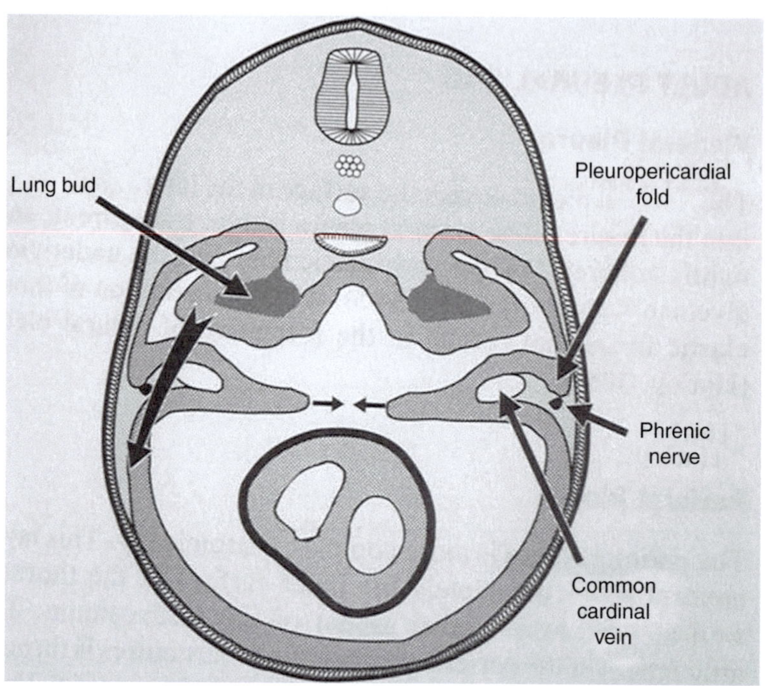

Fig. 3.6 The midline fusion of the pleuropericardial folds

3.3 The Visceral Pleura

The visceral pleura is a thin, transparent membrane which covers all the lung parenchymal surface and extends into the fissures. The visceral pleura is extremely adherent to the underlying lung parenchyma by elastic fibers. There is no plane between the alveolar tissue and the visceral pleura. Indeed the dissection of the visceral pleura, pleurectomy, results in lung damage by tearing the alveolar wall and inducing air leak from the alveoli. The disruption of the elastic fibers results in the formation of pleural blebs.

3.4 The Parietal Pleura

The parietal pleura is more complex anatomically. The parietal pleura almost completely covers the inner surface of the chest wall and the medial aspect of the mediastinum. The attachment of the parietal pleura to these structures is through a fibrous layer known as the endothoracic fascia. The parietal pleura is divided into three parts: the costal pleura, the diaphragmatic pleura, and the mediastinal pleura. The transition between each part produces several pleural sinuses. The first one is the anterior and posterior costomediastinal sinus, the second one is the costophrenic sinus, and the last one is the mediastinophrenic sinuses. The projection of the pleural sinuses is near identical on both sides. Anteriorly, laterally, and posteriorly the lung extends less inferiorly than the pleural sinuses. At the apex of the chest, the pleural space and the lung extend above the bony limits of the thorax (3 cm above the medial part of the clavicle). This data explains why injury in the neck can create pleural intrusion and in turn result in a traumatic pneumothorax.

Anatomically the endothoracic fascia is prominent on the chest ribs. It is absent behind the sternum and on the pericardium. At the level of the thoracic inlet, the fascia is very strong and forms a diaphragm called as the fibrous cervicothoracic fascia of Bourgery. This diaphragm is supported by a number of suspensory ligaments to the surrounding structures – the spine, the clavicle, and the first rib.

3.5   Vascularization of the Pleura

The blood supply of the pleura is complex and originates from different vascular networks depending on the topography of the pleura. Vascularization of the parietal and the visceral pleurae is completely independent.

3.5.1   Arterial Blood Supply

The parietal pleura has a rich vascular supply. The costal pleura is vascularized by the intercostal arteries and from several branches of the internal mammary artery (IMA). The mediastinal pleura is dependent on the bronchial arterial system and upper diaphragmatic arteries with additional supply from branches of the IMA. The pleural dome is completely independent in its blood supply originating from the subclavian arteries.

With respect to the visceral pleura, the bronchial arteries and the pulmonary circulation provide vascularization.

3.5.2   Venous Blood Supply

The venous blood return of the parietal pleura drains into the peribronchial veins and/or directly into the vena cava, while venous blood from the visceral pleura is drained in the pulmonary venous system.

3.5.3   The Lymphatic Drainage

There are two distinct lymphatic systems for the pleura.

Within the visceral pleura, there is a rich network of lymphatics in the subpleural space. These lymphatics are particularly prominent at the origin of the peripheral lobule. All these lymphatics drain to the pulmonary hilum and from there into the pulmonary lymphatic system. There is no communication between the lymphatics of the visceral pleura and the pleural space, but there is a rich connection with the intraparenchymal network.

Conversely, there is a direct communication (stomata) between the pleural space and the parietal pleural lymphatic channels. These stomata (diameter 2–12 μm) were firstly described by Von Recklinghausen in 1863. They are abundant at the base of the pleural cavity especially at the lowest part of the costal pleura ($100/cm^2$) and the diaphragmatic pleura ($8,000/cm^2$). Through these lymphatics the parietal pleura is drained into the intercostal and the internal mammary system.

3.6   The Innervation of the Pleura

The visceral pleural has somatic innervation and therefore is nonsensitive. In contrast, the parietal pleura is innervated through a rich network of somatic, sympathetic, and parasympathetic fibers arising from the intercostal nerves, the phrenic nerve, and also the vagus nerve.

3.7   Pleural Abnormalities

When thoracoscopy was first performed for diagnosis and exploration, it quickly became apparent that this was an excellent therapeutic and minimally invasive tool. Nowadays thoracoscopy permits either pleural or pulmonary biopsy, staging in pulmonary and pleural malignancies, pleurodesis for persistent effusions or pneumothoraces, and even debridement in some cases with empyema (Oakes et al. 1984; Van Schil et al. 1996).

It is not surprising to discover some anatomical variations during thoracoscopy. In fact, altered embryogenesis may explain some of these congenital anomalies within the pleural cavity. These defects are rare and occur in less than 1 % of patients. These anatomical variations are frequently discovered incidentally during the thoracoscopy but should be recognized by the main operator. The most frequent anomaly of the pleura is probably the bullae and blebs (Fig. 3.7). Subpleural blebs or bullae, which are designated

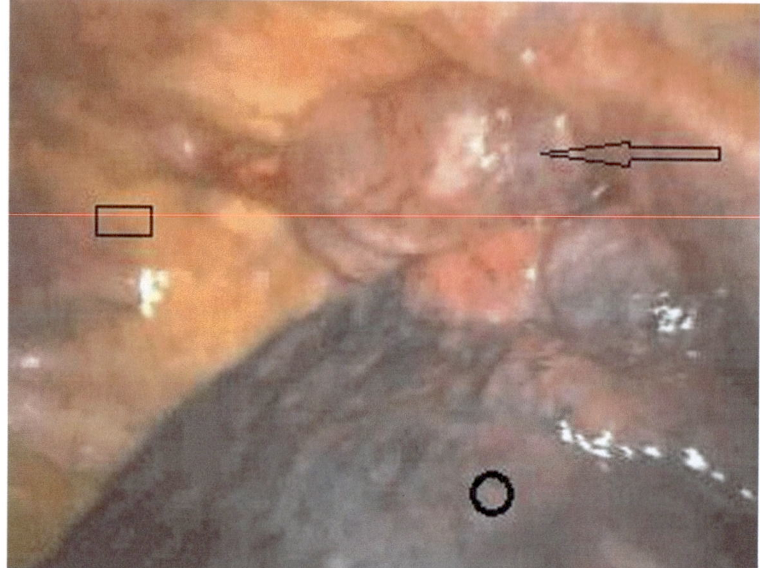

Fig. 3.7 Videothoracoscopic approach in the treatment of primary spontaneous pneumothorax (with the resection of pleural blebs on the apex using staplers), parietal pleura (□), atelectatic lung (O), blebs on the lung apex (*arrow*)

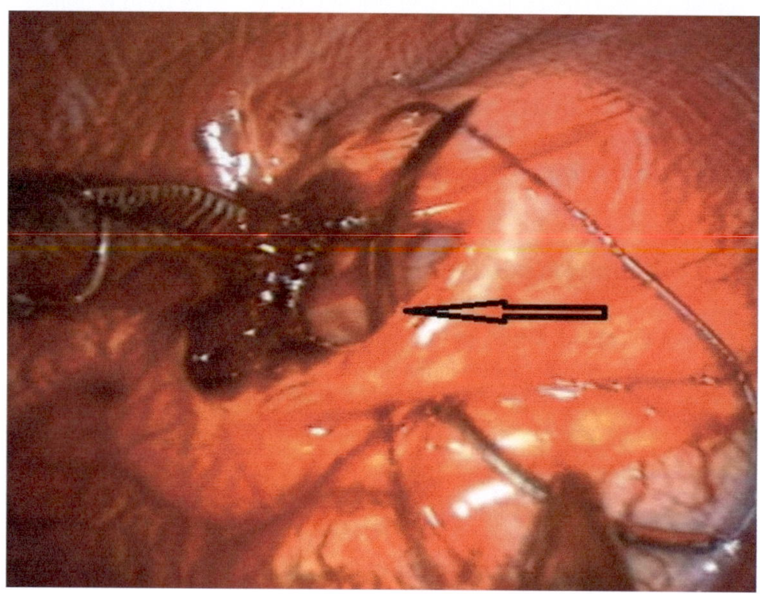

Fig. 3.8 Videothoracoscopic view of a congenital diaphragmatic defect (*arrow*) diagnosed incidentally. Suture under thoracoscopic control with interrupted stitches

as emphysema-like changes, are seen in 75–100 % of patients with primary spontaneous pneumothorax, even in nonsmokers (Ayed et al. 2006). As soon as they are identified, they are either resected with an endostapler by the surgeon or coagulated by the pulmonologist. However there is no guarantee that the visualized blebs are the only factor responsible for the occurrence of the pneumothorax. Controversies remain as to the contribution of these abnormalities to the occurrence of the pneumothoraces, and therefore it is not uncommon for the surgeon to also perform either pleural abrasion or partial parietal pleurectomy at the same time.

Thoracoscopy allows for a perfect exploration of the pleural cavity including the lung, the mediastinum, the parietal pleura, and also the diaphragm. The diaphragmatic surface could have several anomalies recognized as defects or spots. Diaphragmatic defects may be diagnosed incidentally

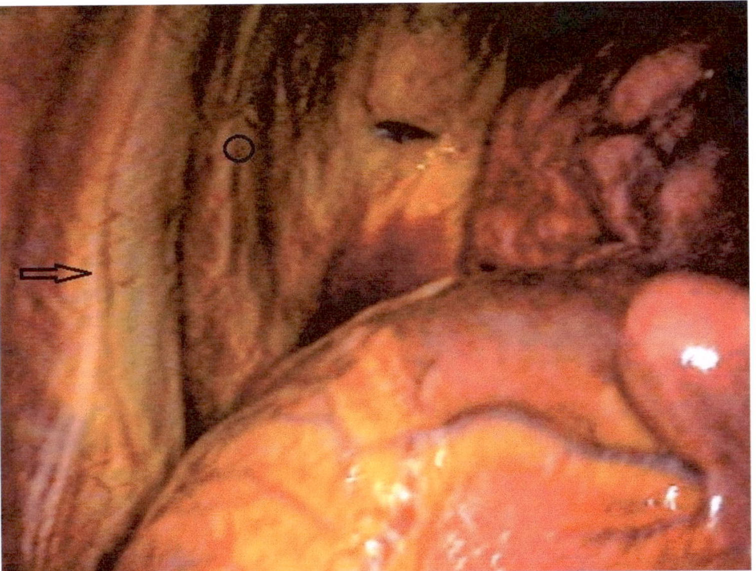

Fig. 3.9 Complete congenital pericardial defect on the left side of the pericardium. Internal mammary vessel (*arrow*), parietal pleural (O)

during thoracoscopy and, if possible, should be repaired (Fig. 3.8). Such diaphragmatic defects may explain part of the pathophysiology of catamenial pneumothorax in women (Korom et al. 2004).

During embryogenesis, an arrest in the development of the transverse septum or pleuroperi-cardial membrane may lead to a partial or complete congenital defect of the pericardium (Fig. 3.9). This abnormality is rare (less than 200 cases published in literature) (Nguyen et al. 2001). Fortunately, in the majority of cases, no symptoms are reported. However, patients may rarely complain of chronic chest pain mimicking coronary artery disease. The diagnosis has also been incidentally made at the time of thoracos-copy (Chapman et al. 1988).

Another frequent congenital anomaly is a cys-tic lesion such as the pleuropericardial cyst. This benign tumor, which is usually asymptomatic, is diagnosed on chest X-ray or computed tomogra-phy. The enlarging volume of the cyst may, in some rare cases, induce chest pain. Surgical exci-sion of the cyst is feasible by video-assisted thora-coscopic surgery but should not be routinely recommended (Hazelrigg et al. 1993).

References

Ayed AK, Chandrasekaran C, Sukumar M (2006) Video-assisted thoracoscopic surgery for primary spontane-ous pneumothorax: clinicopathological correlation. Eur J Cardiothorac Surg 29:221–225

Brizon J, Castaing J (1989) Les feuillets d'anatomie. Fascicule XIV, Thorax, edn. Maloine, Paris

Chapman JE, Rubin JW, Gross CM et al (1988) Congenital absence of the pericardium: an unusual cause of atypi-cal angina. Ann Thorac Surg 45:91–93

Hazelrigg SR, Landreneau SJ, Mack KJ et al (1993) Thoracoscopic resection of mediastinal cysts. Ann Thorac Surg 56:659–660

Korom S, Canyurt H, Missbach A et al (2004) J Thorac Cardiovasc Surg 128:502–508

Lee KF, Olak J (1994) Anatomy and physiology of the pleural space. Chest Surg Clin N Am 4:391–403

Mountain CF (1997) Revisions for the international sys-tem for staging lung cancer. Chest 111:1710–1717

Nguyen DQ, Wilson RF, Bolman RM III et al (2001) Congenital pericardial defect and concomitant coro-nary artery disease. Ann Thorac Surg 72:1371–1373

Oakes DD, Sherck JP, Brodsky JB et al (1984) Therapeutic thoracoscopy. J Thorac Cardiovasc Surg 87:269–273

Van Schil P, Van Meerbeeck J, Vanmaele R et al (1996) Role of thoracoscopy (VATS) in pleural and pulmo-nary pathology. Acta Chir Belg 96:23–27

Wang NS (1998) Anatomy of the pleura. Clin Chest Med 19:229–240

Physiology and Pathophysiology of the Pleural Space

4

Daniella Negrini

The pleural space is a liquid-filled cavity enclosed between the parietal mesothelium located on the inner surface of the thorax, the diaphragm and the mediastinal tissues and the visceral mesothelium present on the lung surface (Fig. 4.1). The pleural space does not simply represent a "separating compartment", but actually plays an essential role in the physiology of the respiratory system. In fact, the intrapleural pressure determines lung expansion during the respiratory cycle. In addition, the small volume and the composition of pleural fluid allows for an almost frictionless continuous sliding of the facing mesothelia during breathing, thus avoiding mechanical damage to the opposing sliding surfaces.

4.1 Morphology of the Parietal and Visceral Pleural Tissue

4.1.1 Mesothelial Cells

Mesothelial cells are flat, squamous-like cells approximately 1–4 µm thick (Wang 1974) with an average diameter of an estimated 25 µm. They contain few organelles, including microtubules and microfilaments, vesicles and vacuoles, a few mitochondria and poorly developed Golgi apparatus and rough endoplasmic reticulum. Cells are connected by tight junctions, adherens junctions in their apical portion (Fig. 4.2), gap junctions and desmosomes at their basal side; the luminar surface of the cells, especially on the visceral side, presents a well-developed microvilli brush (Bernaudin et al. 1991; Wang 1974, 1985). The renewal rate of mesothelial cells is very low (<0.5 % of cells undergo mitosis at any one time); however, cell proliferation greatly increases after injury to the mesothelial surface or after exposure to inflammatory agents suggesting a role for mesothelial cells in wound healing but also in serosal fibrosis and adhesion formation (Foley-Comer et al. 2002; Mutsaers et al. 2002). In spite of its apparent delicacy, mesothelial cells constitute, together with the submesothelial interstitial tissue layer, a protective barrier against mechanical insult. They also synthesise saturated (primarily dipalmitoylphosphatidylcholine) and unsaturated phospholipids (stearoyl linoleoylphosphatidylcholine typically encountered in surfactant lining the alveoli). Unsaturated phospholipids appear functionally more important in the pleural cavity than in the alveolar lining; this is likely due to their specific ability to greatly reduce the coefficient of friction between sliding surfaces compared to saturated phospholipids (Hills et al. 1982, 1992; Mills et al. 2006). Mesothelial cells synthesise hyaluronan (HA) (Wang and Lai-Fook 2000), a large molecular weight (>106 Da) glycosaminoglycan which is a typical constituent of the extracellular tissue fibre matrix and whose most distinctive properties are related to its viscoelastic behaviour.

D. Negrini
Department of Experimental and Clinical Biomedical
Sciences, University of Insubria, Varese, Italy
e-mail: daniela.negrini@uninsubria.it

P. Astoul et al. (eds.), *Thoracoscopy for Pulmonologists*,
DOI 10.1007/978-3-642-38351-9_4, © Springer-Verlag Berlin Heidelberg 2014

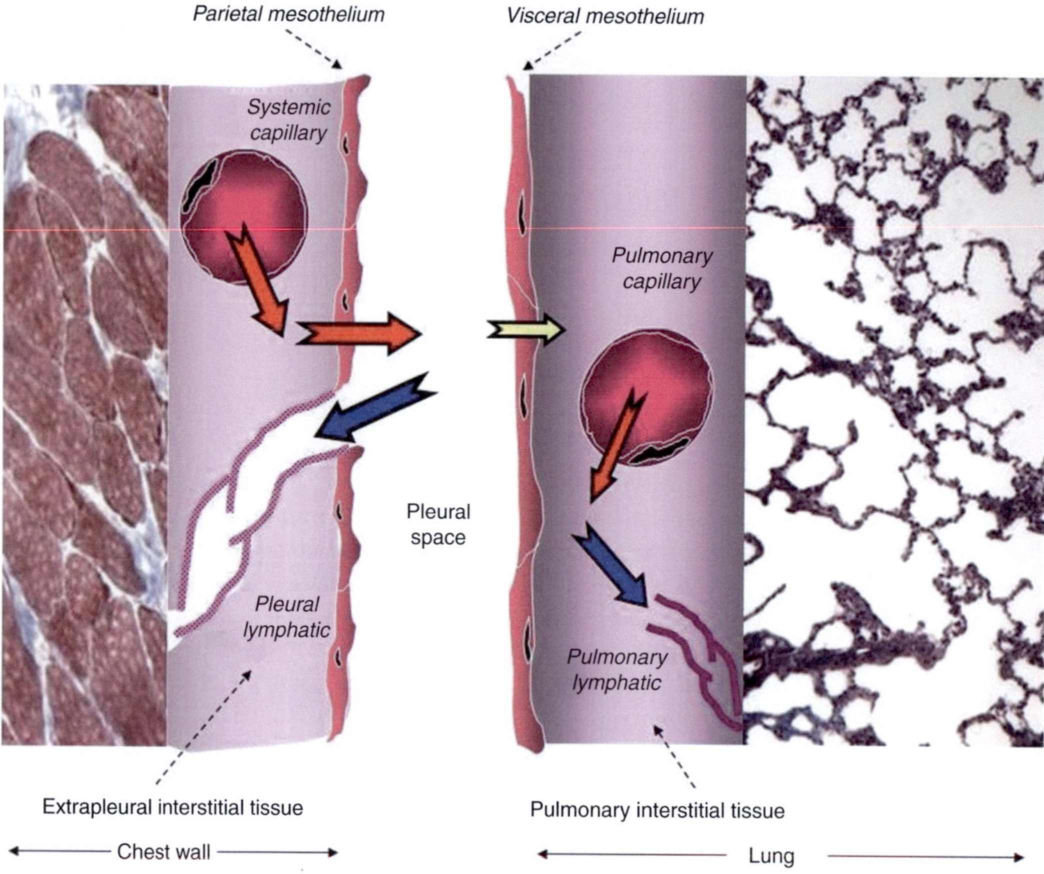

Fig. 4.1 A schematic drawing of the pleuropulmonary compartments involved in the turnover of fluid within the parietal extrapleural interstitium, the pleural space and the pulmonary interstitium. The *red arrows* indicate the fluid filtration across either the systemic, pulmonary endothelium or parietal mesothelium. The *yellow arrow* indicates the absorption of pleural fluid towards the parenchyma. The *blue arrows* represent the absorption of pleural and pulmonary interstitial fluid into the respective lymphatic networks

In fact, since its viscosity is inversely related to the shear rate, or the velocity gradient, it has been proposed that hyaluronan, together with graphite-like phospholipids, may play an important role in lubrication of the pleural surfaces (Andrews and Porter 1973). The cells secrete extracellular fibrous matrix macromolecules such as elastin, fibronectin, glycoproteins, proteoglycans and collagen type I, II and IV (Arai et al. 1975; Bernaudin et al. 1991; Rennard et al. 1985). Finally, mesothelial cells secrete various pro-, anti- and immunomodulatory mediators, such as chemokines, cytokines and growth factors, prostaglandins and prostacyclin, reactive nitrogen and oxygen species and antioxidant enzymes, thus playing an important role in the postinflammatory tissue remodelling (Mutsaers et al. 2002).

4.1.2 Subpleural Interstitial Space and Blood Supply

Mesothelial cells rest on a thin basement membrane supported by a layer of submesothelial interstitial space with a thickness of approximately 10–20 μm on the visceral pulmonary surface and 100–150 μm on the parietal side (Albertine et al. 1982, 1984; Mariassy and Wheeldon 1983). In all mammalian species,

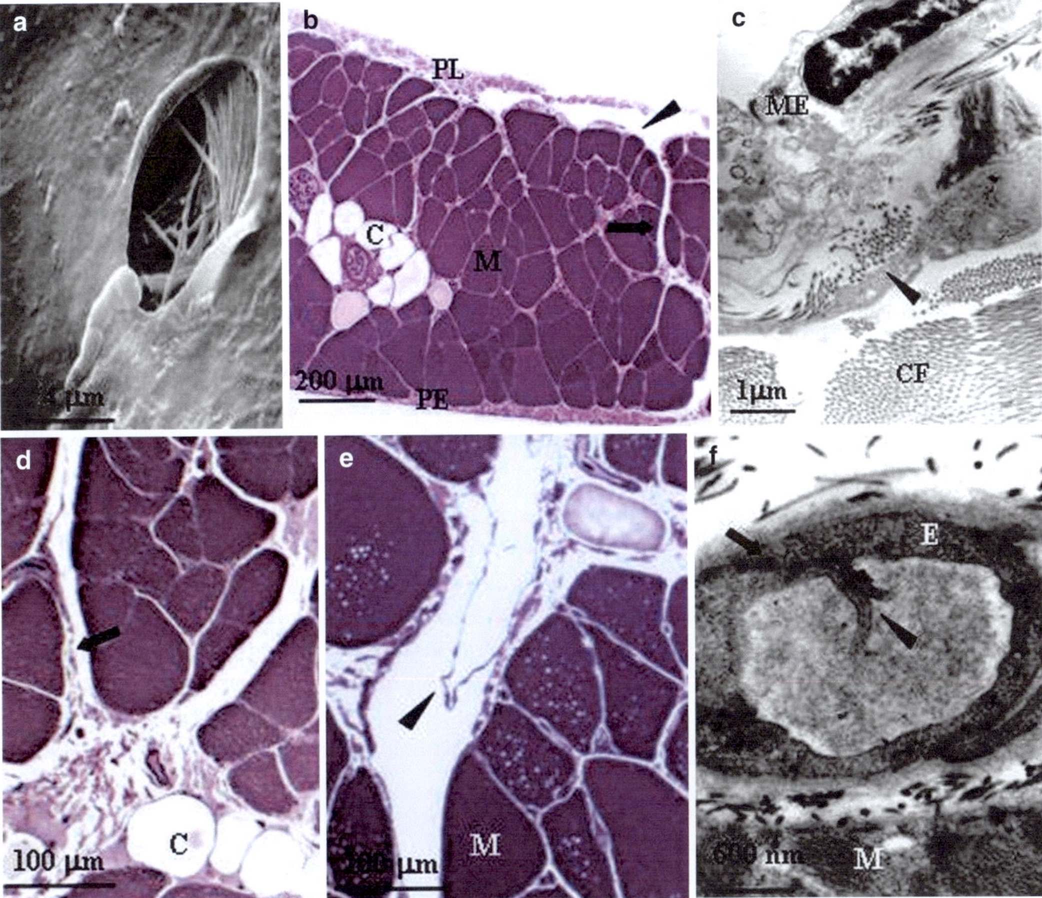

Fig. 4.2 (**a**) Scanning electron microscope photomicrograph of a lymphatic stoma on the tendinous pleural diaphragmatic surface (Modified from Negrini et al. (1991a, b, c)). (**b**) Semithin cross section of rat diaphragm showing the arrangement of the diaphragmatic lymphatic network originating from the pleural (*PL*) and the peritoneal (*PE*) surfaces. Four types of lymphatic structures may be distinguished: submesothelial lacunae (*arrowhead*) within the interstitial space beneath the mesothelial layer; transverse ducts (*arrow*) running perpendicularly to the lacunae through the muscular fibres (*M*); and central collectors (*C*), in the deep diaphragm. (**c**) At transmission electron microscopy (*TEM*), the pleural submesothelial connective tissue layer is composed of loose collagen fibres (*CF*) organised in bundles and contains lymphatic lacunae lined by a discontinuous endothelium (*arrowheads*). *ME* mesothelium. (**d**) Transverse ducts (*arrow*) lined by a discontinuous endothelium and central collector vessels (*C*) lined by a continuous endothelium. (**e**) Transverse lymphatic ducts with intraluminar valves (*arrowheads*) formed by two leaflet attached at opposite sides of the lymphatic vessel walls. (**f**) Primary valves (*arrowheads*) formed by two adjacent endothelial cells of a diaphragmatic initial lymphatic (*arrow*) (**b, c, d, e, f** modified from Grimaldi et al. (2006))

the parietal submesothelial interstitium is supplied by blood capillaries arising from the systemic circulation. In contrast, the blood supply to the visceral submesothelial interstitium may derive either from the bronchial (as in human, sheep, horse and pig) or the pulmonary (as in dog, cat and rabbit) circulation (Agostoni 1986).

4.1.3 The Pleural Lymphatic System

An important and unique feature of the parietal pleura which is not shared by the visceral mesothelium is the presence of so-called stomata (Fig. 4.2a). These are discontinuities of the parietal mesothelium and of the submesothelial interstitial space which form cylindrical-like openings creating the origin of the pleural lymphatic system (Negrini et al. 1991b; Wang 1975). Although widely spread over the diaphragmatic, costal (average density, ~100/cm²) and mediastinal parietal pleura, the greater density is encountered on the diaphragmatic surface (~8,000/cm²), where they are distributed on the tendinous and the muscular region of both the pleural and peritoneal surfaces (Negrini et al. 1991a). The stomata (the average diameter ranges from 0.5 to 20 μm) form at the confluence between the mesothelial cells of the parietal pleura and the lymphatic endothelial cells and empty into an extensive network of lymphatic submesothelial lacunae (Grimaldi et al. 2006; Negrini et al. 1992a), which is located within the interstitial space beneath the mesothelial monolayer (Fig. 4.2b). On the diaphragm, the lymphatic lacunae and the lymphatic capillaries originate directly from the interstitial tissue located amongst the skeletal muscle fibres (Fig. 4.2c) and empty into a system of transverse lymphatic ducts, which depart perpendicularly from the submesothelial lacunae and in turn connect to the deep central collecting system located in the deep interstitial space and surrounded by a continuous endothelial layer (Fig. 4.2d, e). All vessels belonging to this complex network share the same ultrastructural features typical of the so-called initial lymphatic vessels: (a) the basal lamina is discontinuous, (b) anchoring filaments of collagen 3 VII (Schmid-Schöenbein 1990) tightly and directly bond the outer surface of the lymphatic endothelial cells to the fibrous components of the extracellular tissue matrix connective tissue or to muscle fibres and (c) endothelial cells are joined by tight or overlapping junctions. The structure of the lacunae wall, delineated by a discontinuous endothelium and apparently devoid of smooth muscle cells, suggests that these structures do not possess the spontaneous vasomotion that characterises, for instance, the lymphatic mesenteric vessels (Benoit et al. 1989; Zawieja et al. 1993). Initial lymphatic vessels are equipped with two types of unidirectional valves: primary valves in the vessel wall, formed by cytoplasmic extensions of adjacent endothelial cells protruding into the capillary lumen (Fig. 4.2f); this regulates fluid and solute entrance from the interstitial space into the lymphatic lumen. In addition, the intraluminar valves, formed by a leaflet protruding from the lymphatic vessel wall (Fig. 4.2e), direct lymph through the vessel network towards the larger collecting lymphatics. The transverse lymphatic ducts and the central collecting system receive the newly formed lymph from the pleural submesothelial lacunae and from the internal and deeper interstitium and function as a collecting system for the lymph to be carried out of the diaphragm through extra-diaphragmatic collectors, mostly through the right and, to a lesser extent, the left lymphatic ducts.

The pleural lymphatic network is not limited to the diaphragm, but extends to the intercostal and to mediastinal tissues where stomata have also been described (Wang 1975). Conversely, no evidence of stomata has been reported for the visceral pleura, which is supplied by the pulmonary lymphatic network (Albertine et al. 1982; Hainis et al. 1994). Therefore, the lymphatic drainage of the pleural space and of the lung parenchyma occurs through completely independent networks.

4.2 Pleural Surface Pressure

The importance of the pleural space in terms of respiratory physiology depends on two elastic structures: the lung and the chest wall. Like all elastic structures, the lung and the chest tend to passively assume their resting volume, corresponding to the position of minimal mechanical energy. The two structures have different shapes and mechanical properties—the resting volume of the chest is much larger compared to the lung. Therefore, to attain their respective mechanical equilibrium, the chest tends to expand while the lung tends to collapse. The recoil force of the lung and the chest wall per unit pleural surface area, defined as *pleural surface pressure* (P_{pl}), tends to pull apart the two structures, lowering the pressure in the pleural space (intrapleural depression). As a consequence of the effect of gravity on the lung tissue, lung recoil is not uniform, but varies with lung height: in humans, at a volume corresponding to the functional residual capacity (FRC), the average P_{pl} is ~−6 cm H$_2$O at the heart level and decreases by approximately 0.2 cm H$_2$O/cm with increasing lung height (Agostoni 1972, 1986). The P_{pl} gravity distribution is extremely important from the mechanical standpoint, in that it determines local transpulmonary pressure and regional lung expansion (Agostoni 1986; Lai Fook 2004).

4.3 Pleural Fluid Volume and Composition

The mammalian pleural space contains fluid, whose volume (V_{pl}) decreases with body mass, ranging from ~2.5 ml/kg in rats to ~0.04 ml/kg in pigs (Miserocchi et al. 1984), and is 0.26 ml/kg in healthy human subjects (Noppen et al. 2000). The fluid is distributed on an average total pleural surface area of ~90 cm^2/kg of body weight (Miserocchi and Agostoni 1971). Pleural fluid thickness is also very variable amongst different species and within the same species in various regions of the pleural space, ranging between 5 μm over the flat costal surface and 60–100 μm in fluid pools collecting at the lobar margins, at the lung base and in the diaphragmatic apposition zones (Lai-Fook and Kaplowitz 1985). The presence of freely moving fluid into the pleural space is common to all mammals, with the exception of the elephant, whose pleural space is liquid filled only in foetal life, and becomes obliterated by connective tissue at birth and remains obliterated during the animal's entire life (West 2002).

Although the ionic composition of pleural fluid mirrors that of the extracellular extravascular fluid compartment, its physiological protein concentration (C_{pr}) is smaller compared to other interstitial spaces, varying between 2.5 g/dl in rats and 1.2 g/dl in pigs (Miserocchi et al. 1984). The normal concentration of glucose and lactic dehydrogenase (LDH) in pleural fluid is similar or slightly smaller (pleural fluid to serum concentration ratio ~0.9) than the corresponding serum levels (Sahn and Light 1989). However, these parameters usually increase during inflammation when, associated to decreased pleural fluid pH,

they are considered as some of the most important clinical indicators to distinguish between transudative and exudative pleural effusions (Joseph et al. 2001; Sahn and Light 1989).

The pleural fluid also contains saturated and unsaturated phospholipids and hyaluronan, derived from mesothelial cells. While significant levels of HA are found in lung tissue and in the mesothelial microvilli layer (Fraser and Laurent 1996), the normal pleural fluid hyaluronan content (~0.7 μg/ml) (Allen et al. 1992) is not considered significant to contribute to the lubrication of the mesothelial layer. HA dramatically increases in malignant pleural effusions (Thylén et al. 2001) and indeed is a significant prognostic value in malignant mesothelioma. Various cell types, such as detached mesothelial cells, lymphocytes, monocytes and macrophages, are dispersed in the normal pleural fluid at a concentration of 1,500–2,500 cells/mm^3 (Miserocchi and Agostoni 1971; Noppen et al. 2000). However, the concentration and type of cells in pleural fluid does change in several mesothelial and pulmonary pathologies, offering important prognostic tool to differentiate between the various diseases.

4.4 Pleural Fluid Turnover

A direct consequence of the mechanical arrangement of the lung and chest wall and of the existence of the intrapleural depression is that fluid is continuously driven across the mesothelium into the pleural space (see Sect. 4.3); this could potentially lead to a progressive accumulation of pleural fluid and to lung collapse. Therefore, in order to maintain the tight mechanical lung–chest wall coupling, pleural fluid must be continuously removed from the pleural space.

In normal conditions, filtration and corresponding removal of pleural liquid would amount to 0.02–0.09 ml/(h kg body weight) (Miniati et al. 1988; Negrini et al. 1985). Pleural fluid production and its subsequent removal from the pleural space occur through different mechanisms involving not only the pleural mesothelial lining but also in the other compartments schematized in Fig. 4.1.

4.4.1 Filtration of Fluid into the Pleural Space

Fluid and soluble solutes may cross biological barriers, such as the capillary endothelium or the mesothelial layer, through either paracellular pathways between adjacent cells or through vesicular transport (transcytosis) across the cell itself.

4.4.1.1 The Paracellular Transport

Paracellular transport is a passive passage of water and hydrophilic solutes through the intercellular clefts between adjacent cells. The fluid bulk flow (J_v) between any two compartments a and b is set by the hydraulic (P) and colloid osmotic (π) pressure differences across the membrane as described by Starling's law:

$$J_v = L_p \cdot A_m \cdot [(P_a - P_b)$$
$$-\sigma \cdot (\pi_a - \pi_b)] = L_p \cdot A_m \cdot \Delta P \quad (4.1)$$

where L_p is the hydraulic conductivity of the membrane, A_m is the surface area, σ the reflection coefficient of the membrane to plasma proteins and ΔP the net transmembrane pressure gradient.

This equation was derived (Curry and Frøkjaer-Jensen 1984) by viewing the transmembrane fluid fluxes as viscous laminar flows through n parallel intercellular pores of equal radius (r) and length (l), where

$$L_p = \frac{\frac{J_v}{A_m}}{\Delta P} = A_p \cdot r_p^2 8\eta \cdot A_m \cdot l \quad (4.2)$$

A_p and η are the total area of pores and fluid viscosity, respectively, and σ is a pure number ($0 < \sigma < 1$) which in turn depends on the ratio of the radius of a given solute to the radius of the intercellular porous and provides an index of the capability of the solute to cross the intercellular porosity of the membrane. Ions and smallest solutes ($\sigma \to 0$) freely cross the endothelial clefts and equilibrate across both the vascular endothelium and the mesothelium, without providing any osmotic contribution to fluid flux. Vice versa, large molecular weight plasma proteins are restricted in their movement across either the

capillary endothelium ($\sigma \sim 0.8$) or mesothelium ($\sigma \sim 0.2$–0.4) (Negrini et al. 1990, 1991c), generating a colloid osmotic pressure gradient across any two membranes.

A very important parameter appearing in Eq. 4.1 is the hydraulic pressure in compartments a and b or, when examining pleural fluid exchange, in pleuropulmonary compartments described in Fig. 4.1.

Pleural liquid pressure (P_{liq}) has been extensively measured through fluid-filled cannulae and/or micropipettes inserted in various regions of the intact pleural space and at various lung heights in experimental animals (Miserocchi and Agostoni 1980; Miserocchi et al. 1981; Miserocchi et al. 1988). In all pleural regions (costal, diaphragmatic and mediastinal) and at any lung height, P_{liq} is lower than P_{pl}—both at end-expiration (Fig. 4.3a) and at end-inspiration (Fig. 4.3b). This indicates that the mechanism providing pleural fluid removal from the pleural space is capable to decrease the intrapleural pressure below the values set by lung recoil. In addition, because of the significant pressure variability encountered within the space, pleural fluid continuously flows from the costal to the extra-costal (diaphragmatic and mediastinal) regions and within each region in a gravity-dependent fashion (Fig. 4.4b). Extensive measurements performed in experimental animals have shown that the pressures in the interstitial space below the parietal mesothelium (*parietal extrapleural interstitial pressure, P_{epl}*) and the visceral mesothelium (*pulmonary interstitial pressure, P_{pi}*) are also subatmospheric at any lung height (Fig. 4.3a). In particular, P_{pi} is always more subatmospheric than P_{liq}, approximately −10 cm H_2O at heart level and FRC and −22 cm H_2O at end-inspiration (Miserocchi et al. 1990, 1991). According to Eq. 4.1, the flow direction across a membrane is set by ΔP direction: therefore, from the hydraulic (Miserocchi et al. 1984; Negrini et al. 1993; Negrini and Miserocchi 1989) and colloid osmotic (Negrini et al. 2001) pressure values measured in the pleuropulmonary compartments, we may calculate ΔP across the mesothelial and endothelial membranes (Fig. 4.1). Data indicates that fluid filtration into the pleural space depends

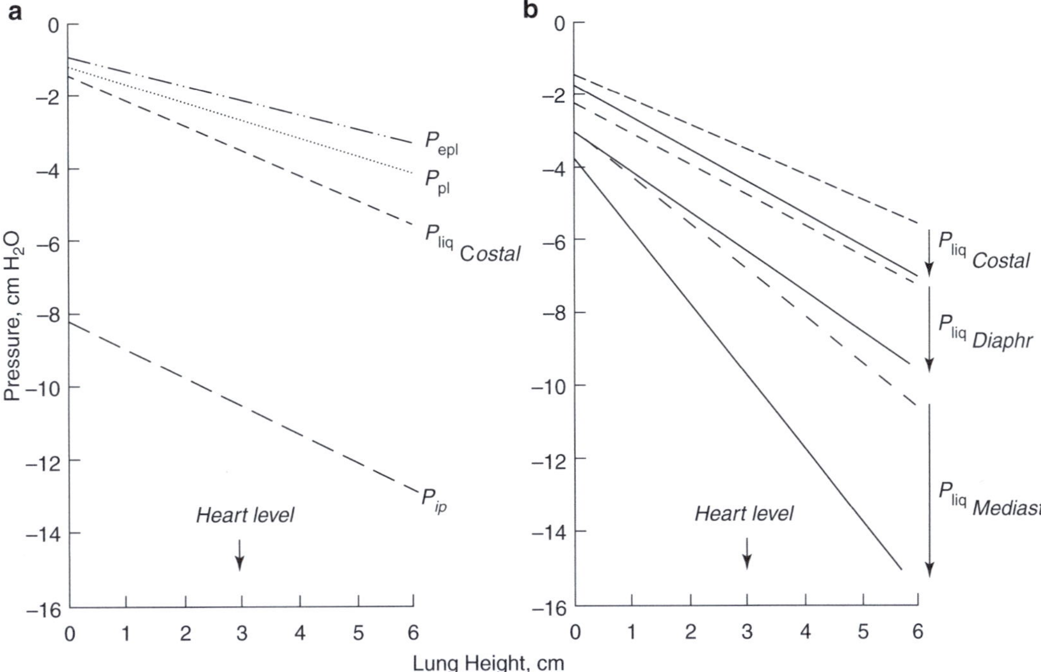

Fig. 4.3 (**a**) The hydraulic pressures in the costal region of the pleural space (P_{liq}, Miserocchi et al. 1983) and in the parietal extrapleural (P_{epl}, Negrini et al. 1987) and pulmonary (P_{pi}, Miserocchi et al. 1993) interstitial spaces as a function of lung height in supine anaesthetised rabbits and at end-expiratory lung volume (FRC). The pleural surface pressure, an index of region lung recoil, is also reported for comparison (*dotted line*, Agostoni 1986). (**b**) The costal, mediastinal and diaphragmatic P_{liq} values at the end-expiratory (*dashes lines*) and end-inspiratory (*continuous lines*) lung volumes (Miserocchi et al. 1981)

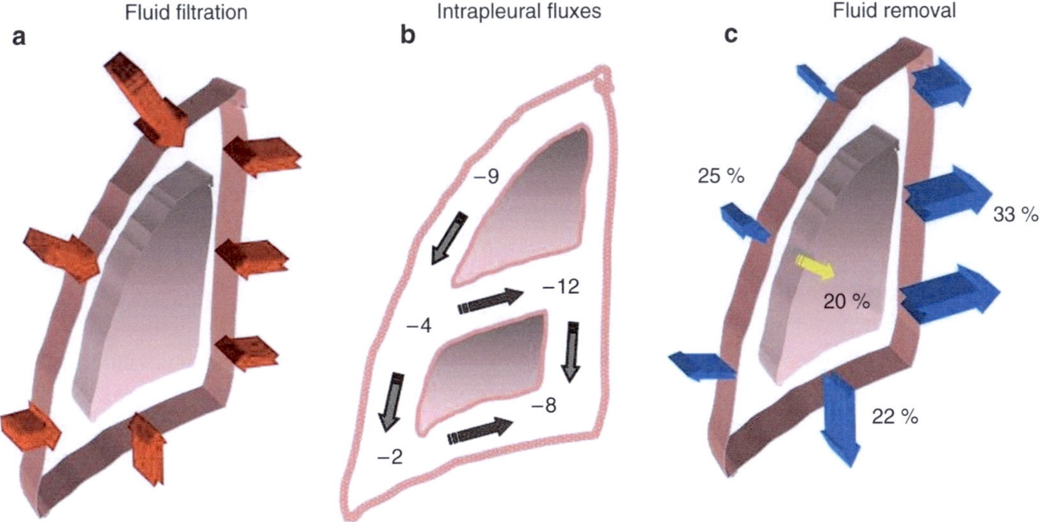

Fig. 4.4 (**a**) The sites of preferential pleural fluid filtration through the parietal mesothelium. (**b**) The top to bottom and costal to extracostal intrapleural flow direction. (**c**) The sites of preferential removal of pleural fluid into the costal, mediastinal and diaphragmatic pleural lymphatic system

upon fluid transfer from the systemic capillaries into the parietal extrapleural interstitial space and from the latter into the pleural space through the parietal mesothelium (Figs. 4.1 and 4.4a). As clearly indicated by Eq. 4.1, the absolute pleural filtration flow per unit surface area is modulated by the L_p of the filtering membranes. In spite of what is commonly reported in studies performed on oedematous or isolated lungs, or on stripped parietal or visceral pleura which suggests that both pleural mesothelia are very permeable to water and even proteins, the L_p of the normal, in situ parietal pleura is relatively low (Negrini et al. 1990, 1991c, 1994) and comparable to that of the endothelium of the systemic capillaries of skeletal muscles (Rippe and Haraldsson 1994; Taylor and Parker 1985). The molecular sieve and the viscous flow resistance of the passive paracellular pathway are likely provided by the fibrous interstitial matrix in the intercellular cleft and by the endothelial cell glycocalyx (Adamson and Michel 1993). The complexity of junctional strands accounts for the fact that less than 10 % of the cell-to-cell contact area is available for microvascular transport and this represents less than 0.04 % of the total capillary surface area (Michel and Curry 1999). At variance with what is observed for the parietal pleura, in normal conditions, the lung parenchyma does not participate to the formation of pleural fluid.

4.4.1.2 Transcytosis

Transcytosis is an energy-dependent process consisting of the transport of water and solutes across the plasmalemma and cytoplasm through small grouped vesicles called caveolae (Bruns and Palade 1968). Transcytosis may consist of endocytosis of a small quantity of fluid followed by transcellular transport or may require recognition of the target macromolecule at the membrane surface through a receptor-mediated mechanism. In the pulmonary endothelium, transcytosis has been described in the transport of albumin, fatty acids and hormones (Schnitzer and Oh 1996; Schnitzer et al. 1995). The process is completely independent upon pressure gradients; therefore, transcytosis might, in principle at least, provide fluid movements either from the extrapleural interstitial space of both the parietal and visceral pleura into the pleural space, thus contributing to fluid filtration, or in the opposite direction, contributing to pleural fluid removal from the pleural space into the adjacent visceral and parietal interstitial space. Data obtained from stripped isolated pleura or isolated pericardium (Bodega et al. 2002) estimates that transcytosis would contribute to approximately 5 % of the interstitial-to-pleural fluid exchange across both mesothelial layers (Agostoni and Zocchi 2007).

4.4.2 Removal of Fluid from the Pleural Space

While pleural fluid production almost completely depends upon passive transmembrane transport across the parietal pleura (Sect. 4.1), fluid egress from the pleural cavity may take place, in normal conditions, through a number of different pathways. These include drainage into the pleural lymphatic system, passive transmesothelial flow, solute-coupled intracellular fluid absorption, intracellular transport through aquaporins and transcytosis.

4.4.2.1 Pleural Lymphatic Drainage

Liquid and solutes enter the pleural lymphatic system through the stomata (Fig. 4.2a) which, as previously discussed, are disseminated throughout the costal, mediastinal and diaphragmatic parietal pleura. While the general principles of lymph formation and accumulation are common to all tissues supplied by the lymphatic system (i.e. all body tissues except the cerebral interstitium and renal medulla), however, stomata are typical of the pleural and peritoneal parietal mesothelia. Entrance of fluid and solutes into the stomata occurs along hydraulic pressure gradients ($\Delta P_{\text{lymph-net}}$) between the pleural space and the lumen of submesothelial lymphatic lacunae when intraluminar lymphatic pressure (P_{lymph}) drops below P_{liq}, as described by the equation

$$\begin{aligned} J_{\text{lymph}} &= K_{\text{lymph}} \cdot (P_{\text{liq}} - P_{\text{lymph}}) \\ &= K_{\text{lymph}} \cdot \Delta P_{\text{lymph-net}} \end{aligned} \tag{4.3}$$

where J_{lymph} and K_{lymph} represents pleural lymph flow and lymphatic conductance, respectively.

The existence, in initial lymphatics, of a lower pressure regime compared to the surrounding compartment is the necessary prerequisite for lymphatic drainage to take place. In non-thoracic tissues, like the mesentery, lymph formation and propulsion is sustained by spontaneous cyclic contractions of a well-organised layer of smooth muscle cells surrounding the lymphatic endothelium (Aukland and Reed 1993). Contractions of the walls of adjacent lymphatic segments, in association with the synchronised opening/closure of the unidirectional leaflets in the lymphatic vessel wall and in the lumen (Bridenbaugh et al. 2003), allow both lymph formation and its subsequent propulsion out of the tissue and towards the venous system. This circumferential support of smooth muscle cells is almost completely absent in the initial lymphatic vessels supplying the intercostal muscles (Moriondo et al. 2006) and the diaphragm (Grimaldi et al. 2006). Therefore, in thoracic tissues and in the pleural space, lymph formation and progression depends upon cyclic expansion and compression of the initial lymphatic vessels which, in turn, is dependent on tissue movements during the cardiac and/or respiratory cycles (Moriondo et al. 2006; Negrini et al. 2004). A similar mechanism, based on extrinsic cardiogenic and respiratory tissue displacement, likely supports the pulmonary lymph flow.

The ability of the pleural lymphatics to drain fluid was proposed more than a century ago by Sir Ernest Starling (Starling and Tubby 1894). However, until recently, in spite of numerous direct and indirect observations in favour of lymphatic function (Allen and Vogt 1937, Bettendorf 1979; Courtice and Simmonds 1954; Miniati et al. 1988, Miserocchi et al. 1982, 1983, 1984; Miserocchi and Negrini 1986; Negrini et al. 1991a; Negrini and Miserocchi 1989), the physiology of lymphatic drainage of the pleural fluid remained controversial. In fact, lymphatics were considered unable to absorb liquid from a compartment set at subatmospheric pressure and instead it was thought to actively absorb proteins but not smaller solutes and water (Agostoni 1972,

Agostoni 1986; Staub et al. 1985; Wiener-Kronish et al. 1984). The definite proof of the ability of pleural lymphatics to generate subatmospheric pressures and to provide an important contribution to pleural fluid drainage came from a series of studies in which P_{lymph} was measured directly in rodent diaphragmatic lymphatics (Negrini and Del Fabbro 1999; Negrini et al. 2004) and in intercostal lymphatics (Moriondo et al. 2006) during spontaneous breathing (Fig. 4.5). Results from these experiments have indicated that lymphatic function in the thoracic tissues and in the pleural cavity depends upon the development of local cyclic tissue stresses associated with the respiratory and cardiac activities that cause P_{lymph} to cyclically oscillate (Fig. 4.5) from values as low as -20 cm H_2O to positive pressure (max P_{lymph} $+10$ cm H_2O). The three-dimensional architecture of matrix macromolecules, their arrangement in the intercostal spaces and their mechanical properties seem to be a determinant in transmitting local tissue stress and in turn play a fundamental role in sustaining and modulating lymph formation in the thoracic tissues and in the pleural space. During spontaneous breathing, based on the recorded P_{liq} and P_{lymph} values, the driving pressure gradient ($\Delta P_{lymph-net}$) promoting pleural fluid entrance into the pleural lymphatics ranges between ≈ -0.5 cm H_2O at end-expiration (Negrini and Del Fabbro 1999; Negrini et al. 2004) and ≈ -24 cm H_2O at end-inspiration (Moriondo et al. 2006), suggesting that removal of pleural fluid occurs throughout the whole respiratory cycle. The P_{lymph} waves attributable to spontaneous contraction of lymphatic smooth muscle cells, commonly observed in dermal or mesenteric lymphatics, are extremely rare in pleural lymphatics, which behave more like those supplying skeletal muscle (Skalak et al. 1984; Trzewik et al. 2001) and the myocardium (Melhorn et al. 1995), i.e. tissues which undergo high tissue stresses. During spontaneous breathing, the entity of tissue stress, and thus the depth of the inspiratory phase, seems to be more effective than respiratory frequency in favouring pleural lymphatic drainage (Moriondo et al. 2006). After the fluid has drained from the pleural

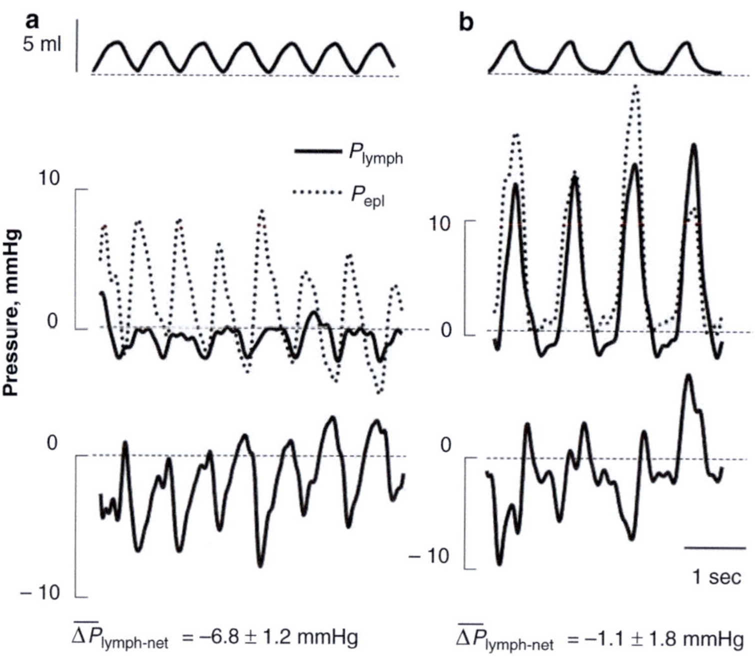

Fig. 4.5 (**a**) Simultaneous recording of tidal volume (*top panel*), lymphatic (P_{lymph}; *middle panel, solid line*) and extrapleural interstitial (P_{epl}; *middle panel, dotted line*) pressure during spontaneous breathing. The negative sign of the pressure gradient, $\Delta P_{lymph\text{-}net} = P_{lymph} - P_{int}$, shown in the bottom panel indicates that, in spontaneous breathing, an interstitial-to-lymphatic fluid flux occurs throughout the whole respiratory cycle. (**b**) Simultaneous recording of P_{lymph}, P_{epl}, and $\Delta P_{lymph\text{-}net}$ during mechanical ventilation in paralysed rats at a breathing frequency of 60 cycles/min (1 Hz). At variance with spontaneous ventilation, both P_{lymph} and P_{int} increase during passive lung inflation. In these conditions, $\Delta P_{lymph\text{-}net}$ and thus lymphatic flow are nullified (Modified from Moriondo et al. (2006))

space, the progression of the newly formed pleural lymph towards larger collecting lymphatic vessels is facilitated by the existence of primary unidirectional flap-like valves (Fig. 4.2e, f) which prevent fluid backflow (Grimaldi et al. 2006). Interestingly, during mechanical ventilation at zero end-expiratory alveolar pressure with muscular paralysis, the $\Delta P_{lymph\text{-}net}$ integrated over the entire respiratory cycle in intercostal lymphatics was essentially nullified (Moriondo et al. 2006), suggesting that active contraction of inspiratory muscles and not simply chest wall expansion is required to enhance lymph formation and progression in thoracic lymphatics. Therefore, because of the importance of the lymphatic system in controlling fluid homeostasis in the thoracic tissues and in particular in the pleural cavity, mechanical ventilation "per se" is expected to determine thoracic tissues overhydration, pleural effusion and, very likely, development of latent pulmonary sub-oedematous conditions in lungs

of patients exposed to positive pressure ventilatory regimes.

Direct measurement of pleural lymphatic flow with closed chest in humans and even in experimental animals is at present very problematic for a series of practical reasons: (a) pleural lymphatics empty principally in the right thoracic duct, but a small proportion (~20 %) also utilises the thoracic duct, mixing with the lymph from distal peripheral and splanchnic tissues. In addition, mediastinal lymphatics may have direct access to the large veins, so that an accurate evaluation of all distinct components would be very difficult to attain; (b) direct cannulation of the right thoracic duct requires an invasive surgical approach and thoracoscopy, which, per se, substantially alters lymphatic flow. Therefore, determination of pleural lymphatic flow in normal conditions is actually based on indirect estimates on various mammalian species (Miniati et al. 1988, Negrini et al. 1991c, 1985). Data indicate that, in conditions as close as possible to the physiological one, approximately 70–80 % of the total pleural fluid turnover rate is accounted for by mediastinal (30 % of total drainage), diaphragmatic (22 %) and costal (25 %) lymphatics (Miserocchi et al. 1986). Therefore, as witnessed by the complex P_{liq} distribution within the pleural regions (Fig. 4.3), fluid filtered through the parietal pleura (Fig. 4.4a) recirculates to the extrapleural compartments (Fig. 4.4b) to leave the cavity through regional lymphatic vessels (Fig. 4.4c).

4.4.2.2 Passive Transmesothelial Fluid Flow

In spite of the low capillary pressure in the visceral subpleural capillaries ($P_c \sim 10$ cm H_2O) (Negrini et al. 1992b) and very negative pressure values ($P_{pi} \sim -10$ cm H_2O) (Miserocchi et al. 1990, 1991) in the normal pulmonary interstitium, a net pressure gradient is maintained in favour of fluid filtration from the pulmonary capillaries into the surrounding interstitial space (Figs. 4.1 and 4.4a). The permeability of the pulmonary endothelium, in particular the alveolar endothelium, to water and proteins is extremely low (Kelly et al. 1998; Parker 2006), a feature that provides an efficient safety factor which limits, for a given trans-endothelial ΔP, fluid transfer into the normal lung parenchyma.

The fluid filtered from pulmonary capillaries into the adjacent lung interstitium is promptly removed by the pulmonary lymphatics (Hainis et al. 1994), which set and maintain the subatmospheric P_{pi} value (Miserocchi et al. 1990; Negrini et al. 1992b). Therefore, in the setting of a continuous filtration from the capillaries into the parenchyma, a pressure gradient is maintained across the visceral pleura providing a potential route for fluid removal from the pleural space into the lung. However, the presence of tight and adherent junctions between mesothelial cells (Bernaudin et al. 1991; Wang 1974, 1985), the tight arrangement of extracellular matrix fibres and the thickness of the submesothelial interstitium (Albertine et al. 1982), plus indirect functional evidence (Miniati et al. 1988; Negrini et al. 1985), all suggest that the permeability to water

is even lower, under normal conditions, in the visceral than in the parietal pleura, so that only a small share (about 20 %, Figs. 4.1 and 4.4) of total pleural fluid egress may actually take place through the visceral mesothelium.

The role of pulmonary capillaries and of lung parenchyma in formation/absorption of the pleural fluid may dramatically change in pathophysiological conditions, as discussed in Sect. 5.1.2.

4.4.2.3 Active Solute-Coupled Pleural Fluid Absorption

An active solute-coupled absorption of pleural fluid into the visceral and parietal mesothelium has been proposed on the basis of results obtained in vitro on isolated parietal or visceral pleural mesothelium or in vivo, from the rate of disappearance of a large hydrothorax containing Na+ transport inhibitors (Agostoni and Zocchi 2007). These studies suggested on one hand that Na+ and K+ inhibitors increase (by ~10 %) the electrical resistance of the mesothelia and, on the other hand, that active solute-coupled fluid absorption would account for ~30 % of the total pleural fluid absorption. Although very interesting from a conceptual standpoint, these conclusions still deserve to be adequately confirmed when applied to the actual physiological condition. Indeed while active ion transports are thought to be important for mesothelial cell function, the net fluid flux attributed to ion transfer from the pleural space into the cell and from the latter into the submesothelial interstitium remains to be accurately determined, yet mesothelial cell behaviour is very sensitive to mechanical stress, a parameter which was not controlled for in the in vitro studies of pleural mesothelia. Finally, the quantitative contribution of active solute-coupled fluid transport under physiological condition has not been evaluated yet.

4.4.2.4 Intracellular Transport Through Aquaporins

In addition to the paracellular route for water transfer, exclusive water channels (aquaporins, AQP) have been recently described in many cell types, including alveolar type I (AQP5) and pulmonary endothelial (AQP1) cells (Borok and

Verkman 2002) and in the parietal pleura of wild-type mice (Song et al. 2000). However, in spite of their recognised role in osmotically driven water transport across both the epithelial and endothelial membranes, aquaporins do not seem to provide any significant contribution to regulation of tissue fluid volume in normal or pathological conditions (Borok and Verkman 2002; Song et al. 2000).

4.4.2.5 Transcytosis

It has been indirectly estimated that transcytosis might contribute for close to 10 % of the pleural-to-interstitial fluid removal in controlled pleural effusions (Agostoni and Zocchi 2007), while the actual role in normal pleural fluid turnover is yet unknown. It is worth noting that the quantitative contribution of transcytosis to total transmembrane fluid flux is, in general, still highly controversial. In fact unlike fluid flux, transcytosis is independent on pressure gradients, and in caveolin-depleted knockout mice, transport of macromolecules and water was in fact further enhanced (Rosengren et al. 2004, Rosengren et al. 2006). Hence, one may conclude that, although the drainage of pleural fluid cannot be attributed to one single mechanism, the most important egress route is represented by the pleural lymphatics which not only maintain pleural fluid volume and pressure in normal conditions but may also, as described in Sect. 5.2, offset pathophysiological pleural fluid loads.

4.5 Pathophysiology of Pleural Effusion

The maintenance of normal pleural fluid volume depends on the capability of the pleural lymphatic system to drain any filtered fluid in excess to normal fluid production. In fact, although other mechanisms may be involved in the removal of pleural fluid, it appears that these mechanisms play a secondary role when compared to the lymphatic system under normal conditions. In addition, it is likely that these mechanisms are unable to be or do not seem modulated when there are increased draining requirements.

4.5.1 Increased Pleural Fluid Filtration

A pleural effusion can be expected to develop when fluid filtration, either through the parietal or visceral pleura, overcomes its absorption.

4.5.1.1 Abnormal Pleural Fluid Production Through the Parietal Pleura

According to Eq. 4.1, increased fluid filtration may occur as a result of a number of factors. These include increased ΔP across the parietal pleura due to systemic hypertension and elevation of P_c in systemic pleural capillaries and P_{epl} in extrapleural interstitium. An elevated trans-endothelial ΔP can occur when plasma C_{pr} and corresponding π decreases as observed, for example, in liver pathologies. However, systemic hypertension or hypoproteinaemia may not necessarily be accompanied by a pleural effusion. In fact, the low hydraulic permeability of the normal parietal pleura efficiently counteracts a potential increase in transmesothelial pressure gradient, limiting fluid filtration. An increased hydraulic permeability (L_p in Eq.4.1) of the parietal pleura may also result in the development of an effusion. Significant (up to 100-fold) increases of the L_p of the pulmonary endothelium and, very likely, of the mesothelial layers may be caused by inflammatory conditions of different etiology (Taylor and Parker 1985).

4.5.1.2 Abnormal Pleural Fluid Production Through the Visceral Pleura

Normal conditions within the visceral pleura do not result in pleural fluid production, but, if any, contribute to its drainage. This has been discussed in detail in Sect. 4 of this chapter. However, the visceral pleural surface might become a source of pleural fluid production in pathological conditions associated with pulmonary oedema.

The fibrous scaffold of the lung parenchyma is provided by large macromolecules such as insoluble fibrous collagen, elastin and the "non-fibrillar" component hyaluronan (HA), the most abundant glycosaminoglycans (GAG) in the lung and proteoglycans (PGs). While inextensible collagen types I and III specifically account for tensile strength and elastin is important for the recoil properties of the lung tissue, HA and PGs fill the porous mesh of the matrix and contract bonds with collagen and elastin, stabilising the architecture of the pulmonary matrix. In the lung tissue, the most represented PG families are chondroitin sulphate-containing PGs (CS-PG, versican) and heparan sulphate-containing PGs (HS-PG, perlecan). The high molecular weight versican forms aggregates with HA, fibronectin and various collagens in the walls of airways and pulmonary vessels (Crouch et al. 1997; Li et al. 2000), stabilises the structure of the tissue fibres and provides the typical mechanical stiffness of the pulmonary parenchyma. HS-PGs form the basement membranes of the vascular endothelium (Yurchenko 1990) or the epithelial cells in the alveolar wall (Zhao et al. 1999). In the vascular basal membrane, a mesh of HS-PGs and collagen IV is thought to fill the clefts between adjacent endothelial cells, thus modulating the viscous resistance to movement of water and solutes across the capillary wall (Farquhar 1981). Hence, pulmonary PGs are important components of the matrix, essential in determining the mechanical properties of the solid tissue matrix as well as the permeability of the pulmonary vascular endothelium to water and solutes.

The development of either hydraulic (Miserocchi et al. 1993; Negrini et al. 1996; Passi et al. 1998) or lesional oedema (Negrini et al. 1998, 2006) is characterised by increased fluid filtration from pulmonary capillaries into the pulmonary interstitial space as a result of an increased ΔP (Eq. 4.1). However, since pulmonary matrix architecture provides a stiff framework around the pulmonary microvasculature (mechanical compliance ~0.05 ml H_2O/ mmHg·g^{-1} dry tissue) (Miserocchi et al. 1993), an increased fluid filtration determines a sudden P_{pi} shift from negative to positive values (Miserocchi et al. 1993; Negrini et al. 1996). Such a response is of great functional importance: indeed, as demonstrated in Eq. 4.1, a positive P_{pi} reduces the pulmonary capillary to

interstitial ΔP, thus decreasing fluid filtration and retarding, or even counteracting, oedema progression. Therefore, provided the pulmonary matrix framework remains intact, and at the onset of pulmonary oedema, an increased fluid filtration into the lung parenchyma is limited by the mechanical response of the stiff matrix. This limits the increase in extravascular lung water and prevents interstitial oedema. In addition, it is worth noting that, based on Eq. 4.3, an increased P_{pi} also enhances pulmonary lymph flow, favouring pulmonary interstitial fluid clearance.

However, severe oedema eventually occurs when the fibrous matrix loses its normal stiffness and therefore becomes more compliant. The abrupt change in the mechanical properties of the matrix depends upon the progressive fragmentation of the PG macromolecules and the loss of the intermolecular bonds between the PGs and other ECM components (Miserocchi et al. 1993; Negrini et al. 1996, 1998, 2006). Fragmentation of PGs is triggered by the activation of a family of matrix metalloproteinases (gelatinase A, MMP-2 and gelatinase B, MMP-9) expressed in ciliated and endothelial cells, pneumocytes and smooth muscle cells (Galis et al. 1994), which are able to selectively cleave large pulmonary CS-PGs (Passi et al. 1999). These can degrade type IV collagen, fibronectin and elastin (Ohnishi et al. 1998); Woessner 1991). MMPs are harmless to the normal lung due to the presence of aspecific antiproteases (e.g. α2 macroglobulin) and of specific MMPs tissue inhibitors; however, direct activation of MMPs by tissue stress or by acute or chronic inflammation may overwhelm the antiprotease protection, shifting the dynamic equilibrium in favour of PG degradation. MMPs may also be triggered by mechanical tissue stress, as demonstrated by the increased synthesis and activation of MMP-2 expressed by pulmonary interstitial fibroblasts after 4 h of low volume mechanical ventilation (Negrini et al. 2006). Degradation of pulmonary matrix macromolecules triggers a cascade of events that involve not only the lung interstitial tissue but also the pulmonary microvasculature and lymphatics.

This cascade includes rupture of CS-PGs and increased tissue compliance which leaves the tissue more expandable; in this scenario, the P_i drops from positive to atmospheric values, and, as expected, from Eq. 4.1, the protective effect against fluid accumulation is greatly nullified. In addition, the cleavage of HS-PG molecules greatly increases the permeability of the endothelial layer and, at later stages, epithelial barriers to fluid and solutes. This greatly enhances fluid filtration movements towards the lung interstitial tissue. Finally, the disorganisation of the matrix architecture is likely to depress pulmonary lymphatic function, whose efficiency in adapting to increased fluid accumulation largely depends upon the integrity of the filaments anchoring the outer lymphatic endothelial surface to the surrounding matrix macromolecules.

The combined effect of these profound changes is a complete perturbation of the physiological steady state and progressive evolution towards severe lung oedema. The latter may interfere with pleural fluid turnover by inducing a recruitment of the visceral pleura as a source of pleural fluid. In fact, because pulmonary P_{pi} increases in both interstitial and severe pulmonary oedema, in agreement with Eq. 4.1, the pulmonary tissue to pleural space ΔP nullifies or even reverses with respect to the physiological condition. Such a reversed pathological process would be facilitated by a greatly increased endothelial and mesothelial L_p which would depend upon activation of systemic and pulmonary MMPs. Interestingly, the effect of MMPs on the pleural mesothelia is limited and/or retarded by antiproteases specific of the pleural fluid (Bieth 1985). In addition, since both the parietal and the visceral pleural surfaces are involved in fluid production at this stage of oedema, filtration flux into the pleural cavity would occur through a larger surface area, potentially increasing Am (Eq. 4.1) by ~ twofold.

In spite of the potential contribution of the visceral mesothelium to pleural fluid production in oedematous lung disease, severe oedema is only rarely associated with clinically relevant pleural effusion. This finding may be explained in part, on one hand, by the fact that even in lung disease, the visceral mesothelium is not as permeable to water as previously commonly assumed and, on the other hand, by the great capability of the pleural lymphatic system to modulate its own drainage to cope with the draining requirements of the tissue.

4.5.2 Pleural Lymph Flow Modulation and Lymphatic Saturation

The lymphatic system can be greatly modulated up to 20 times its physiological value (Taylor and Parker 1985) when interstitial (or pleural) fluid volume and pressure increases.

The modulatory behaviour of pleural lymphatics may be explained mathematically by the equation:

$$J_1 = J_{1_{max}} \cdot \left(1 - e^{\frac{K_i (P_{liq} - P_{lymph})}{J_{1_{max}}}} \right) \tag{4.4}$$

where $J_{1_{max}}$ is maximal pleural lymph flow (Miserocchi and Negrini 1997). When this equation is applied to the pleural space, it states that, for a given P_{lymph} in pleural lymphatics, pleural lymph flow (J_1) depends entirely upon P_{liq}. Thereby, J_1 will progressively increase with increasing P_{liq} when filtration of fluid into the pleural space increases in conditions that would favour the development of a pleural effusion. The capability of pleural lymphatics to adapt their drainage to pleural fluid volume is however limited and indeed saturates when $J_1 = J_{1_{max}}$. In cases where fluid filtration overwhelms $J_{1_{max}}$, a pleural effusion will develop despite the presence of a perfectly functioning lymphatic removal system. Therefore, the pleural lymphatic function is designed to maintain pleural fluid volume in conditions close to the normal physiological state, whereas they are inefficient in counteracting large volume shifts. The same process occurs in the lung, which is primarily drained by the pulmonary lymphatics (Schraufnagel et al. 2005) and which may progress towards interstitial and/ or alveolar oedema, depending on the severity of the pathology, above the threshold of pulmonary lymphatic saturation. Such condition may occur as a consequence of increased filtration from the vascular compartment (see Eq. 4.1), but may also develop during mechanical ventilation. In fact, even at low tidal volumes, mechanical ventilation has been shown to impair both pulmonary (Schraufnagel et al. 2005) and intercostal (Moriondo et al. 2006) lymphatics. Lymphatic flow adjustment might depend, at least partially, upon the release of inflammatory mediators and nitric oxide (NO) which are known to increase local lymph flow by strengthening the contraction force and pumping frequency of the smooth muscle cells in larger lymphatic conduits (Gasheva et al. 2006).

4.5.3 Pleuroperitoneal Fluid and Solutes Exchanges Through the Diaphragmatic Lymphatic Network

The unique structure of the lymphatic system within the diaphragm and the common clinical observation that pleural effusions may develop in ascitic patients may support the existence of a functionally relevant transfer of fluid and solutes from the peritoneal to the pleural cavity. This may occur directly through the diaphragmatic lymphatic network (Lai Fook et al. 2005). In fact, since peritoneal fluid pressure P_{abd} in the sub-diaphragmatic region is only slightly negative or even positive during inspiratory diaphragmatic contraction, a ΔP exists, even in physiological conditions (Fig. 4.6). This may potentially drive fluid across the diaphragm. However, experiments performed in spontaneously breathing rats where small aliquots of fluorescent dextrans were injected in the peritoneal cavity (Moriondo et al. 2007) showed that, in spite of a favourable trans-diaphragmatic ΔP, the great majority of the tracer was absorbed from the peritoneal cavity into the deeper diaphragmatic collecting lymphatics without moving into the opposite diaphragmatic pleural side. In fact, at 30 min after peritoneal injection of dextrans, the majority of the tracer was still localised in the transverse lymphatic ducts proximal to the site of injection while less than 0.5 % of dextrans stained the pleural submesothelial lacunae. The majority of

the tracer remained in the lymphatic transverse ducts (84 %) on the peritoneal side or accumulated towards the larger lymphatic located deeper in the diaphragm. This suggests that, in normal conditions, fluid is removed from the peritoneal cavity, not on the basis of the peritoneal-to-pleural ΔP but rather down ΔP which appears to develop between the pleural and peritoneal spaces and the lumen of the diaphragmatic lymphatics during the respiratory cycle. Indeed, as mentioned in Sect. 4.2.1, the diaphragmatic P_{lymph} is much lower when compared to P_{liq} and P_{abd}: this explains the confluence of the tracer, irrespective to the injection site, towards the deeper collecting duct. Based on the distribution of the tracer in the diaphragmatic network, the lymphatic drainage appears more efficient on the pleural rather than on the peritoneal side, a difference that might be necessary to the maintenance of a "dry" pleural cavity, at least in the physiological steady state.

Therefore, in normal conditions, diaphragmatic lymphatics create a diffuse network to optimise the lymphatic drainage of the pleural and peritoneal cavities while maintaining their functional separation. In normal conditions, the tracer distributes preferentially to lymph vessels located in the muscular diaphragmatic portion, suggesting that active muscle contraction, rather than passive tendon stretch, is more efficient in enhancing local diaphragmatic lymph flow. This observation may have important clinical relevance; progressive fluid accumulation into the peritoneal and, more importantly, the pleural space might be expected in mechanically ventilated patients whose active diaphragmatic contraction is abolished or impaired.

A more diffuse invasion of the whole diaphragmatic lymphatic network, in particular of the medial tendinous region, was observed in experimentally induced peritoneal ascites or pleural effusion (Moriondo et al. 2007), i.e. conditions that increase the peritoneal-to-pleural ΔP or generate a transient pleural-to-peritoneal ΔP, respectively (Fig. 4.6). However, even in these cases, only less than 1 % of the injected tracer in either the peritoneal or the pleural space was recovered in the contralateral diaphragmatic side (Table 4.1). The drainage increased through

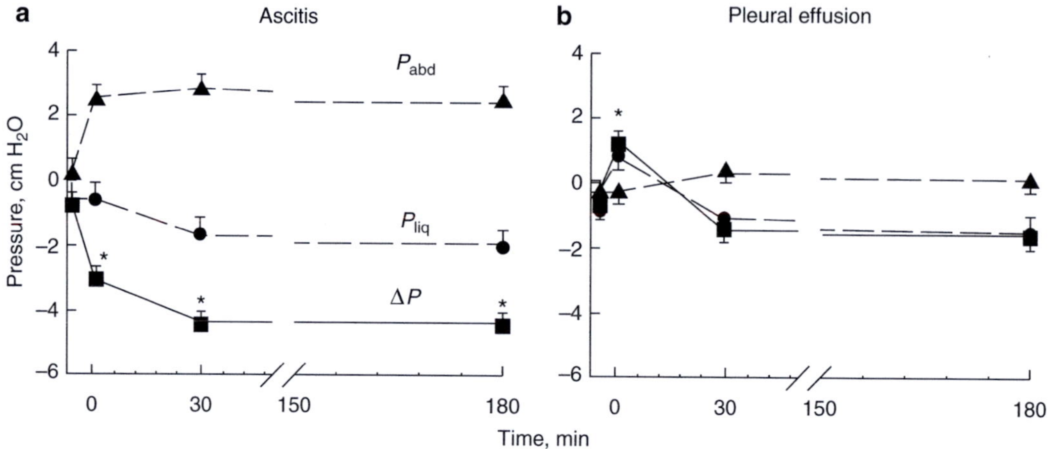

Fig. 4.6 The average sub-diaphragmatic abdominal pressure (P_{abd}, *triangles*) and P_{pl} (*circles*) and trans-diaphragmatic (ΔP, *squares*, calculated as $\Delta P = P_{liq} - P_{abd}$) pressure in control pre-injection baseline ($t < 0$) and after dextrans injection into the peritoneal (panel **a**) or pleural (panel **b**) spaces. The injection was performed at time = 0. A negative ΔP would sustain potential fluid flow from the peritoneal to the pleural space. In experimental ascites, the peritoneal-to-pleural ΔP further increases with respect to the pre-injection baseline value and remains stable for up to 180 min after intraperitoneal injection. Vice versa, pleural effusion reversed the pre-injection ΔP value causing the development of a transient pleural-to-peritoneal ΔP that was completely nullified at 30 min from injection (panel **b**) (Modified from Moriondo et al. 2007). * significantly different ($p < 0.05$) from pre-injection baseline values

Table 4.1 Distribution of fluorescent dextrans in the pleural or peritoneal submesothelial lymphatic lacunae of the diaphragm after induction of acute experimental ascitis or pleural effusion, respectively

	Pleural submesothelial lacunae		Peritoneal submesothelial lacunae	
	30 min	180 min	30 min	180 min
Ascites			1.2 %	0.06 %
Pleural effusion	2.3 %	1.9 %		

From Moriondo et al. (2007)

Data are expressed as percentage of total dextrans observed in the diaphragmatic lymphatic network at either 30 or 180 min from dextrans injection in either the peritoneal (in case of experimental ascites) or pleural (in case of experimental pleural effusion) cavity

greater recruitment of the tendinous lymphatics, which is likely to ensure a greater volume capacity and a faster removal into the deeper collecting ducts. This recruitment strategy suggests that the diaphragmatic lymphatic system is specifically designed as an extrinsic mechanism to efficiently exploit the local changes in tissue stress and thereby support lymph formation and propulsion both under normal and pathophysiological circumstances.

Hence, provided the diaphragmatic structure is maintained, the passage of fluid and solute across the diaphragm is prevented by the ΔP favouring liquid movement towards the deeper collecting lymphatics and by the primary and intraluminar lymphatic valves which drive fluid centripetally towards the deeper collecting ducts. However, one cannot exclude that, in compromised pathological conditions, the diaphragmatic lymphatics might lose their functional properties, allowing fluid and solute to cross the diaphragm. Such a condition might occur when the diaphragm, and thus its lymphatic network, is overstretched, as in cases of excessive fluid accumulation in the abdomen, and/or in obese patients or when it is impaired, like during passive mechanical ventilation.

Conclusions

The pleural space represents an interesting interstitial tissue compartment which, in physiological conditions, is particularly well protected from perturbations that might disturb the steady-state turnover rate. In fact, an increase in intrapleural fluid volume would progressively pull apart the lung from the chest wall, interfering with normal lung expansion and in turn leading to respiratory inefficiency. The factors contributing to the maintenance of normal pleural fluid volume are (a) a low permeability to water and solutes of the pleural mesothelial and submesothelial interstitial spaces; (b) an efficient removal of fluid and large molecular weight solutes through the specifically developed and adjustable pleural lymphatic network; and (c) the structure and function of the diaphragmatic lymphatics that, while providing efficient drainage of both pleural and peritoneal cavities, guarantee their complete functional separation. The adaptation of the pleural lymphatic system in the setting of increased tissue fluid volume suggests that perturbations to pleural fluid volume due to an increased pleural fluid filtration may be satisfactorily controlled by lymphatic removal. Inefficiency of the lymphatic pump due to impairment of intercostal or diaphragmatic muscular contraction, valve incontinence or the saturation of lymphatics may lead to an uncontrolled increase of pleural fluid volume and, ultimately, the development of a clinically severe pleural effusion.

References

Adamson R, Michel C (1993) Pathways through the intercellular cleft of frog mesenteric capillaries. J Physiol 466:303–327

Agostoni E (1972) Mechanics of the pleural space. Physiol Rev 52:57–128

Agostoni E (1986) Mechanics of the pleural space. In: Macklem P, Mead J (eds) Handbook of physiology section 2: the respiratory system, vol 3. Mechanics of breathing, Part 2. The American Physiological Society, Bethesda, pp 531–559

Agostoni E, Zocchi L (2007) Pleural liquid and its changes. Respir Physiol Neurobiol 159:311–323

Albertine KH, Wiener-Kronish JP, Roos PJ et al (1982) Structure, blood supply and lymphatic vessels of the sheep's visceral pleura. Am J Anat 165:277–294

Albertine KH, Wiener-Kronish JP, Staub NC (1984) The structure of the parietal pleura and its relationship to pleural liquid dynamics in sheep. Anat Rec 208:401–409

Allen L, Vogt E (1937) A mechanisms for lymphatic absorption from serous cavities. Am J Physiol 119:776–782

Allen S, Fraser R, Laurent U et al (1992) Turnover of hyaluronan in the rabbit pleural space. J Appl Physiol 73:1457–1460

Andrews P, Porter K (1973) The ultrastructure morphology and possible functional significance of the mesothelial microvilli. Anat Rec 177:409–426

Arai H, Endo M, Sasai Y et al (1975) Histochemical demonstration of hyaluronic acid in a case of pleural mesothelioma. Am Rev Respir Dis 111:699–702

Aukland K, Reed RK (1993) Interstitial-lymphatic mechanisms in the control of extracellular fluid volume. Physiol Rev 73:1–78

Benoit JN, Zawieja DC, Goodman AH et al (1989) Characterization of intact mesenteric lymphatic pump and its responsiveness to acute edemagenic stress. Am J Physiol 257:2059–2069

Bernaudin JF, Jaurand MC, Fleury J et al (1991) Mesothelial cells. In: Crystal RG, West JB (eds) The lung scientific foundation. Raven Press, New York, pp 31–638

Bettendorf U (1979) Electronmicroscopic studies on the peritoneal reabsorption of intrapleurally injected latex particles via the diaphragmatic lymphatics. Lymphology 12:20–38

Bieth J (1985) Proteinase and proteinase inhibitors. Marcel Dekker Inc, New York

Bodega F, Zocchi L, Agostoni E (2002) Albumin transcytosis in mesothelium. Am J Physiol Lung Cell Mol Physiol 282:L3–L11

Borok Z, Verkman A (2002) Invited review: role of aquaporin water channel in fluid transport in lung and airways. J Appl Physiol 93:2199–2206

Bridenbaugh EA, Gashev AA, Zawieja DC (2003) Lymphatic muscle: a review of contractile function. Lymphat Res Biol 1:147–158

Bruns R, Palade G (1968) Studies on blood capillaries. General organization of blood capillaries in muscle. J Cell Biol 37:244–276

Courtice FC, Simmonds WJ (1954) Physiological significance of lymph drainage of the serous cavities and lungs. Physiol Rev 34:419–448

Crouch E, Martin G, Brody J et al (1997) Basement membrane. In: Crystal R, West J, Weibel E (eds) The lung: scientific foudation. Lippincott-Raven, Philadelphia, pp 767–786

Curry FE, Frøkjaer-Jensen J (1984) Water flow across the walls of single muscle capillaries in the frog, Rana pipiens. J Physiol 350:293–307

Farquhar M (1981) The glomerular basement membrane. A selective macromolecular filter. In: Hay E (ed) Cell biology of extracellular matrix. Plenum Press, New York, pp 335–378

Foley-Comer AJ, Herrick SE, Al-Mishlab T et al (2002) Evidence for incorporation of free-floating mesothelial cells as a mechanism of serosal healing. J Cell Sci 115:1383–1389

Fraser J, Laurent T (1996) Hyaluronan. In: Comper W (ed) Extracellular matrix, vol 2. Harwood academic publishers, Amsterdam, pp 141–199

Galis ZS, Muszynski M, Sukhova GK (1994) Cytokine-stimulated human vascular smooth muscle cells synthesize a complement of enzymes required for extracellular matrix digestion. Circ Res 75:181–189

Gasheva OY, Zawieja DC, Gashev AA (2006) Contraction-initiated NO-dependent lymphatic relaxation: a self-regulatory mechanism in rat thoracic duct. J Physiol 575:821–832

Grimaldi A, Moriondo A, Sciacca L et al (2006) Functional arrangement of rat diaphragmatic initial lymphatic network. Am J Physiol Heart Circ Physiol 291:H876–H885

Hainis K, Sznajder J, Schraufnaugel D (1994) Lung lymphatics cast from airspace. Am J Physiol Lung Cell Mol Physiol 267:L199–L205

Hills BA (1992) Graphite-like lubrication of mesothelium by oligolamellar pleural surfactant. J Appl Physiol 73:1034–1039

Hills BA, Butler BD, Barrow RR (1982) Boundary lubrication imparted by pleural surfactants and their identification. J Appl Physiol 53:463–469

Joseph J, Badrinath B, Basran G, Sahn S (2001) Is the pleural fluid transudate or exudate? A revisit of the diagnostic criteria. Thorax 56:867–870

Kelly J, Moore T, Babal P et al (1998) Pulmonary microvascular and macrovascular endothelial cells: differential regulation of Ca2+ and permeability. Am J Physiol Lung Cell Mol Physiol 274:L810–L819

Lai Fook S (2004) Pleural mechanics and fluid exchanges. Physiol Rev 84:385–410

Lai-Fook SJ, Kaplowitz MR (1985) Pleural space thickness in situ by light microscopy in five mammalians species. J Appl Physiol 59:603–610

Lai-Fook SJ, Houtz PK, Jones PD (2005) http://www.ncbi.nlm.nih.gov/pubmed/16099890 Transdiaphragmatic transport of tracer albumin from peritoneal to pleural liquid measured in rats. J Appl Physiol 99:2212–2221

Li R, D'Souza AJ, Laird BB et al (2000) Effects of solution polarity and viscosity on peptide deamidation. J Pept Res 56:326–334

Mariassy AT, Wheeldon EB (1983) The pleura: a combined light microscopy, scanning and transmission electron microscopy study in the sheep. Exp Lung Res 4:293–313

Melhorn U, Davis K, Burke E et al (1995) Impact of cardiopulmonary bypass and cardioplegic arrest on myocardial lymphatic function. Am J Physiol 268:H178–H183

Michel C, Curry F (1999) Microvascular permeability. Physiol Rev 79:703–716

Mills P, Chen Y, Hills Y, Hills BA (2006) Comparison of surfactant lipids between pleural and pulmonary lining fluids. Pulm Pharmacol Ther 19:292–296

Miniati M, Parker JC, Pistolesi M et al (1988) Reabsorption kinetics of albumin from the pleural space in dogs. Am J Physiol 255:H375–H385

Miserocchi G, Agostoni E (1971) Contents of the pleural space. J Appl Physiol 30:208–218

Miserocchi G, Agostoni E (1980) Pleural liquid and surface pressure at various lung volumes. Respir Physiol Neurobiol 39:315–326

Miserocchi G, Negrini D (1986) Contribution of Starling and lymphatic flows to pleural liquid exchange in anesthetized rabbits. J Appl Physiol 61:325–330

Miserocchi G, Negrini D (1997) Pleural space: pressures and fluid dynamics. In: West JB, Crystal R, Weibel E, Barnes P, Berger L (eds) The lung: scientific foundations, 2nd edn. Lippincott-Raven Press, Philadelphia, pp 1217–1225

Miserocchi G, Nakamura T, Mariani E et al (1981) Pleural liquid pressure over the interlobar, mediastinal and diaphragmatic surfaces of the lung. Respir Physiol Neurobiol 46:61–69

Miserocchi G, Mariani E, Negrini D (1982) Role of the diaphragm in setting liquid pressure in serous cavities. Respir Physiol Neurobiol 50:381–392

Miserocchi G, Negrini D, Mariani E et al (1983) Reabsorption of a saline or plasma induced hydrothorax. J Appl Physiol 54:1574–1578

Miserocchi G, Negrini D, Mortola J (1984) Comparative features of Starling-lymphatic interaction at the pleural level in mammals. J Appl Physiol 56:1151–1156

Miserocchi G, Negrini D, Para AF et al (1986) Kinetics of the intrapleural distribution of a radioactive bolus. Respir Physiol 65:13–27

Miserocchi G, Kelly S, Negrini D (1988) Pleural and extrapleural interstitial liquid pressure measures by cannulas and micropipettes. J Appl Physiol 65:555–562

Miserocchi G, Negrini D, Gonano C (1990) Direct measurements of interstitial pulmonary pressure in in-situ lung with intact pleural space. J Appl Physiol 69:2168–2174

Miserocchi G, Negrini D, Gonano C (1991) Parenchymal stress affects interstitial and pleural pressures in in-situ lung. J Appl Physiol 71:1967–1972

Miserocchi G, Negrini D, Del Fabbro M et al (1993) Pulmonary interstitial pressure in intact in situ lung: the transition to interstitial edema. J Appl Physiol 74:1171–1177

Moriondo A, Mukenge S, Negrini D (2006) Transmural pressure in rat initial subpleural lymphatics during spontaneous or mechanical ventilation. Am J Physiol Heart Circ Physiol 289:H263–H269

Moriondo A, Grimaldi A, Sciacca L et al (2007) Regional recruitment of rat diaphragmatic lymphatics in response to increased pleural or peritoneal fluid load. J Physiol 579:835–847

Mutsaers SE, Whitaker D, Papadimitriou JM (2002) Stimulation of mesothelial cell proliferation by exudate macrophages enhances serosal wound healing in a murine model. Am J Pathol 160:681–692

Negrini D, Capelli C, Morini M et al (1987) Gravity-dependent distribution of parietal subpleural interstitial pressure. J Appl Physiol 63:1912–1918

Negrini D, Del Fabbro M (1999) Subatmospheric pressure in the rabbit pleural lymphatic network. J Physiol 520:761–769

Negrini D, Miserocchi G (1989) Size related differences in parietal extrapleural and pleural liquid pressure distribution. J Appl Physiol 67:1967–1972

Negrini D, Pistolesi M, Miniati M et al (1985) Regional protein absorption rates from the pleural cavity in dogs. J Appl Physiol 58:2062–2067

Negrini D, Townsley MI, Taylor AE (1990) Hydraulic conductivity and osmotic reflection coefficient of canine parietal pleura in vivo. J Appl Physiol 69:438–442

Negrini D, Ballard ST, Benoit JN (1991a) Contribution of lymphatic myogenic activity and of respiratory movements to pleural lymph flow. J Appl Physiol 76:2267–2274

Negrini D, Mukenge S, Del Fabbro M, Gonano C, Miserocchi G (1991b) Distribution of diaphragmatic lymphatic stomata. J Appl Physiol 70:1544–1549

Negrini D, Reed RK, Miserocchi G (1991c) Permeability-surface area product and reflection coefficient of parietal pleura in dogs. J Appl Physiol 71:2543–2547

Negrini D, Del Fabbro M, Gonano C et al (1992a) Distribution of diaphragmatic lymphatic lacunae. J Appl Physiol 72:1166–1172

Negrini D, Gonano C, Miserocchi G (1992b) Microvascular pressure profile in intact in-situ lung. J Appl Physiol 72:332–339

Negrini D, Del Fabbro M, Venturoli D (1993) Fluid exchanges across the parietal and pleural mesothelia. J Appl Physiol 74:1779–1784

Negrini D, Venturoli D, Townsley MI, Reed RK (1994) Permeability of the parietal pleura to liquid and proteins. J Appl Physiol 76:627–633

Negrini D, Passi A, De Luca G et al (1996) Pulmonary interstitial pressure and proteoglycans during development of pulmonary edema. Am J Physiol 270(Heart Circ. Physiol.39):H2000–H2007

Negrini D, Passi A, De Luca G et al (1998) Proteoglycan involvement during development of lesional pulmonary edema. Am J Physiol Lung Cell Mol Physiol 274:L203–L211

Negrini D, Passi A, Bertin K et al (2001) Isolation of pulmonary interstitial fluid in rabbits by a modified wick technique. Am J Physiol Lung Cell Mol Physiol 280:L1057–L1065

Negrini D, Moriondo A, Mukenge S (2004) Transmural pressure during cardiogenic pressure oscillations in rodent diaphragmatic lymphatic vessels. Lymphat Res Biol 2:69–80

Negrini D, Tenstad O, Passi A et al (2006) Differential degradation of matrix proteoglycans and edema development in rabbit lung. Am J Physiol Lung Cell Mol Physiol 290:L470–L477

Noppen M, De Waele M, Li R et al (2000) Volume and cellular content of normal pleural fluid in humans examined by pleural lavage. Am J Respir Crit Care Med 162:1023–1026

Ohnishi K, Takagi M, Kurokawa Y et al (1998) Matrix metalloproteinase-mediated extracellular matrix protein degradation in human pulmonary emphysema. Lab Invest 78:1077–1087

Parker J (2006) Hydraulic conductance (Lp) of lung endothelial phenotypes and Starling safety factors against edema. Am J Physiol Lung Cell Mol Physiol 292:L378–L380

Passi A, Negrini D, Albertini R et al (1998) Involvement of lung interstitial proteoglycans in development of hydraulic and elastase induced edema. Am J Physiol 275(3 Pt 1):L631–L635

Passi A, Negrini D, Albertini R et al (1999) The sensitivity of versican from rabbit lung to gelatinase A (MMP-2) and B (MMP-9) and its involvement in the development of hydraulic lung edema. FEBS Lett 456:93–96

Rennard SI, Jaurand MC, Bignon J et al (1985) Connective tissue matrix of the pleura. In: Chretien J, Bignon J, Hirsh A (eds) The pleural in health and disease. Marcel Dekker Inc, New York

Rippe B, Haraldsson B (1994) Transport of macromolecules across microvascular walls: the two pore theory. Physiol Rev 74:163–219

Rosengren B, Carlsson O, Venturoli D et al (2004) Transvascular passage of macromolecules into the peritoneal cavity normo and hypo-thermic rats in vivo: active or passive transport ? J Vasc Res 41:123–130

Rosengren B, Rippe A, Rippe C et al (2006) Transvascular protein transport in mice lacking endothelial caveolae. Am J Physiol Heart Circ Physiol 291:1371–1377

Sahn S, Light R (1989) The sun should never set on a parapneumonic effusion. Chest 95:945–947

Schmid-Schöenbein GW (1990) Microlymphatics and lymph flow. Physiol Rev 70:987–1019, New York, pp 69–85

Schnitzer J, Oh P (1996) Acquapori-1 in plasma membrane and caveole provides mercury -sensitive water channels across lung endothelium. Am J Physiol Heart Circ Physiol 270:H416–H422

Schnitzer J, Oh P, Jacobson B et al (1995) Caveolae from luminar plasmalemma of rat lung endothelium: microdomains enriched in caveolin, Ca2+ –ATPase and inositol trisphosphate receptor. Proc Natl Acad Sci U S A 92:1759–1763

Schraufnagel D, Agaram N, Faruqui A et al (2005) Pulmonary lymphatics and oedema accumulation after brief lung injury. Am J Physiol Lung Cell Mol Physiol 289:L685–L695

Skalak T, Schmid-Schöenbein G, Zweifach B (1984) New morphological evidences for a mechanism of lymph formation in skeletal muscle. Microvasc Res 28:95–112

Song Y, Yang B, Matthay MA et al (2000) Role of aquaporin water channels in pleural fluid dynamics. Am J Physiol Cell Physiol 279:C1744–C1750

Starling EH, Tubby AH (1894) On absorption from and secretion into the serous cavities. J Physiol 16: 140–155

Staub N, Wiener-Kronish J, Albertine K (1985) Transport through the pleura. In: Chretien J, Bignon J, Hirsch A (eds) The pleura in health and disease. Dekker, New York, p 188

Taylor AE, Parker JC (1985) Pulmonary interstitial space and lymphatics. In: Fishman AP, Fisher AB (eds) Handbook of physiology. The respiratory system circulations and non respiratory functions, vol 1, Chapter 4. The American Physiological Society, Bethesda, pp 167–230

Thylén A, Hjerpe A, Martensson G (2001) Hyaluronan content in pleural fluid as a prognostic factor in patients with malignant pleural mesothelioma. Cancer 92:1224–1230

Trzewik J, Millipatty S, Artmann G et al (2001) Evidence for a second valve system in lymphatic endothelial microvalves. FASEB J 15:1711–1717

Wang NS (1974) The regional differences of pleural mesothelial cells in rabbits. Am Rev Respir Dis 110:623–633

Wang N (1975) The preformed stomata connecting the pleural cavity and the lymphatics in the parietal pleura. Am Rev Respir Dis 111:12–20

Wang NS (1985) Mesothelial cells in situ. In: Chretien J, Bignon J, Hirsh A (eds) The pleura in health and disease. Marcel Dekker, Inc, New York, pp 23–42

Wang PM, Lai-Fook SJ (2000) Pleural tissue hyaluronan produced by postmortem ventilation in rabbits. Lung 178:1–12

West J (2002) Why doesn't the elephant have a pleural space? News Physiol Sci 17:47–50

Wiener-Kronish J, Albertine K, Licko V et al (1984) Protein egress and entry rates in pleural fluid and plasma in sheep. J Appl Physiol 56:459–463

Woessner JF Jr (1991) Matrix metalloproteinases and their inhibitors in connective tissue remodeling. FASEB J 5:2145–2154

Yurchenko P (1990) Molecular architecture of basement membrane. FASEB J 4:1577–1590

Zawieja DC, Davis KI, Schuster R et al (1993) Distribution, propagation and coordination of contractile activity in lymphatics. Am J Physiol 264:H1283–H1291

Zhao J, Sime P, Bringas PJ et al (1999) Adenovirus – mediated decorin gene transfer prevents TGF-beta-induced inhibition of lung morphogenesis. Am J Physiol Lung Cell Mol Physiol 277:L412–L422

Ultrasound for Medical Thoracoscopy

5

Cyrus Daneshvar, Saiyad A. Sarkar, and David P. Breen

5.1 Introduction

The method for thoracoscopy described since Jacobaeus performed his first routine medical thoracoscopies depends upon being able to access the pleural space, which if absent relies upon the induction of a pneumothorax (Marchetti et al. 2011). Inducing a pneumothorax was frequently performed immediately prior to the procedure or more classically on the preceding day. This was followed by a chest radiograph to confirm the presence of a free pleural cavity thus allowing safe access and subsequent optimal inspection. Although induction of a pneumothorax is a safe procedure, it does require further intervention of the pleural space and therefore, theoretically at least, increase the risk of complications – especially iatrogenic pleural infection. Further, it requires the patient to be admitted for an additional day at an associated increase in cost.

One of the primary reasons for the failure of thoracoscopy is the inability to obtain safe access to the pleural cavity. This may be due to minimal pleural fluid, pleural adhesions, multiple septations or an absent pleural space (e.g. when previous pleurodesis has been performed).

In the past, it was felt that ultrasound did not have a significant role in pulmonology. This was partly because ultrasound is not useful for visualising normal aerated lung, due to its failure to penetrate air. However, over time, it became apparent that ultrasound could contribute to the assessment, diagnosis and management of thoracic disease (Medford and Entwisle 2010). This included chest wall disease, pleura, pleural effusions, empyemas and peripheral parenchymal lung disease.

The seminal paper by Diacon et al. emphasised the important role of thoracic ultrasound in selecting the safest position for thoracocentesis in patients with radiographic evidence of a pleural effusion (Diacon et al. 2003b). The recognition of the limitations of clinical examination in identifying the location for thoracocentesis was clearly demonstrated and has led to the widespread use of ultrasound in the management of pleural diseases. However, thoracic ultrasound can also provide additional diagnostic information including fluid and pleural space characteristics, pleural thickening and diaphragmatic disease and underlying lung abnormalities. Such features are useful in the diagnostic pathway and interpretation of the pleural space, but are not adequately sensitive to preclude further diagnostic investigations (Qureshi et al. 2009).

In thoracoscopy, the assessment of the pleural space using thoracic ultrasound may not only allow the thoracoscopist to identify a safe port of entry but may also allow them to recognise potential procedural difficulties and therefore consider alternative diagnostic strategies (e.g. CT-guided biopsies). Therefore, both procedures complement

C. Daneshvar (✉) • D.P. Breen
Department of Respiratory Medicine,
Galway University Hospitals, Galway, Ireland
e-mail: cyrus.daneshvar@hse.ie; david.breen@hse.ie

S.A. Sarkar
Pulmonary and Critical Care Department,
Franklin Square Hospital Center,
9000 Franklin Square Dr,
Baltimore, MD 21237, USA

P. Astoul et al. (eds.), *Thoracoscopy for Pulmonologists*,
DOI 10.1007/978-3-642-38351-9_5, © Springer-Verlag Berlin Heidelberg 2014

one another, and thoracoscopists should be able to perform, or at least have real-time access to, thoracic ultrasound.

5.2 Description of Ultrasound Procedure

Ultrasound, as used pre-thoracoscopy, does not differ from the procedure performed in the assessment of pleural disease. Therefore, the same technique and training requirements are necessary. A detailed description of thoracic ultrasound is beyond the scope of this chapter but has been covered in depth elsewhere (Koegelenberg et al. 2012). However, some important principles are highlighted below.

5.2.1 Equipment

The primary transducer for performing thoracic ultrasound in thoracoscopy is a curvilinear probe with a frequency range of 2–5 MHz (Fig. 5.1) (Light and Lee 2008; McLoud and Flower 1991). The lower frequency allows a balance between accurate assessment of both proximal and deep structures, but higher frequency probes (7.5 MHz) may be used to assess the superficial soft tissues and pleural surfaces (Evans and Gleeson 2004). For use during the sterile phases of the procedure, for example, at the time of thoracoscopy or in the setting of a small pleural collection (e.g. minithoracoscopy), additional equipment including a sterile probe sheath and sterile gel is required (Fig. 5.2).

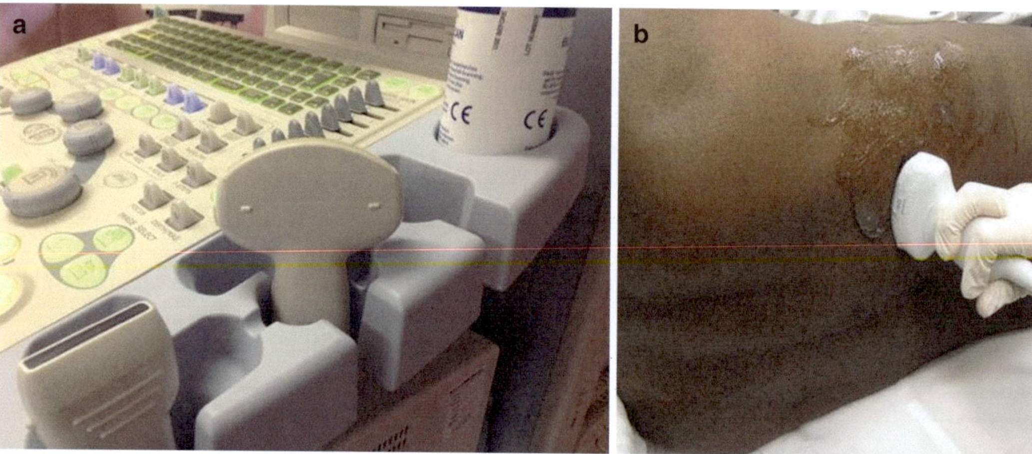

Fig. 5.1 Panel (**a**) curvilinear ultrasound probe with a frequency range of 2–5 MHz. Panel (**b**) thoracic ultrasound performed pre-thoracoscopy with the patient in the lateral decubitus position

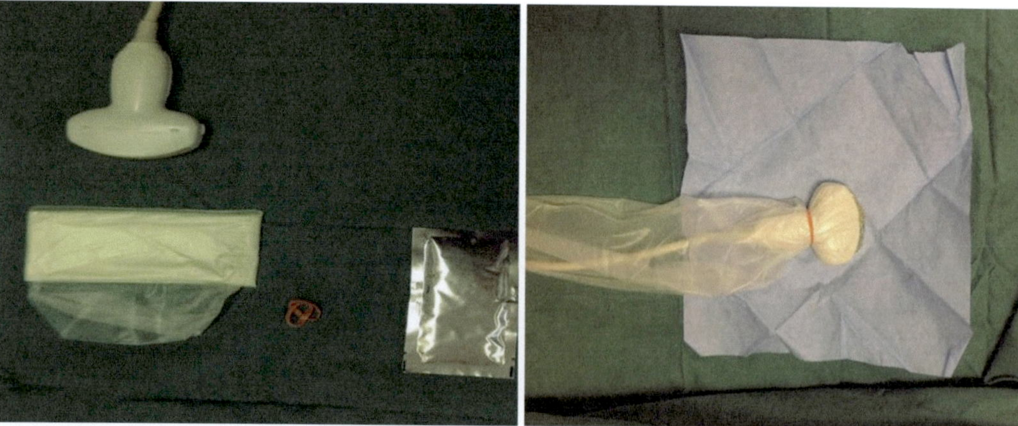

Fig. 5.2 Sterile sheath for ultrasound probe

5.3 Procedure at Thoracoscopy

Positioning of the patient differs from that preferred in the usual thoracic ultrasound assessment where patients are sat upright with their arms outstretched anteriorly. In thoracoscopy, the patient must be in the planned position for the port entry. Usually, this is the lateral decubitus position since this is the preferred position for medical thoracoscopy (and other pleural procedures under direct ultrasound guidance). Once the patient is correctly positioned, the transducer is held like a pen between the thumb and first fingers, with the medial aspect of the palm resting against the chest wall to enable the sonographer to remain steady and have a tactile awareness of their position whilst adjusting the images on the ultrasound machine to optimise their quality. The probe position should be orientated with the marker pointing towards the patients head, as is standard in sonography.

To ensure accurate orientation, a systematic approach is necessary where solid organs below the diaphragm should be identified first. Having identified the kidney, the probe is moved cranially to visualise the liver or spleen. Next, the costophrenic angle should be identified. The diaphragm should be examined by asking the patient to take deep breaths or sniff to ascertain the presence of paradoxical movement or any unexpected significant lung/organ excursions. Following this, the presence of pleural fluid is assessed. The ultrasonographic features of the space should be recorded, including the dimensions and characteristics of the pleural fluid. The position for trocar placement is then identified, and that location is further interrogated by tilting the transducer caudally and cranially to ascertain a three-dimensional representation of the area. This helps to ensure the absence of tethered viscera, septations, significant lung excursion on inspiration and interposition of subdiaphragmatic organs. Furthermore, this entry position should preferably still remain within the classical safe triangle (Laws et al. 2003). The site should be marked and the patient must maintain their position. If any adjustment is made, the site should be reassessed. By performing thoracic ultrasound using sterile conditions at the start of the procedure, the time between confirming position and port entry is minimised and in our opinion is the safest method.

5.4 Ultrasound Features

5.4.1 General Appearance

In thoracic ultrasound of the normal thorax, sound waves do not penetrate the lung due to the interface between the soft tissue and lung (predominantly air) having a poor acoustic impedance match leading to most of the sound waves being reflected back to the transducer. However, information can be obtained by confirming the presence of a pleural stripe which represents the acoustic reflection from the solid parietal and visceral pleura. At the costophrenic angle, the subdiaphragmatic organ will be obscured by the lung during respiration, whilst the diaphragm will not be fully visualised due to obscuring by the normal lung (Fig. 5.3). The normal movement of the lung is inferred by the presence of the sliding lung sign, which actually represents the movement between the parietal and visceral pleural surfaces. The absence of this sign may indicate pleurodesis or a pneumothorax, the two being distinguished by the presence or absence of comet tails (distal reverberation echoes), respectively. If previous pleurodesis has been performed, absence of the lung sliding sign would suggest that the lung may not fully deflate upon trocar insertion. In such cases, an alternate diagnostic approach may be considered.

5.4.2 Pathological Changes

Collections within the pleural cavity can be observed by the presence of echogenic regions bordered by the parietal pleura, diaphragm and underlying lung (Fig. 5.3). However, the ultrasonographic images are highly variable and therefore experience is required to interpret complex pleural spaces (Figs. 5.4, 5.5, and 5.6). Finally, the intercostal arteries have been shown to be variable in their position in relation to the superior rib, especially in

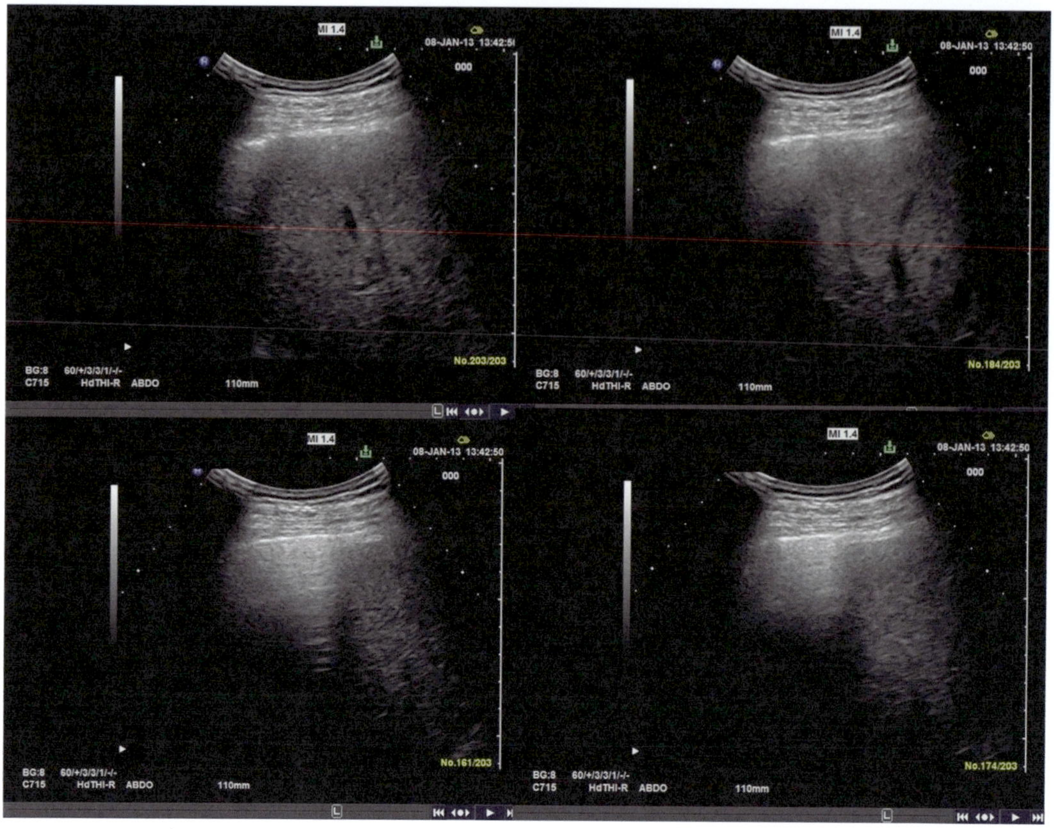

Fig. 5.3 Appearances of normal pleural cavity without fluid. The lung progressively obscures the liver during the respiratory cycle

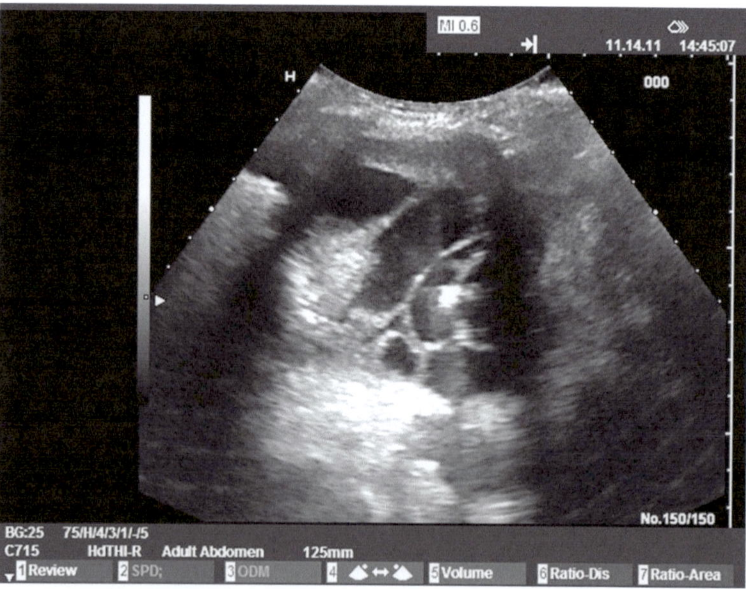

Fig. 5.4 A complex multiloculated pleural space secondary to malignancy

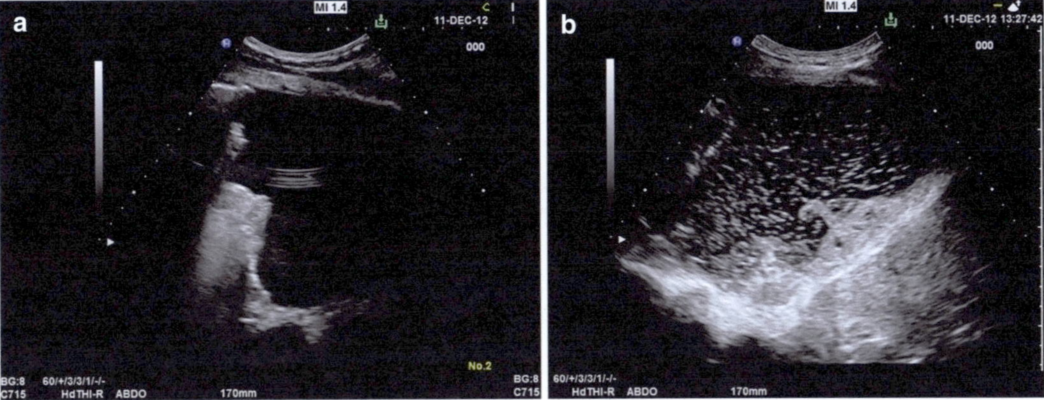

Fig. 5.5 A malignant pleural effusion secondary to oesophageal cancer (panel **a**). The space is highly echogenic and this is accentuated with patient movement (panel **b**). In addition, an indwelling pleural catheter can be seen crossing the space in panel (**a**)

Fig. 5.6 A malignant pleural space secondary to lung cancer. There is evidence of swirling within the fluid. In addition, the underlying lung is atelectatic

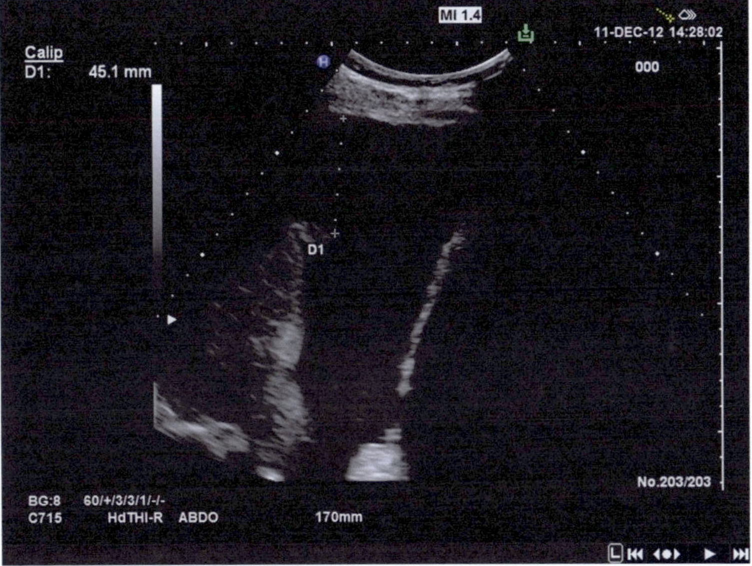

the paravertebral region of the posterior ribs and in more elderly patients with ectatic vessels (Dewhurst et al. 2012; Yoneyama et al. 2010). Even within the safe triangle, Doppler signals may be utilised to identify aberrant vasculature underlying the area of port of entry.

Identifying abnormalities during assessment with thoracic ultrasound may lead the clinician to identify alternative diagnostic strategies. Quereshi et al. noted features of malignant and benign pleural effusions, showing a sensitivity of 79 % and specificity of 100 % (Qureshi et al. 2009). Features supporting malignant disease included parietal pleural thickening >1 cm, parietal pleural nodularity, visceral pleural thickening/nodularity and nodular or thickened diaphragms. Skilled assessment with the thoracic ultrasound may lead to alternative diagnostic pathways that are less invasive. Further, the poor ability to predict adhesions or septations and predict the complexity of the pleural space by CT scanning makes this a useful modality (Kearney et al. 2000).

Probably the most important role of thoracic ultrasound in medical thoracoscopy is to ensure successful entry into the pleural space (Hersh et al. 2003). Studies have demonstrated the role of ultrasound in identifying adhesions which could limit access to the pleural cavity and possibly result in procedural-related complications. Ultrasound has been shown to be superior to CT scanning in identifying pleural adhesions. Medford et al. demonstrated that ultrasound pre-thoracoscopy allowed for the identification of adhesions in all cases compared to a rate of detection of only 12.5 % by CT scanning in the non-ultrasound group (Medford et al. 2010). Further, in their study, there was no failure to access the pleural space in the ultrasound group compared to a failure rate of 16.7 % in the non-ultrasound group. Additional important features were revealed by ultrasound in 43 % of cases. Other authors have reported similar results. Cassanelli et al. in a surgical series reported that thoracic ultrasound had a sensitivity of 80.6 % (95 % confidence interval, 0.740–0.872) and specificity of 96.1 % (95 % confidence interval, 0.949–0.973) for the detection of adhesions – confirmed at VATS (Cassanelli et al. 2012). Wei et al. also demonstrated a sensitivity of 88 % and specificity of 82.6 % for the detection of adhesions and showed there to be good agreement between ultrasonographers (Wei et al. 2012).

5.4.3 Practical Considerations

Practical concerns over pre-thoracoscopy ultrasound may be the perceived lengthening of procedure time as a result of performing a scan. Macha et al. reported on a case series of 687 patients with pleural disease and found that ultrasound used prior to thoracoscopy saved the usual 20–30 min of time needed to induce a pneumothorax (Macha et al. 1993). This is supported by a further study suggesting that thoracic ultrasound adds only minutes to the length of the procedure (Hersh et al. 2003).

5.4.4 Additional Roles of Ultrasound

In the patients undergoing a diagnostic thoracoscopy, post procedure ultrasound may have a role in ensuring complete evacuation of air from the pleural cavity. This has a number of advantages over chest radiograph, i.e. portable, bedside with no radiation risks, thus facilitating "on-the-table" removal of the chest drain. This may allow further cost saving but has not been formally evaluated.

In the setting of therapeutic thoracoscopy, where the chest drain remains in situ for a number of days, thoracic ultrasound can allow ongoing evaluation of the pleural cavity to assess the efficacy of pleurodesis as characterised by the absence of the lung sliding sign (Leo et al. 2005). It may also have an important role in the detection of early post thoracoscopy complications such as residual pleural fluid, failure of pleurodesis, empyema, air leak, pneumothorax or trapped lung.

Future utilisation of ultrasound during thoracoscopy may include intra-procedural ultrasound for the localisation and/or biopsy/fine needle aspiration (FNA) of peripheral nodules and mediastinal lymph nodes assessment (Matsumoto et al. 2004; Hida et al. 1996; Friedel et al. 1998). The role for use during minithoracoscopy where small volume pleural spaces are accessed is clear (Tassi et al. 2011).

5.4.5 Cost Benefit

The routine use of thoracic ultrasound pre-thoracoscopy will initially add additional expense to an interventional pulmonology programme. For example, in a paper by Hersh et al., such an approach was shown to be unlikely cost-effective if the machine was used just at the time of thoracoscopy itself (Hersh et al. 2003). Within the United Kingdom, this cost has been estimated to be between £13,500 and £22,000 lb sterling (Medford 2010). However, as the authors stated in their discussion, it is likely that the use of the ultrasound machine will quickly expand to routine clinical practice such as pleural space assessment, thoracocentesis, drain insertion as well as non-thoracic indications such as neck and vascular interrogation.

Later studies have assessed the cost-effectiveness of using thoracic ultrasound in pleural disease, including Patel et al. who reported on the cost-effectiveness of ultrasound prior to thoracocentesis (Patel et al. 2012). The reduction in cost seen could in part be accounted for by a reduction in complications including haemorrhage and pneumothorax. In the setting of thoracoscopy, it is estimated that the cost saving will be obtained by reducing hospital stay, as may be required for induction of pneumothorax, and by reducing failure to access the pleural cavity thus reducing the requirement for further procedures – CT-guided biopsy or VATS.

5.4.6 Training

A survey of programme directors in the United States of America was undertaken in 2010 (Eisen et al. 2010). Although the majority of programmes offered sonographic training in vascular access, only three out of four programmes trained fellows in pleural and/or lung ultrasound. A number of barriers were identified, particularly the lack of faculty with adequate experience. As training has expanded to incorporate thoracic ultrasound, it seems likely that the new generation of pulmonologists will be skilled in this imaging technique. In the United Kingdom, the Royal College of Radiologists (RCR) guidelines were published in 2005 and updated in 2012 that set out the minimal requirements for trainees to be competent in basic thoracic ultrasound for the identification of normal and abnormal anatomy and guidance of pleural procedures (The Royal College of Radiologists 2012). If using thoracic ultrasound pre-thoracoscopy, we believe that competency through formal training as set out in the RCR document or equivalent is essential. In addition, it is essential to gain specific experience in thoracic ultrasound pre-thoracoscopy. Although the technique is identical to that used in the non-thoracoscopy patient, a number of important points need to be highlighted. As mentioned previously, most ultrasound imaging and basic sampling of the pleural cavity is performed in the sitting position. Therefore, it is recommended that the pulmonologist becomes familiar with the postural effects of patients in the lateral decubitus position. It should be emphasised that although the guidelines state a minimum number of procedures to be observed and performed, it is our opinion that a period of mentoring is best – for instance, an attachment with a chest radiologist or a pulmonologist with accredited experience in thoracic ultrasound.

Conclusion

Thoracic ultrasound is an easy-to-learn skill for pulmonologists that has now become an essential tool in pleural pathology and more recently premedical thoracoscopy. There is evidence to support its use in improving the decision-making process. The ultrasound assessment may suggest an alternative diagnostic strategy. In patients who undergo thoracoscopy, it improves pleural access, limits complications, reduces the length of patient hospital stay and has healthcare cost benefits. Guidelines now exist to ensure competency in the technique.

References

Cassanelli N, Caroli G, Dolci G et al (2012) Accuracy of transthoracic ultrasound for the detection of pleural adhesions. Eur J Cardiothorac Surg 42:813–818

Dewhurst C, O'Neill S, O'Regan K, Maher M (2012) Demonstration of the course of the posterior intercostal artery on CT angiography: relevance to interventional radiology procedures in the chest. Diagn Interv Radiol 18:221–224

Diacon AH, van de Wal BW, Wyser C et al (2003a) Diagnostic tools in tuberculous pleurisy: a direct comparative study. Eur Respir J 22:589–591

Diacon AH, Brutsche MH, Soler M (2003b) Accuracy of pleural puncture sites: a prospective comparison of clinical examination with ultrasound. Chest 123: 436–441

Eisen LA, Leung S, Gallagher AE, Kvetan V (2010) Barriers to ultrasound training in critical care medicine fellowships: a survey of program directors. Crit Care Med 38:1978–1983

Evans AL, Gleeson FV (2004) Radiology in pleural disease: state of the art. Respirology 9:300–312

Friedel G, Hurtgen M, Toomes H (1998) Intraoperative thoracic sonography. Thorac Cardiovasc Surg 46:147–151

Hersh CP, Feller-Kopman D, Wahidi M et al (2003) Ultrasound guidance for medical thoracoscopy: a novel approach. Respiration 70:299–301

Hida Y, Kato H, Nishibe T et al (1996) Value of intraoperative intrathoracic ultrasonography during video-assisted thoracoscopic pulmonary resection. Surg Laparosc Endosc 6:472–475

Kearney SE, Davies CW, Davies RJ, Gleeson FV (2000) Computed tomography and ultrasound in parapneumonic effusions and empyema. Clin Radiol 55:542–547

Koegelenberg CFN, von Groote-Bidlingmaier F, Bolliger CT (2012) Transthoracic ultrasonography for the respiratory physician. Respiration 84:337–350

Laws D, Neville E, Duffy J (2003) BTS guidelines for the insertion of a chest drain. Thorax 58(suppl 2):ii53–ii59

Leo F, Dellamonica J, Venissac N, Pop D, Mouroux J (2005) Can chest ultrasonography assess pleurodesis after VATS for spontaneous pneumothorax? Eur J Cardiothorac Surg 28:47–49

Light RW, Lee YCG (2008) Textbook of pleural diseases. Hodder Arnold, London

Macha HN, Reichle G, von Zwehl D et al (1993) The role of ultrasound assisted thoracoscopy in the diagnosis of pleural disease. Clinical experience in 687 cases. Eur J Cardiothorac Surg 7:19–22

Marchetti GP, Pinelli V, Tassi GF (2011) 100 years of thoracoscopy: historical notes. Respiration 82:187–192

Matsumoto S, Hirata T, Ogawa E et al (2004) Ultrasonographic evaluation of small nodules in the peripheral lung during video-assisted thoracic surgery (VATS). Eur J Cardiothorac Surg 26:469–473

McLoud TC, Flower CD (1991) Imaging the pleura: sonography, CT, and MR imaging. AJR Am J Roentgenol 156:1145–1153

Medford AR (2010) Additional cost benefits of chest physician-operated thoracic ultrasound (TUS) prior to medical thoracoscopy (MT). Respir Med 104:1077–1078

Medford ARL, Entwisle JJ (2010) Indications for thoracic ultrasound in chest medicine: an observational study. Postgrad Med J 86:8–11

Medford AR, Agrawal S, Bennett JA (2010) Thoracic ultrasound prior to medical thoracoscopy improves pleural access and predicts fibrous septation. Respirology 15:804–808

Patel PA, Ernst FR, Gunnarsson CL (2012) Ultrasonography guidance reduces complications and costs associated with thoracentesis procedures. J Clin Ultrasound 40:135–141

Qureshi NR, Rahman NM, Gleeson FV (2009) Thoracic ultrasound in the diagnosis of malignant pleural effusion. Thorax 64:139–143

The Royal College of Radiologists (2012) Ultrasound training recommendations for medical and surgical specialties, in Appendix 6. Thoracic ultrasound training, 2nd edn. London, p 3

Tassi GF, Marchetti GP, Pinelli V (2011) Minithoracoscopy: a complementary technique for medical thoracoscopy. Respiration 82:204–206

Wei B, Wang T, Jiang F et al (2012) Use of transthoracic ultrasound to predict pleural adhesions: a prospective blinded study. Thorac Cardiovasc Surg 60:101–104

Yoneyama H, Arahata M, Temaru R, Ishizaka S, Minami S (2010) Evaluation of the risk of intercostal artery laceration during thoracentesis in elderly patients by using 3D-CT angiography. Intern Med 49:289–292

Anaesthesiology for Thoracoscopy

6

Antoine Delage and Charles-Hugo Marquette

6.1 Introduction

Medical thoracoscopy is often performed by respiratory physicians in the setting of undiagnosed pleural effusion or malignant pleural disease. Traditionally, thoracoscopy was performed during several procedures to avoid the use of general anaesthesia. It later was done under general anaesthesia using separate lung ventilation. However, it has been shown that thoracoscopy can be safely done in a spontaneously breathing subject under conscious sedation and analgesia. Generally speaking, medical thoracoscopy, mostly done for diagnostic purposes, can be performed under local anaesthesia in the endoscopy suite. In contrast, video-assisted thoracoscopic surgery (VATS) which is commonly done for therapeutic purposes is often performed in the operating room, requiring general anaesthesia with one-lung ventilation (Buchanan and Neville 2004; Horswell 1993). We will review here the different anaesthetic techniques used for thoracoscopy and VATS, as well as the adequate preoperative and postoperative patient management for this procedure. A review of the physiology pertaining to thoracoscopy is also discussed in order to guide the appropriate choice of anaesthesia in patients undergoing this procedure.

6.2 Physiology of Thoracoscopy and the Lateral Decubitus Position

Understanding the physiological repercussions of thoracoscopy is of key importance in making a rational decision regarding anaesthesia (Horswell 1993). It has been demonstrated that in spontaneously breathing patients undergoing thoracoscopy under local anaesthesia, although the lung is partially deflated during the procedure, patients show surprisingly little change in their arterial oxygen (PaO_2) and carbon dioxide ($PaCO_2$) tensions, as well as cardiac rhythm (Faurschou et al. 1983; Oldenburg and Newhouse 1979). This can be mainly explained by the physiological changes occurring in the lateral decubitus position (LDP). In an awake subject with a closed chest lying in the LDP, gravity will cause a vertical gradient in blood flow, preferentially to the dependent lung, as well as higher pleural pressures and an increased curvature of the dependent hemidiaphragm. This will result in the lower, dependent lung being better ventilated and receiving better perfusion than the upper, nondependent lung.

When the nondependent hemithorax is opened during thoracoscopy, the negative pleural pressure causes air to enter the pleural cavity, creating a pneumothorax. The open-chest lung, exposed to atmospheric pressure, tends to collapse because of unopposed elastic recoil. During spontaneous ventilation, this collapse is accentuated during inspiration, because of increased negative pleural pressure, and decreased during

A. Delage (✉) • C.-H. Marquette
Department of Pulmonology, Thoracic Oncology,
and Intensive Care, Hôpital Pasteur, Nice, France
e-mail: antoine@delage.com; marquette.ch@chu-nice.fr

P. Astoul et al. (eds.), *Thoracoscopy for Pulmonologists*,
DOI 10.1007/978-3-642-38351-9_6, © Springer-Verlag Berlin Heidelberg 2014

expiration. This reversal of lung movement during respiration has been termed *paradoxical respiration* (Horswell 1993). The dependent, closed-chest, lung pleural pressure is also negative during inspiration, creating an imbalance between the two sides of the mediastinum which shifts toward the dependent lung during inspiration. The tidal volume of the closed-chest lung is thus reduced by this amount of mediastinal shift. This mediastinal shift can also decrease venous return to the right heart, creating a clinical picture similar to shock, with a concomitant activation of the sympathetic system. However, as mentioned above, these changes have surprisingly little effect on the physiological and clinical parameters measured during the procedure, partly owing to the fact that the dependent lower lung is better perfused and ventilated and therefore compensates for its open-chest counterpart.

In a patient with an open chest who is anaesthetised and paralysed, positive pressure ventilation can rectify the problems of mediastinal shift and paradoxical respiration which are described above. However, in this situation, ventilation in the nondependent, open-chest lung is increased when compared to an awake and spontaneously breathing subject whereas perfusion remains the same, being governed mainly by gravity. Also, pneumothorax does not develop during positive pressure ventilation in a patient with an open chest and single-lung ventilation techniques may be required for adequate visualisation of the pleural cavity, although this has been challenged by some authors (Cerfolio et al. 2004).

6.3 Preoperative Assessment

A detailed medical and drug history as well as physical examination are essential before the procedure. Imaging, such as chest radiographs (posteroanterior, lateral and decubitus views), pleural ultrasonography or chest computed tomography (CT), is essential in choosing the appropriate insertion sites for the instruments. Additional preoperative evaluation for the patient undergoing thoracoscopy includes pulmonary function testing, electrocardiogram

Table 6.1 Preferred anaesthesia as used in different settings for thoracoscopy

Preferred anaesthesia	Indication for thoracoscopy
Local anaesthesia	Undiagnosed pleural effusion
	Pleural biopsy
Local or general anaesthesia	Spontaneous pneumothorax
	Empyema (early stage)
	Bullectomy
	Chemical pleurodesis
	Pulmonary biopsy (forceps)
General anaesthesia	Sympatholysis
	Chronic empyema
	Pulmonary biopsy (stapler)

Modified from Rodriguez-Panadero et al. 2006

(ECG), blood gas analysis and routine blood chemistry analysis, including coagulation studies, complete blood count and studies of renal and liver function (Buchanan and Neville 2004; Horswell 1993; Rodriguez-Panadero et al. 2006; Lee et al. 2007; Mathur et al. 1995). Most experts recommend preoperative evaluation for patients undergoing general anaesthesia by an anaesthesiologist. The choice of general anaesthesia or conscious sedation will depend on the patient's preoperative status as well as indication and planned procedure. General indications for the choice of anaesthesia for thoracoscopy are listed in Table 6.1.

The only absolute contraindication to perform thoracoscopy under local anaesthesia is lack of a pleural space due to pleural adhesions. Severe hypoxemia, end-stage pulmonary fibrosis and unstable cardiovascular status are relative contraindications that border on the absolute. In patients with advanced pulmonary fibrosis, the loss of elasticity of lung tissue may make lung reexpansion difficult and lead to prolong air leakage after surgery. Other relative contraindications to medical thoracoscopy are listed in Table 6.2. For patients with bleeding diathesis or taking anticoagulant medication, the international normalised ratio (INR) should be <2.0. As a general rule, patients undergoing medical thoracoscopy under local anaesthesia should be able to lie immobile in the decubitus position for at least 1 h (Buchanan and Neville 2004; Lee et al. 2007; Mathur et al. 1995). In some circumstances, it

Table 6.2 Contraindications to medical thoracoscopy

Contraindications to medical thoracoscopy
Inability to visualise the pleural space (*absolute*)
Severe hypoxemia
End-stage pulmonary fibrosis
Respiratory insufficiency requiring mechanical ventilatory assistance
Unstable cardiovascular status (hypotension, unstable coronary artery disease, arrhythmias)
Uncontrolled bleeding disorder
Uncontrolled cough
Severe pulmonary hypertension
Superior vena cava obstruction
Poor general performance status
Inability to lie in decubitus for more than 1 h

may be preferable to perform thoracoscopy under general anaesthesia or to wait for the patient's status to improve before attempting the procedure.

6.4 Preoperative Preparation

The patient's respiratory and cardiovascular status should be optimised before the procedure. This may include chest physiotherapy, bronchodilators, antibiotics and corticosteroids for patients with chronic obstructive pulmonary disease. Current medications are usually continued except for anticoagulant medications. The role of preoperative medication has not been studied prospectively in randomised trials. Some authors administer atropine 0.4–0.8 mg prior to the procedure to prevent vasovagal reactions (Rodriguez-Panadero et al. 2006; Mathur et al. 1995; Gravino et al. 2005; Smit et al. 1998). Benzodiazepines, such as midazolam or lorazepam, are commonly used to produce anxiolysis and sedation before the procedure is started.

6.5 Monitoring

Currently, there are no specific guidelines for monitoring requirements during thoracoscopy. Thoracoscopy, especially when done under local anaesthesia, is a short procedure and does not warrant invasive intraoperative monitoring. An intravenous peripheral line should be inserted to administer fluids and medication during the procedure. Oxygen is given via nasal canula or face mask. Basic mandatory monitoring, when sedation and analgesia is administered, should include continuous electrocardiographic monitoring, digital pulse oximetry and regular non-invasive blood pressure measurements (at least every 5 min). General anaesthesia should be undertaken in the presence of trained personnel, and additional monitoring is required including capnography or capnometry, blood pressure monitoring and continuous or regular temperature measurements. The American Society of Anesthesiologists publishes a standard of care for basic intraoperative monitoring (Standards for basic anesthetic monitoring - http://www.asahq.org/publicationsAndServices/sgstoc.htm).

6.6 Thoracoscopy Under Local Anaesthesia

Many authors have confirmed that thoracoscopy for the diagnosis of pleural disease can be performed safely under local anaesthesia (Oldenburg and Newhouse 1979; Gravino et al. 2005). The procedure can be performed using local anaesthesia with "conscious sedation" (Loddenkemper 1998; Boutin et al. 1991; Menzies and Charbonneau 1991). This widely used term, also known as diaz-analgesia, refers to a patient who remains awake or arousable and spontaneously breathing while having been administered small doses of anxiolytics and analgesics. This is distinguished from sedation, during which the patient is unconscious and spontaneously breathing and not intubated (Smit et al. 1998; Danby et al. 1998; Migliore et al. 2002). These techniques contrast to general anaesthesia, during which the airway is fully controlled by the insertion of an endotracheal tube or laryngeal mask.

The most commonly used drugs for sedation are midazolam and propofol. Benzodiazepines, such as midazolam or diazepam, are more widely used because they cause less hemodynamic instability and respiratory depression than propofol.

Analgesia is given concurrently, most commonly in the form of short-acting synthetic opiates such as fentanyl, remifentanil or sufentanil. Sedatives and analgesics can be given either as continuous IV perfusions or as boluses. Only one small randomised trial compared the use of sufentanil given in boluses and continuous remifentanil during thoracoscopy and found no difference between the two techniques (Gravino et al. 2005). The choice of analgesic and sedative drugs should thus be based on local expertise and policy.

The simplest way to perform local anaesthesia is by local anaesthetic infiltration of the lateral thoracic wall and parietal pleura (Buchanan and Neville 2004; Horswell 1993; Boutin et al. 1991). Lidocaine or mepivacaine with epinephrine is infiltrated at the sites of proposed trocar insertion before the incision is made. Some authors have also used ropivacaine instead of lidocaine (Gravino et al. 2005; Migliore et al. 2002). In addition to the skin, the intercostal muscle, neurovascular bundle and underlying pleura of the chosen intercostal space should be extensively anaesthetised. The addition of epinephrine to the anaesthetic mixture reduces the amount of blood oozing on the pleural side of the port, making visualisation easier and, in addition, reducing blood contamination of the thoracoscope (Rodriguez-Panadero et al. 2006; Horswell 1993). Once a pneumothorax is established, local anaesthetic may be nebulised or sprayed with a catheter on the parietal pleura for further anaesthesia. This technique of spray catheter pleural anaesthesia has been shown to reduce pain prior to talc poudrage for spontaneous pneumothorax (Lee and Colt 2007b). Intercostal nerve blocks or thoracic epidural anaesthesia is other means of providing more complete analgesia but should be done by a trained physician (Horswell 1993).

6.7 Thoracoscopy Under General Anaesthesia

General anaesthesia is widely used in the surgical literature to perform thoracoscopy. In a paralysed patient under positive pressure ventilation, pneumothorax will not develop in the open-chest lung and paradoxical respiration will not occur, potentially making adequate visualisation of the pleural space more difficult. To counteract this limitation, ventilation of the two lungs may be separated by various techniques during the procedure (Horswell 1993; Cohen 2004).

The double-lumen endotracheal tube has evolved as the technique of choice for one-lung ventilation during surgery. Double-lumen tubes are essentially two catheters bonded together side by side, with each lumen intended to ventilate one of the lungs. They are made as left-sided or right-sided depending on which mainstem bronchus the tip of the catheter is meant to be inserted into. Adequate positioning of the double-lumen tube should be confirmed by fiberoptic bronchoscopy (Horswell 1993; Smith et al. 1986). Clinical signs alone are unreliable in ascertaining that the tube is correctly positioned and bronchoscopy has revealed malpositioning of the tube in up to 48 % of cases and this can lead to intraoperative problems in 25 % of cases (Smith et al. 1986; Read et al. 1977). The position of the double-lumen tube is usually determined upon initial intubation in the supine position and again when the patient is turned to the lateral decubitus position.

Selective mainstem bronchial blockade is another method to obtain lung separation for thoracoscopic surgery. It is most commonly used in children and small adults in which double-lumen tubes are too large to be inserted or in patients with a difficult airway (Horswell 1993; Cohen 2004). The most commonly used endobronchial blocker is a Fogarty embolectomy catheter with a 3–6 ml balloon. A snare-guided endobronchial blocker also exists, and this can be positioned into the desired bronchus with the loop of the snare tied around the fiberoptic bronchoscope. Endobronchial blockers have several drawbacks which include difficulty in positioning the blocker into the desired airway, inability to suction the airway distal to the blocker and displacement during the surgery which may lead to tracheal obstruction. Overall, endobronchial blockage requires intense monitoring and cumbersome manipulation, thus making double-lumen tubes the preferred method for lung separation.

The use of double-lumen endotracheal tubes and endobronchial blockers is associated with costs and complications. Recently, Cerfolio and colleagues reported a series of 376 patients who underwent VATS for pleural effusion or pleural biopsies using a technique of single-lumen endotracheal tube anaesthesia and lower tidal volumes (Cerfolio et al. 2004). During the procedure, the tidal volume was reduced to 150–250 ml by the anaesthesiologist. Using this technique, adequate visualisation of the pleural space was possible in most cases, thereby preventing the need for separate lung ventilation.

6.8 Choosing the Type of Anaesthesia

No consensus exists in the literature on the appropriate choice of anaesthesia for thoracoscopy. Usually, the choice between local and general anaesthesia will be guided by multiple factors, including the planned procedure and its underlying indication, as well as patient-related factors. For example, a child or a patient who is afraid of the procedure or unable to lie on his/her side for an hour should undergo the procedure under general anaesthesia. In addition, if thoracoscopy is expected to be prolonged or painful (e.g. multiloculated empyema), general anaesthesia is probably preferable. During thoracoscopy performed for the management of spontaneous pneumothorax by pleurodesis, the insufflation of a pleurodesis agent may be quite painful for the sedated patient and may necessitate the administration of additional analgesia for maintenance of patient comfort. General anaesthesia may be preferable in these cases. Suggestions for anaesthetic agent according to the indication for thoracoscopy are listed in Table 6.1.

From our experience, certain comorbidities may warrant caution in the choice of local anaesthesia. One particular case is the elderly subject with a history of cardiac insufficiency. In these patients, the vasoplegic and myocardial depressant properties associated with certain sedative and analgesic drugs, especially propofol, as well as the diminution of the sympathetic tone by these agents may lead to hypotension and shock. One should use smaller incremental doses of sedation and analgesia in these patients. Also, sedation must be undertaken prudently in obese patients and patients with known obstructive sleep apnea-hypopnea syndrome. In addition to having a decreased respiratory reserve when lying down, these subjects tend to obstruct their upper airway and become apnoeic when given sedatives and analgesics. As a consequence, they tend to desaturate easily. They also can be difficult to ventilate and may have difficult airways if intubation is necessary, a situation which can be greatly exacerbated by the fact that the patient is lying in the lateral decubitus position.

It should always be remembered before undertaking a thoracoscopic procedure under local anaesthesia that, if it became necessary to urgently intubate the patient during the procedure, the lateral decubitus position makes airway access and intubation quite difficult. Whenever uncertain, an anaesthesiologist should be consulted and general anaesthesia should be considered as the airway is controlled during the procedure and physiological parameters can be better monitored and corrected if needed.

6.9 Post-thoracoscopy Pain Management

Post-thoracoscopy pain can be controlled in most cases with the use of mild oral analgesics or non-steroidal anti-inflammatory drugs (NSAIDs). The amount of post-procedural pain is determined by factors intrinsic to the patient as much as procedure-related factors. For example, procedures that involve decortication or pleurodesis will cause more pain than simple biopsies. In patients where the pain is inadequately controlled by NSAIDs or mild analgesics, other methods should be used, for example, intravenous analgesics, patient-controlled delivery systems or epidural or spinal anaesthesia. In all cases, there are enormous benefits for aggressive pain control methods for patients, their families and the health-care personnel (Mulder 1993).

Conclusion

Thoracoscopy can be done under local or general anaesthesia. Generally speaking, more simple procedures such as parietal pleural biopsies or pleurodesis with talc can be done under local anaesthesia with sedation. Patients requiring more complex thoracoscopic interventions (e.g. decortication for multiloculated empyema, sympathectomy), those with certain comorbidities (e.g. heart failure, obesity) or those unable to lie on their side for more than an hour will require general anaesthesia. Adequate preoperative assessment and preparation is of key importance. For patients undergoing general anaesthesia, the procedure is usually done using separate lung ventilation, although pleural biopsies and pleurodesis can also be safely done with a single-lumen endotracheal tube using lower tidal volumes.

References

Boutin C, Viallat JR, Aelony Y (1991) Diagnostic thoracoscopy for pleural effusions. In: Boutin C, Viallat JR, Aelony Y (eds) Practical thoracoscopy. Springer, Berlin, pp 51–64

Buchanan DR, Neville E (2004) Thoracoscopy for physicians: a practical guide. Arnold Publishers, London, p 166

Cerfolio RJ, Bryan AS, Sheils TM et al (2004) Video-assisted thoracoscopic surgery using single-lumen endotracheal tube anesthesia. Chest 126:281–285

Cohen E (2004) Methods of lung separation. Minerva Anestesiol 70:313–318

Danby CA, Adebonojo SA, Moritz DM (1998) Video-assisted talc pleurodesis for malignant pleural effusion utilizing local anesthesia and IV sedation. Chest 113:739–742

Faurschou P, Madsen F, Viskum K (1983) Thoracoscopy: influence of the procedure on some respiratory and cardiac values. Thorax 38:341–343

Gravino E, Griffo S, Gentile M et al (2005) Comparison of two protocols of conscious analgosedation in video-assisted talc pleurodesis. Minerva Anestesiol 71:157–165

Horswell JL (1993) Anesthetic techniques for thoracoscopy. Ann Thorac Surg 56:624–629

Lee P, Colt HG (2007a) State of the art: pleuroscopy. J Thorac Oncol 2:663–670

Lee P, Colt HG (2007b) A spray catheter technique for pleural anesthesia: a novel method for pain control before talc poudrage. Anesth Analg 104:198–200

Lee P, Hsu A, Lo C et al (2007) Prospective evaluation of flex-rigid pleuroscopy for indeterminate pleural effusion: accuracy, safety and outcome. Respirology 12:881–886

Loddenkemper R (1998) Thoracoscopy: state of the art. Eur Respir J 11:213–221

Mathur PN, Astoul P, Boutin C (1995) Medical thoracoscopy: technical details. Clin Chest Med 16:479–486

Menzies R, Charbonneau M (1991) Thoracoscopy for the diagnosis of pleural disease. Ann Intern Med 114:271–276

Migliore M, Giuliano R, Aziz T et al (2002) Four-step local anesthesia and sedation for thoracoscopic diagnosis and management of pleural diseases. Chest 21:2032–2035

Mulder DS (1993) Pain management principles and anesthesia techniques for thoracoscopy. Ann Thorac Surg 56:630–632

Oldenburg FA, Newhouse MT (1979) Thoracoscopy. A safe, accurate diagnostic procedure using the rigid thoracoscope and local anesthesia. Chest 75:45–50

Read R, Friday C, Eason C (1977) Prospective study of the Robert-Shaw endobronchial catheter in thoracic surgery. Ann Thorac Surg 24:156–161

Rodriguez-Panadero F, Janssen JP, Astoul P (2006) Thoracoscopy: general overview and place in the diagnosis and management of pleural effusion. Eur Respir J 28:409–421

Smit HJ, Schramel FM, Sutedja TG et al (1998) Video-assisted thoracoscopy is feasible under local anesthesia. Diagn Ther Endosc 4:177–182

Smith G, Hirsch N, Ehrenwerth J (1986) Placement of double-lumen endobronchial tubes. Correlation between clinical impressions and bronchoscopic findings. Br J Anaesth 58:1537–1542

Thoracoscopy: Equipment and Technique

7

Philippe Astoul and David P. Breen

7.1 Introduction

Although Jacobaeus is credited with the development of thoracoscopy, the first documented report of thoracoscopy in the literature appeared in 1866. Samuel Gordon described the exploration of a pleural cavity of an 11-year-old girl with empyema. This first procedure was performed in 1865 by the Irish physician Francis Richard Cruise (Cruise 1865). However, it was Jacobaeus who made the procedure more operator friendly by improving the endoscopic view through the induction of a pneumothorax at the onset of the procedure (Jacobaeus 1910).

The term "medical thoracoscopy" appeared in the literature approximately 15 years ago to distinguish it from the newly developed operation of "video-assisted thoracoscopic surgery" (VATS).

Medical thoracoscopy is usually performed by pulmonologists in the endoscopy suite under local anesthesia and with intravenous conscious sedation/analgesia, while VATS requires general anesthesia and double-lumen tracheal intubation.

P. Astoul (✉)
Division of Thoracic Oncology, Pleural Diseases, and Interventional Pulmonology, Hôpital NORD, Marseille, France
e-mail: pastoul@ap-hm.fr

D.P. Breen
Department of Respiratory Medicine, Galway University Hospitals, Galway, Ireland
e-mail: david.breen@hse.ie

It is usually undertaken by thoracic surgeons in the operating room. The range of indications and interventions performed differs between the two procedures. Medical thoracoscopy is frequently indicated for diagnostic purposes (pleural effusions) and/or talc pleurodesis ("poudrage") to prevent recurrence of persistent pleural effusions or pneumothorax.

In this chapter, we will describe the equipment and technique necessary for a successful thoracoscopy.

7.2 Equipment

7.2.1 Standard

The standard required equipment for thoracoscopy includes a pleural needle (Fig. 7.1a, b), a trocar – consisting of an obturator and a cannula (Fig. 7.2) – a direct-viewing and angle-viewing optical telescope (Fig. 7.3a, b), an optical forceps (Fig. 7.4), and a light source.

Additional essential instruments include an insulated trocar (Fig. 7.2) that can be used to create a second port of entry and through which electrocautery can be performed. Recently new sets are available for single puncture thoracoscopy allowing minimally invasive diagnostic treatment with one small incision. With a 5.5-mm trocar, the procedure is possible under local anesthetics and without painful stress for the patient (Fig. 7.5).

P. Astoul et al. (eds.), *Thoracoscopy for Pulmonologists*,
DOI 10.1007/978-3-642-38351-9_7, © Springer-Verlag Berlin Heidelberg 2014

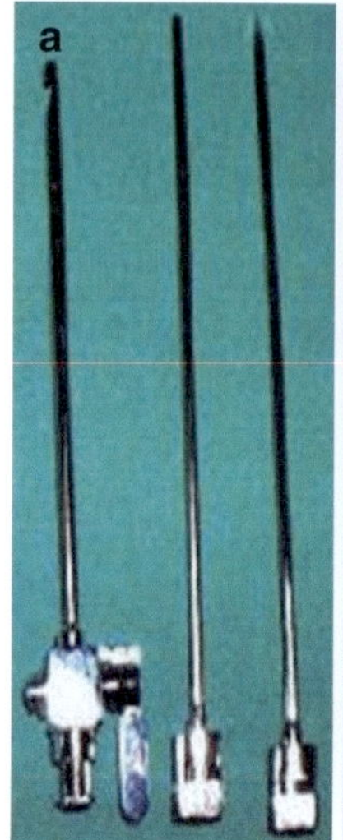
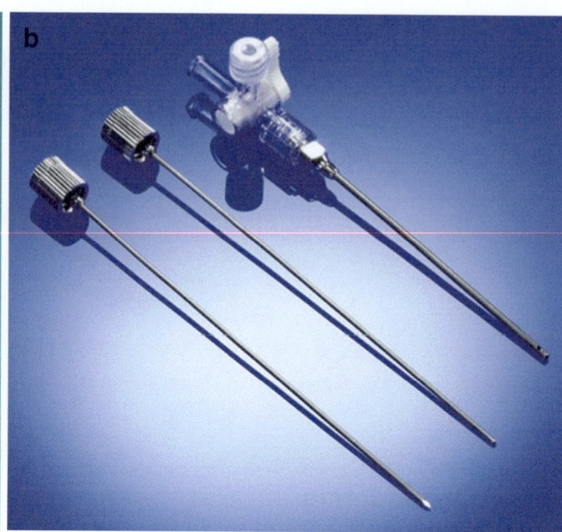

Fig. 7.1 A metallic (**a**) and single-use (**b**) pleural needle. The pleural trocar, 2–3 mm in diameter, 100 mm in length, with tap. A pointed obturator to penetrate the skin and the intercostal tissue and subsequently changed to a blunt obturator to pass through the parietal pleura

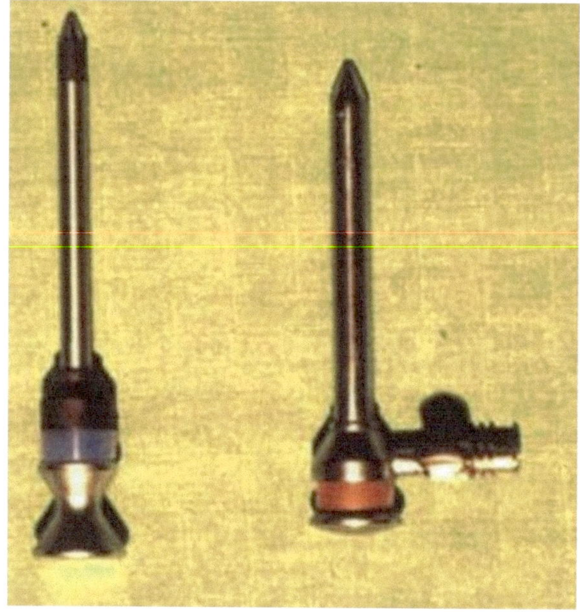
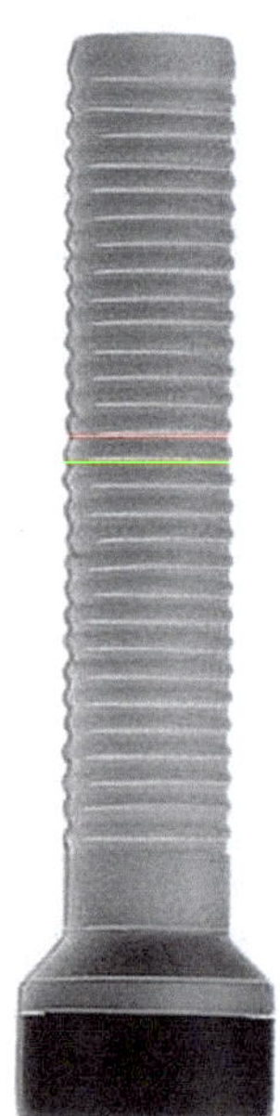

Fig. 7.2 Trocars. From the *left to the right*. 7-mm diameter metallic trocar consisting of an obturator and a cannula. 5-mm diameter insulated trocar allowing the use of coagulating forceps. 10-mm diameter plastic trocar

The optimal diameter of the thoracoscope (trocar and telescope) is 7 mm (Fig. 7.3a), as originally developed by Boutin in conjunction with the Wolf Corporation (Wolf Company, Knittlingen, Germany) (Boutin et al. 1981b). Larger telescopes (diameter 10–12 mm) are available, but they have been developed with the surgeon in mind, where the procedure will be performed under general anesthesia and double-lumen intubation. However, their large size makes them impractical for a procedure performed under local anesthesia.

In addition, equipment with a smaller diameter is also available, the so-called minithoracoscopy (please refer to the dedicated chapter in Part VI of this textbook).

Both 3- and 5-mm optical biopsy forceps (Fig. 7.4) are available and frequently provide adequate biopsies for a definitive diagnosis of the underlying pathology.

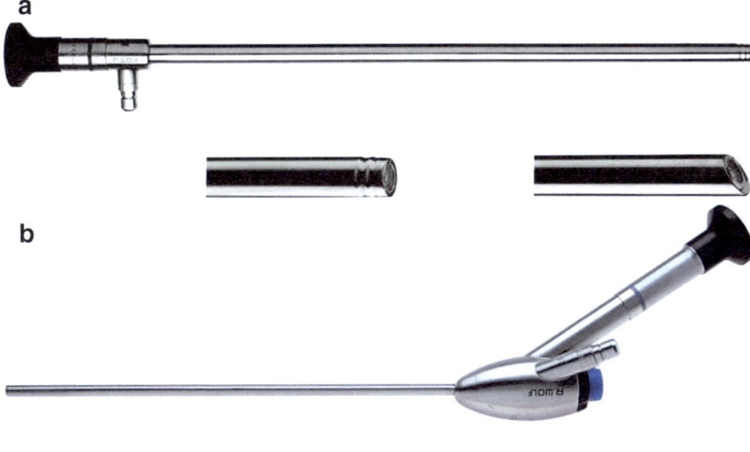

Fig. 7.3 A direct-viewing (0°) and angle-viewing (50° oblique angle of view) optical telescope. (**a**) Examination telescope, Panoview, 7 mm in diameter and 350 mm in length, allows for high-quality exploration. (**b**) A new telescope is available which includes a working channel for suction catheter, grasping forceps, and coagulating forceps with a single point of entry (Richard Wolf, Knittlingen, Germany)

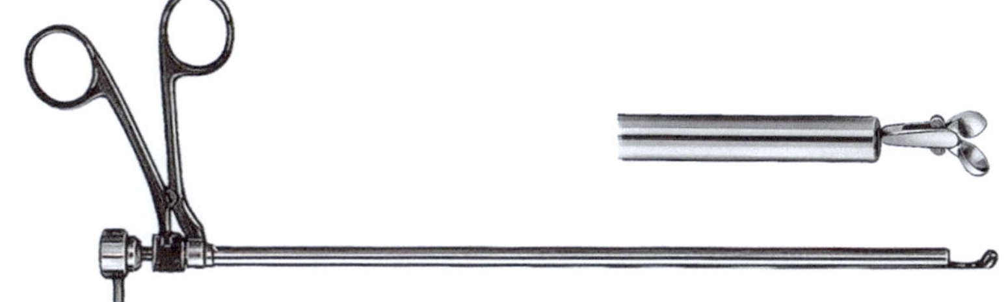

Fig. 7.4 Optical biopsy forceps. This is mainly used for biopsies of the parietal pleura. Coagulation is not possible with this instrument (Richard Wolf, Knittlingen, Germany)

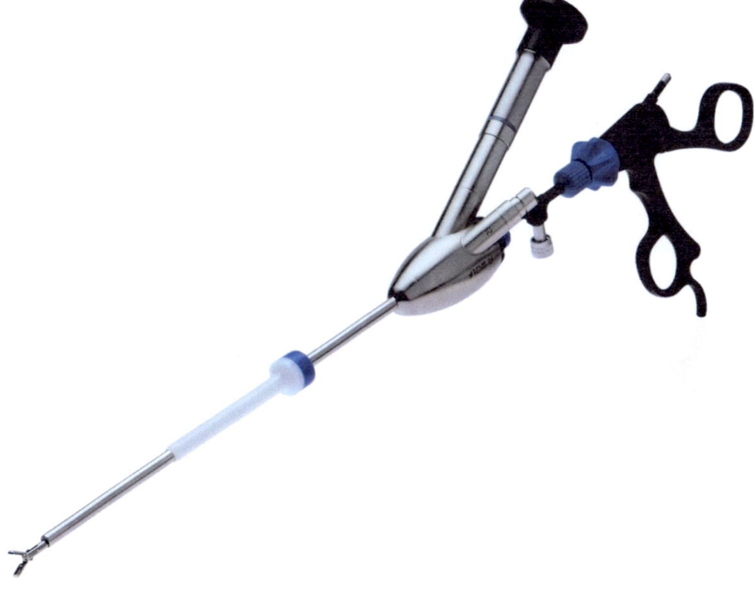

Fig. 7.5 A new generation optical biopsy forceps with working channel for instruments including the coagulating forceps (Richard Wolf, Knittlingen, Germany)

7.2.2 Other Required Equipment

- A suitable area for surgical scrubbing, sterile gowns, sheets, and gloves
- An endoscopy room (Fig. 7.6)
- A thoracoscopy table
- Separate mobile carts
- A mayo stand, which can be covered with sterile sheets, for the instruments (Fig. 7.7)
- Anesthetic equipment

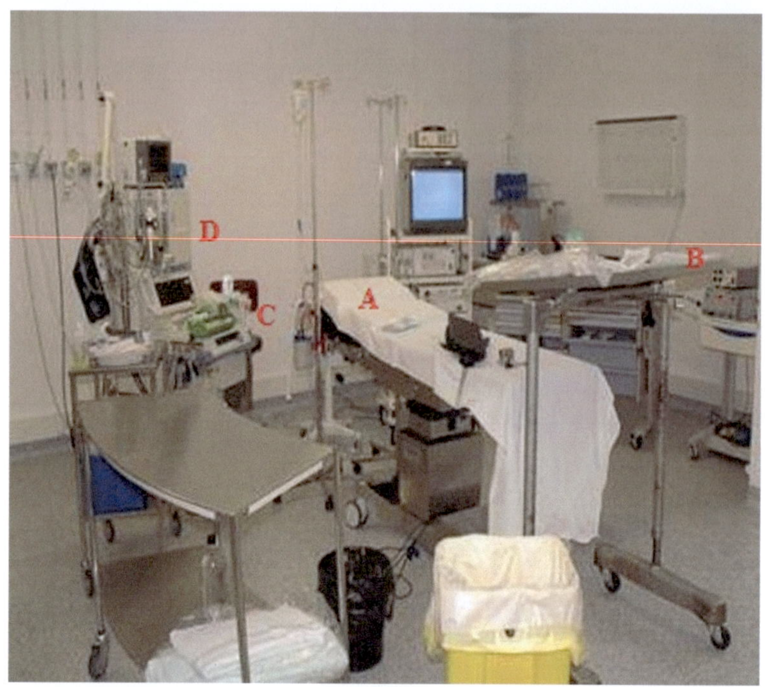

Fig. 7.6 A general view of an endoscopy room

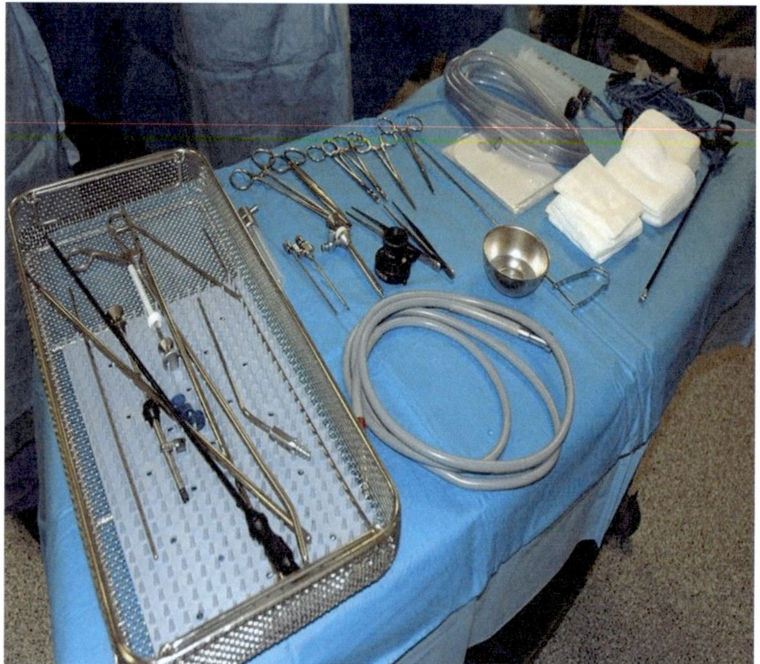

Fig. 7.7 A Mayo stand covered with sterile sheets for the instruments

- Monitoring equipment including ECG, blood pressure, and saturation probes
- Needles – 24G and 21G for the administration of local anesthetic agents
- 10- and 50-mm syringes
- Surgical swabs
- Scalpel
- Clamps

- Grasping forceps and a swab holder
- Electrocautery and loop to divide adhesions and control hemorrhage – if it occurs
- Sterile covers for the cables used to attach the optics and camera to the lighting source
- Plastic sterile aspiration tubes, 4 and 6 mm in diameter
- Aspiration tubing and collection bottles of at least 2 l capacity which can be connected to negative pressure
- Cupulas for local anesthetic (LA), warm saline – used to prevent fogging of the optics – and soap
- Chest drains ranging from size 20 to 32 Fr
- A guide for the chest drain or a self-contained chest tube set with an inner stylet

7.3 Practical Considerations

It is mandatory that the operator is skilled with a good knowledge of pleural anatomy and the associated landmarks. The physician should be well acquainted with all the equipment used during the procedure. When setting up for the procedure prior to the commencement of the intervention, it is necessary to ensure that all necessary equipment is available. We advise that the drain and underwater seal is prepared and the patient is earthed for electrocautery before starting the intervention. This will allow for a rapid response to complications should they arise. In addition, the physician must be skilled in the postoperative management of patients including pain control and chest drain assessment and removal.

The light source should be of a high quality to maximize the quality of the images. Care must be taken to ensure that the connecting cables between the light and power sources and the thoracoscope are attached correctly. Sterility of these cables must be maintained at all times to reduce postoperative infectious complications. Although not essential for the procedure, we recommend that the physician invests in equipment that will allow the capture of images and/or movie clips. This provides an objective record of the pleural space especially if redo thoracoscopy is planned to access the response to therapy (Breen et al. 2008).

A compromise must be made when choosing the optimal trocar size. Large trocars allow for the insertion of large telescopes which will improve the quality of the procedure. However, the larger the trocar, the greater the discomfort to the patient. We believe that a 5- or 7-mm trocar is optimal for thoracoscopy (Fig. 7.2), allowing good visualization of the pleural space and biopsy through a single port of entry when using an optical forceps (Fig. 7.4). A conically shaped tip on the trocar reduces the risk of trauma to the intercostal neurovascular bundle during introduction.

The vast majority of procedures including talc poudrage can be performed through a single port of entry – if the initial trocar size is at least 5 mm in diameter. A second port of entry is occasionally indicated. This point of entry is located one intercostal space superior or inferior to the primary port of entry or, in the setting of hemorrhage, located to allow electrocoagulation of the site of bleeding

7.3.1 Second Port of Entry

A second port of entry is necessary in some scenarios. These include situations where the movement of the trocar is sufficiently painful to prevent a full inspection of the area of interest. This complication can be minimized by choosing the position carefully at the outset with the aid of available radiographs, CT, and pre-thoracoscopy ultrasound (see Chap. 4).

However, in some cases it may be due to simple geographical issues between the entry point and the lesion or secondary to a narrow intercostal space that prevents complete maneuverability of the trocar. Although the LA provides excellent anesthesia to the immediate area of entry, it has no effect on the ribs which, if they are forcefully pushed up or down by the movement of the thoracoscope, may induce pain. Another scenario requiring a second port of entry is when large adhesions are present that require cutting or circumnavigation. This is particularly important if the adhesions are vascularized and require coagulation to safely separate them (Fig. 7.8).

Fig. 7.8 Large adhesions can be severed using an electro-cautery loop (**a**) (in this case, on the *left side*, through a second point of entry) or coagulating forceps (**b**). This is particularly important if the adhesions are highly vascularized requiring coagulation to safely separate them. Vascularized adhesion (*arrow*), parietal pleural side (*square*), lung (*circle*)

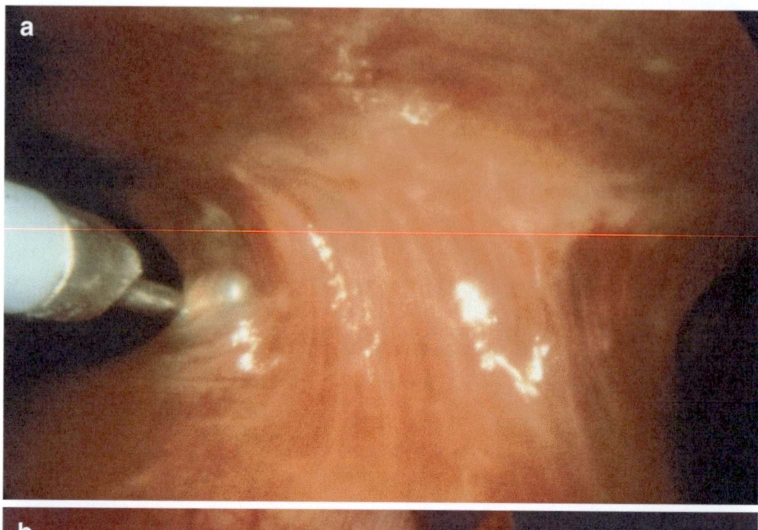

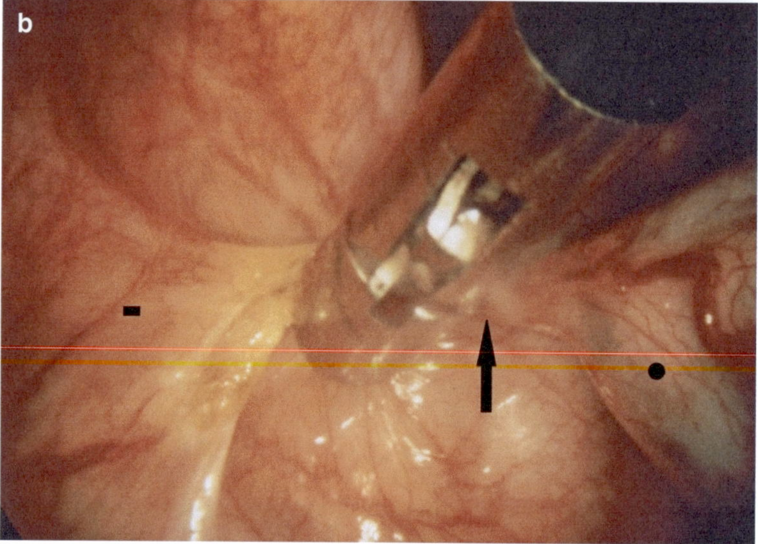

If a thoracoscopy is performed, it is paramount that a full inspection of the cavity is undertaken from the apex to the diaphragm. If this is not feasible through a single port, then a second access point should be created. As previously discussed, if electrocautery is needed for control of hemorrhage, then the physician must be able to create a second port of entry rapidly. This second port can be placed rapidly under direct vision. The chosen site is viewed through the primary port with the optic while the assistant depresses on the chest wall at the second site of entry. The external compression can be easily visualized on the internal chest wall (Fig. 7.9a, b). The trocar can then be placed rapidly under direct vision as described later in this chapter.

7.3.2 Alternative Equipment

Thoracoscopy can be performed using alternative equipment apart from that described above. Indeed a flexible bronchoscope has been used for inspection of the pleural cavity! Recently, a dedicated semirigid/flexible thoracoscope has been developed (Chap. 26). There are advantages and disadvantages associated with this equipment. The rigid thoracoscope provides excellent vision, large

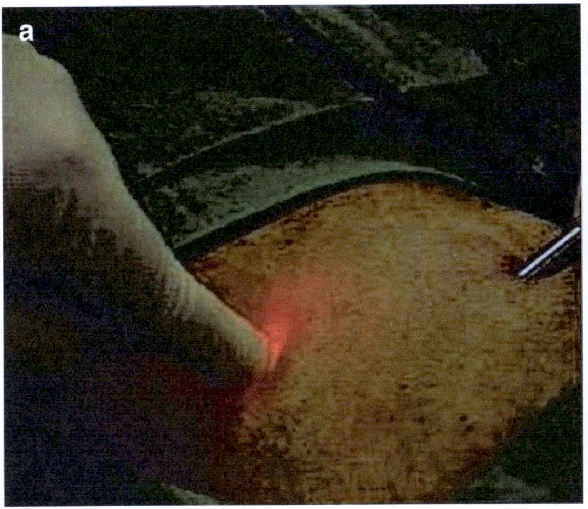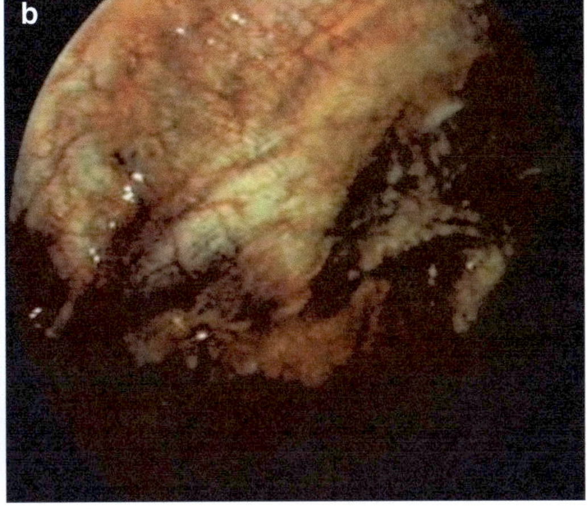

Fig. 7.9 A 5-mm trocar can be placed rapidly under direct vision through a second point of entry. (**a**) The chosen site is viewed through the primary port with the optic, while the assistant depresses on the chest wall at the second site of entry. (**b**) The external compression can be easily visualized on the internal chest wall

biopsy samples via a single port of entry, ease of biopsy from harder lesions, and easy orientation inside the pleural cavity. However, physicians who are skilled with the flexible bronchoscope may feel more comfortable with the semirigid thoracoscope. The flexible equipment allows lateral vision or retro visualization (this would require a separate oblique view telescope if using rigid instruments) (Ishida et al. 2011).

However, when compared with rigid instruments, the control of the working end of the flexible thoracoscope is limited due to its flexibility. In addition, the biopsy size is small which in turn limits its diagnostic yield, especially in the setting of malignant mesothelioma. Finally, the initial access to the pleural space still requires placement of a trocar which is the same diameter as that used for rigid equipment. Therefore there is no reduction in the discomfort experienced by the patient during the procedure.

Therefore, despite the obvious attraction of the semirigid thoracoscope to respiratory physicians – because of its similarity to the bronchoscope – it is limited by the inherent disadvantages of flexible instruments including the fragility of the instruments, sterilization requirements, high maintenance costs, and small size of the biopsies. We believe that there are no clear advantages of the flexible thoracoscope over the rigid equipment.

Smaller equipment, so-called minithoracoscopy, has also been developed as an alternative for diagnostic thoracoscopy under local anesthesia. This consists of rigid equipment using either a 2- or 3-mm thoracoscope. Tassi et al. obtained a diagnostic yield of 93 % using a 3-mm thoracoscope. In a paper comparing 2-mm, 3-mm, and standard thoracoscopes, the authors obtained a diagnostic yield of 40, 100, and 100 % for the 2-, 3-, and 7-mm equipment, respectively (Tassi et al. 2011).

One of the disadvantages of the mini equipment is that it is necessary to create a second port of entry in order to obtain biopsies. This compares to the standard equipment where all procedures can be performed through a single port of entry.

7.4 Technique

7.4.1 Preparation of the Patient

Although thoracoscopy is a safe and relatively simple procedure – if the performing physician is well trained and familiar with the endoscopic anatomy of the thorax – a few simple rules, which apply to all endoscopic procedures, should be followed carefully.

7.4.1.1 Preoperative Discussion with the Patient

Although this is a basic requirement for informed consent, it is especially important when the procedure is performed under local anesthesia as the patient will be more confident during the intervention if he or she knows the details of the procedure in advance.

7.4.1.2 Preoperative Assessment

The patient's medical status should be optimized prior to the thoracoscopy. The procedure should be deferred for subjects with uncontrolled cough. This makes the procedure very difficult for both the patient and physician alike and results in complications (subcutaneous emphysema). Great care should be taken with patients with a poor performance status, hypoproteinemia, or diffuse neoplastic infiltration of the chest wall. Ultimately physicians should try to balance the benefits with the risks of the procedure. As with all interventions the procedure should not be performed unless there is a definite benefit to the patient.

7.4.1.3 Preoperative Investigations

All patients undergoing thoracoscopy should have a preoperative ECG. Patients with unstable angina or a history of a recent myocardial infarction should be rejected for thoracoscopy. Coagulation and blood gas analysis should be performed preoperatively. Extreme care should be taken with patients with hypercapnia especially if the $PaCO_2$ is greater than 55 mmHg. Hematological abnormalities should be corrected, if possible, prior to the intervention. Patients with pancytopenia or coagulation disorders are at an increased risk of complications, and indeed thoracoscopy is contraindicated if the platelet levels are below 60,000/mm^3. The INR should be less than 2.0. The use of aspirin may prolong bleeding time, but is not an absolute contraindication to biopsy.

Radiological assessment includes chest radiography, computed tomography (CT), and preferably ultrasonography (US) prior to the procedure – depending on the local facilities. Historically a posteroanterior and lateral chest X-ray film was mandatory in order to evaluate the best port of entry, to exclude the presence of contralateral pulmonary lesions (these could lead to acute respiratory insufficiency at the time of pneumothorax induction), and to evaluate the size and shape of the pleural effusion to be explored. However the role for preoperative chest X-ray is less important in current practice as most centers will perform pre-thoracoscopy US. A contrast-enhanced CT (delayed pleural enhancement) is recommended in the workup of all patients with a pleural effusion of unclear origin. This may provide additional information such as areas of loculation, pleural nodules, and adenopathy.

7.4.1.4 Premedication for Thoracoscopy

Preoperative preparation should include chest physiotherapy. Bronchodilators, antibiotics, and corticosteroids should be prescribed if indicated to optimize pulmonary function. Routine prophylactic antibiotics are not indicated, unless the patient is neutropenic. The role of preoperative medication has not been subjected to randomized studies. In some centers, 0.4–0.8 mg of atropine (intramuscular or subcutaneous), is administered prior to the procedure to prevent vasovagal reactions. Details of drugs used during the procedure have been discussed in detail in Chap 5. Briefly, sedation during the procedure is performed using incremental doses of a narcotic agent and a benzodiazepine. Drugs to antagonize the effects of both morphine and benzodiazepines should be available if oversedation/analgesia occurs.

The choice of anesthetic technique takes a number of considerations into account including the mental status of the patient, the age of the patient, the expected duration of the procedure, the indication for the thoracoscopy, and the proposed intervention during the procedure.

Patients should have an intravenous cannula placed. Basic monitoring includes ECG and pulse oximetry. Supplementary oxygen should be provided to the patient to maintain oxygen saturation above 90 %. All patients should be treated with prophylactic heparin during their hospital stay.

7.4.2 Technique

7.4.2.1 Patient Preparation

The patient is placed in the lateral decubitus position with the healthy lung down. The positioning of the patient is essential – especially if the procedure is performed under local anesthetic. He/she must remain in the one position for the duration of the procedure, and therefore this must be as comfortable as possible. Two techniques can be used to widen the intercostal space during the procedure. A round bolster can be placed underneath the thorax, thus arching the vertebral column superiorly and in turn enlarging the intercostal space. Secondly, the upper arm can be raised over the head and placed on a metal cradle (Fig. 7.10). Both these maneuvers increase the size of the intercostal space and in turn provide more space for the instruments and therefore reduce the degree of discomfort for the patient as there is less pressure on the ribs when manipulating the rigid instruments during inspection of the cavity and/or performing biopsy.

Patients have been placed in other positions for thoracoscopy including dorsal decubitus and ventral decubitus.

Once the patient is positioned and the operating field is sterilized (Fig. 7.11), the operator and assistant place sterile drapes over the patient and the operating tables. The only uncovered area

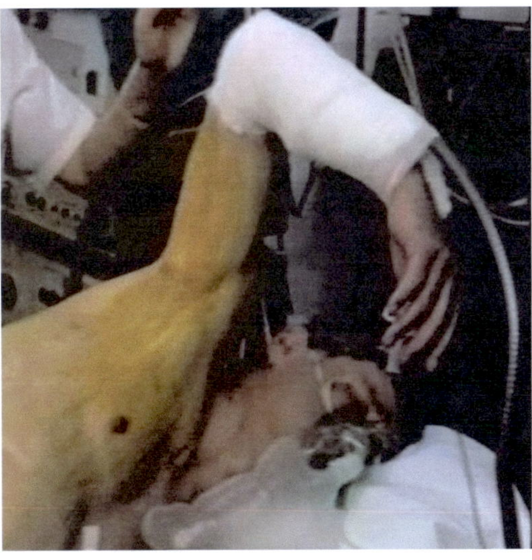

Fig. 7.10 The patient usually lies with the healthy side down. A round bolster is slipped under the thorax to arch the vertebral column convexly upward, thus enlarging the intercostal spaces. The upper arm is raised at a right angle with the forearm attached to a gutter

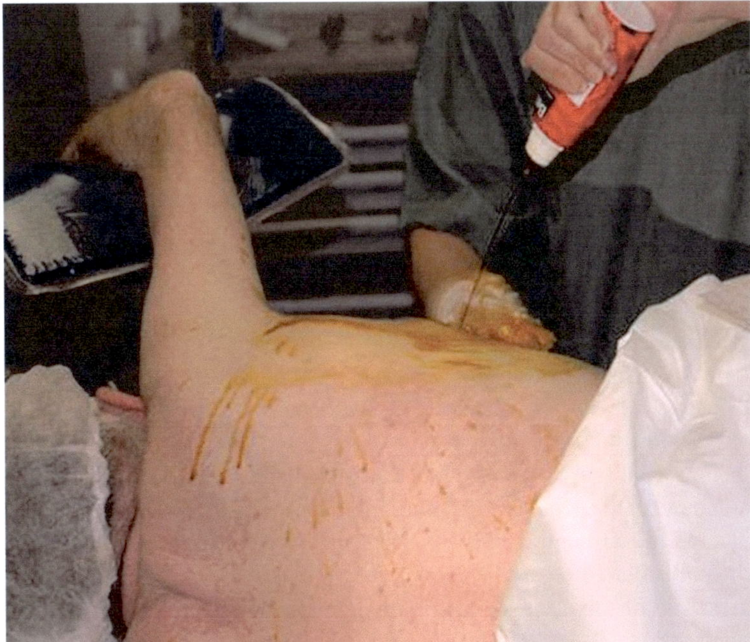

Fig. 7.11 Preparation of the operating field

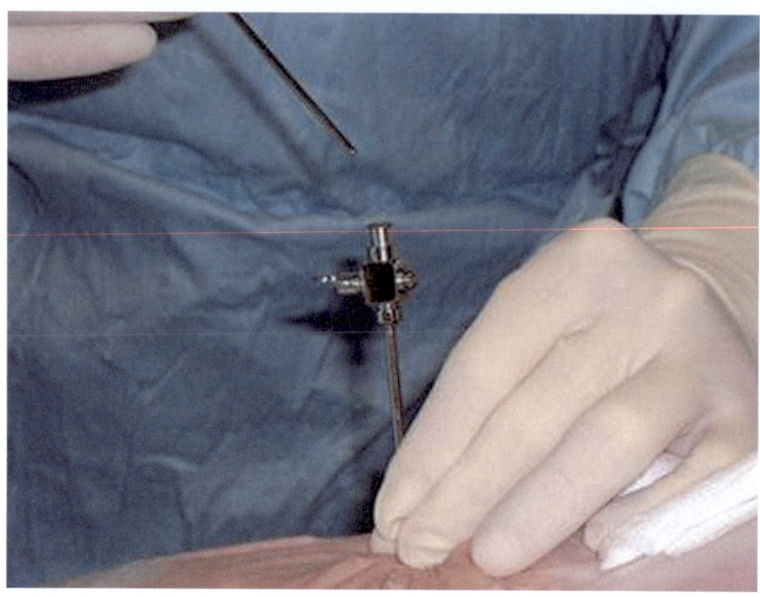

Fig. 7.12 Induction of the pneumothorax using the pleural needle

should be the area of operation which should remain exposed to allow for the insertion of the instruments. By applying sterile drapes to the patients and tables, the operators now have a safe environment to arrange all the equipment needed for the procedure.

The first step in the operation is to choose the most suitable location for the pleural puncture. It is essential that the physician performing the procedure is fully aware of thoracic anatomy and surface landmarks. The choice of puncture depends on the nature of the suspected underlying pathology and in addition after interrogation of the available radiological images and US scan prior to the procedure. For pleural effusions, the optimal point of entry depends on the patient's suspected disease; for pneumothorax a higher point of entry is chosen (third or fourth intercostal space), as most abnormalities in this disease (blebs and bullae) can be found at the apex of the lung and can be best visualized from a high point of entry. In cases with suspected malignancy, a lower point of entry is preferred (sixth or seventh intercostal spaces), as most pleural malignancies are found in the posterior and inferior areas of the pleura. The optimal point of entry is localized in the midaxillary line, as there are no large muscle groups in this region that need to be transversed by the trocar.

7.4.2.2 Local Anesthesia (LA)

Even if the procedure is performed under general anesthesia, it is mandatory to apply LA to the skin, subcutaneous tissues, and pleura before introducing the trocar into the pleural space.

At the designated point of entry, 15–30 mL of 1 % lidocaine is injected perpendicularly into the skin, subcutaneous tissues, intercostal muscles, and the parietal pleura. When the procedure is performed under heavy sedation, 15 mL of 1 % lidocaine is used; 30 mL is optimal with light sedation. The addition of adrenaline may reduce the amount of blood oozing from the intercostal or pleural vessels, thus minimizing contamination of the optical telescope.

After the administration of LA, a small incision is made in the skin to allow easy passage of the pleural needle through the skin and subcutaneous tissues. The pleural needle is used to induce the pneumothorax (Fig. 7.12).

7.4.2.3 Induction of Pneumothorax

The space between the lung and chest wall must be of a sufficient size to visualize the area of abnormality and to allow easy movement of the instruments within the pleural space. Therefore, a pneumothorax must be induced. Some centers create a pneumothorax a few hours or even the day before thoracoscopy. In theory, this may

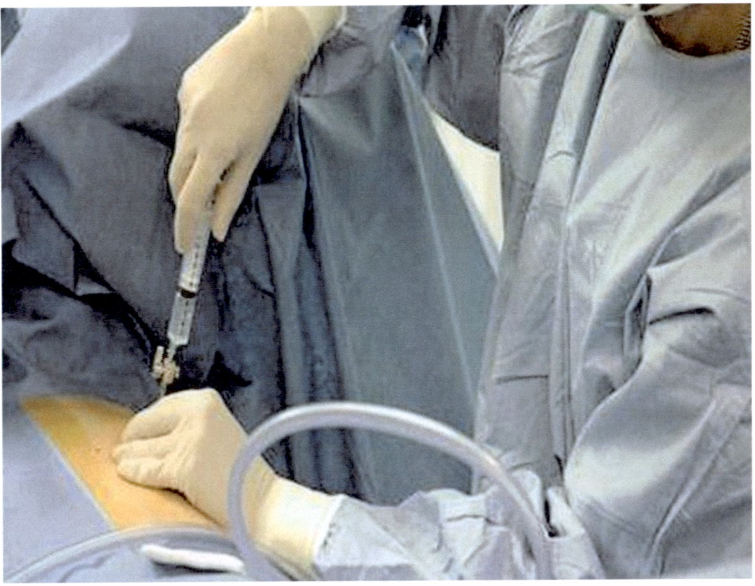

Fig. 7.13 The presence of pneumothorax can be confirmed by attaching a syringe to the needle and aspirating a quantity of air

reduce blood flow to the periphery of the lung, which in turn may prevent damage to the underlying lung during exploration of the pleural space. However, in our experience, the direct introduction of a trocar, with a conical tip, into the thoracic wall, without prior induction of a pneumothorax, is safe and effective – if there is sufficient pleural fluid. Very occasionally, the introduction of the trocar can be troublesome, for example, in cases of pleural adhesions. Therefore, the trocar must be introduced slowly and carefully. The inner part of the trocar must be withdrawn when a reduction of resistance is felt which suggests that the operator has transversed the parietal pleura. A previously induced pneumothorax can be useful to assess pleural lesions and lung collapsibility in advance. However, a contrast-enhanced CT will be helpful in this assessment as well.

The pleural needle consists of three separate components (Fig. 7.1a, b). The needle is 2 or 3 mm in diameter and 100 mm in length. It consists of a hollow outer component and two obturators, one blunt and one sharp. The sharp obturator is used to pass through the skin and subcutaneous tissues, and this can be removed and replaced by the blunt obturator to "pop" through the pleura into the thoracic cavity. The use of a blunt obturator reduces the risk of

damage or laceration to the lung, diaphragm, or intercostal neurovascular bundle. The correct position of the needle can be confirmed by aspirating pleural fluid (effusion) through the hollow outer core. Once the position is confirmed, the needle is opened to atmospheric pressure and air is allowed to enter the pleural space (Fig. 7.12). A characteristic whistle of air can be heard as it passes through the needle with each respiratory cycle. When an equal amount of air is heard entering on inspiration as leaving on expiration, a state of equilibrium is created between the pleural space and the cavity. The pneumothorax can be further confirmed by attaching a syringe to the needle and aspirating a quantity of air (Fig. 7.13).

Once a sufficient pneumothorax is obtained, the needle is removed, and an incision is made in the skin – this should be up to 8 to 10 mm (Fig. 7.14). This incision should be big enough to allow the passage of the trocar for thoracic inspection and the chest drain at the end of the procedure. If too large, the incision will require additional sutures for closure. The incision should be made only in the skin and not through deeper structures in an attempt to maintain a bloodless field. The incision is followed by blunt dissection with scissors down to the level of the pleura (Fig. 7.15). It is essential that this is blunt and not cutting to prevent damage to the intercostal

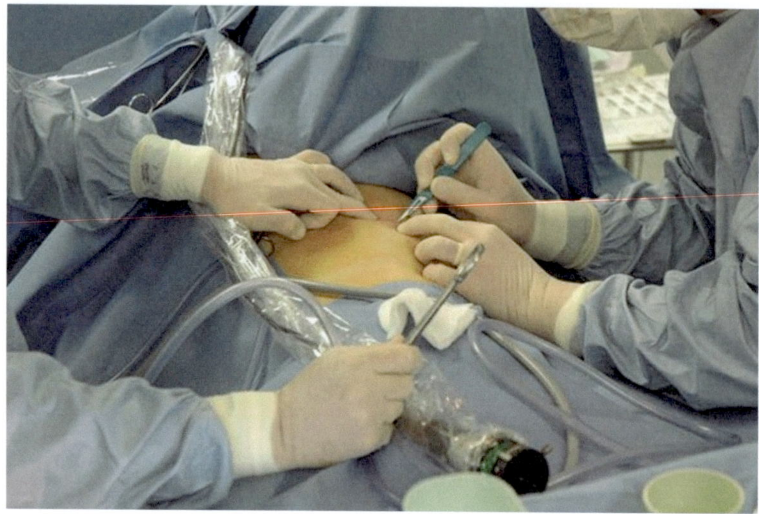

Fig. 7.14 Skin incision. When the pneumothorax is obtained, the needle is removed and an incision is made in the skin – this should be up to 8–10 mm. This incision should be big enough to allow the passage of the trocar for thoracic inspection and the chest drain at the end of the procedure

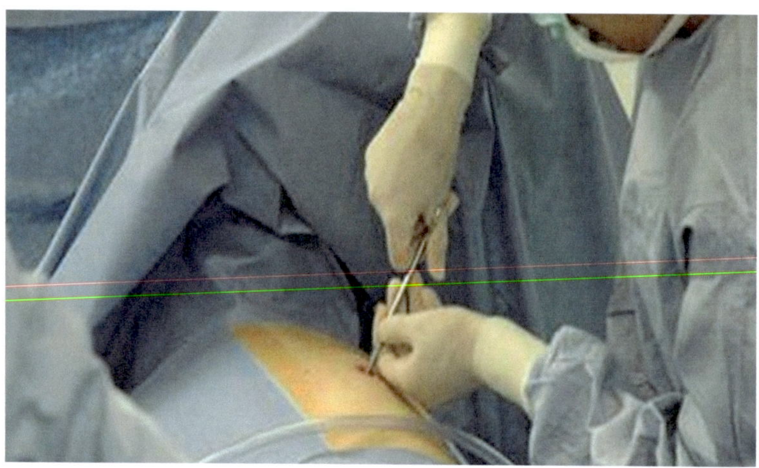

Fig. 7.15 Dissection of the chest wall

neurovascular bundle during dissection. Once dissection reaches the pleural space, the trocar can be inserted and the obturator removed. The trocar should always be inserted perpendicularly to the chest wall with a slow and careful rotating motion (Fig. 7.16). It is safer to locate the tip over the inferior rib in the chosen port of entry, in order to prevent damage to the intercostal vessels and nerves. Occasionally, introduction of the trocar can be troublesome in the setting of pleural adhesions. If resistance is met or adhesions are present, a number of techniques can be performed to increase the size of the pleural space to allow visual exploration. Firstly, the incision can be increased to allow the physician's finger to enter

the pleural space. Then the operator can perform a slow circular rotation with the finger to break down any adhesions in the near vicinity of the incision (Janssen and Boutin 1992). At this stage the tract made by the trocar in the chest wall can be explored with the telescope. Further adhesions can be severed with the biopsy forceps or cautery. This should be performed at the parietal level to prevent bleeding (Fig. 7.8).

The cavity is now ready for drainage of fluid, if present, and inspection. Fluid evacuation can be performed gently with an aspiration catheter attached to negative pressure. The technique for pleural fluid aspiration should ensure that the suction catheter is in continuous motion which helps

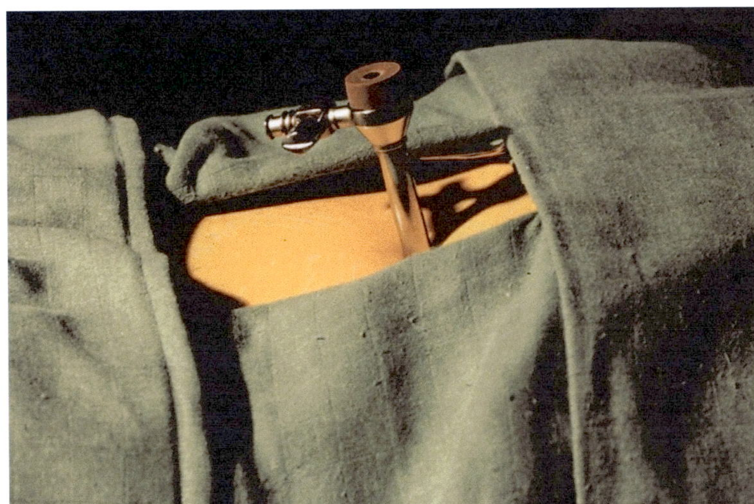

Fig. 7.16 Insertion of the 7-mm trocar

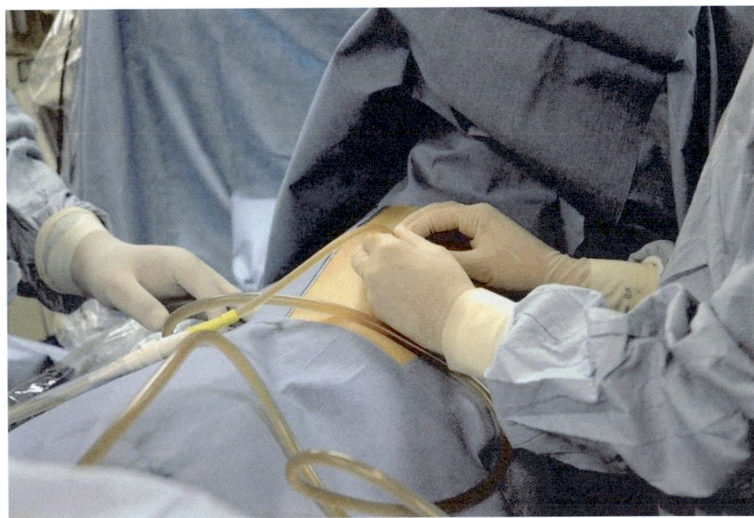

Fig. 7.17 Pleural fluid aspiration

to prevent coughing that could be provoked by the attachment of the catheter to the visceral pleura and the underlying lung (Fig. 7.17). With fluid removal, air enters the pleural cavity passively.

Once all fluid is removed, inspection should be performed systematically. With the direct-viewing optic, the operator should commence with visualization of the posterior costophrenic gutter and diaphragm. Then, with slow movement, the posterior pleural surface should be visualized in the direction of the apex, then the apex and the anterior surface until reaching the anterior diaphragm (Fig. 7.18). An operator and an assistant can perform the procedure (Fig. 7.19). In addition, the surface of the lung, visceral pleura, fissures, and, if the left cavity, the pericardium and pericardial fat should be visualized. This technique allows for the maximal surface of the cavity to be observed (right side, Fig. 7.20a–g; left side, Fig. 7.21a–h).

For the complete exploration of the pleural cavity, a slow circular motion of the scope is recommended. The optic should remain in the anatomical position at all times to allow for easy identification of the internal structures. In addition, certain characteristics are observed – the diaphragm shows respiratory movements, the lung has a transmitted pulsating motion, and the costal pleura appears to be motionless.

Fig. 7.18 Using the direct-viewing optic, the operator should commence with visualization of the posterior costophrenic gutter and diaphragm. Then, with a slow movement, the posterior pleural surface should be visualized in the direction of the apex, then the apex and the anterior surface until reaching the anterior diaphragm

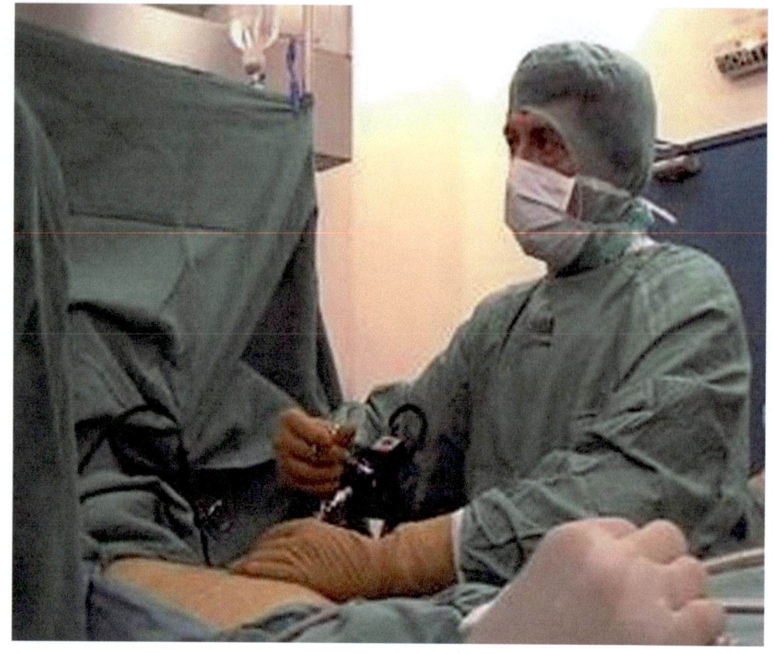

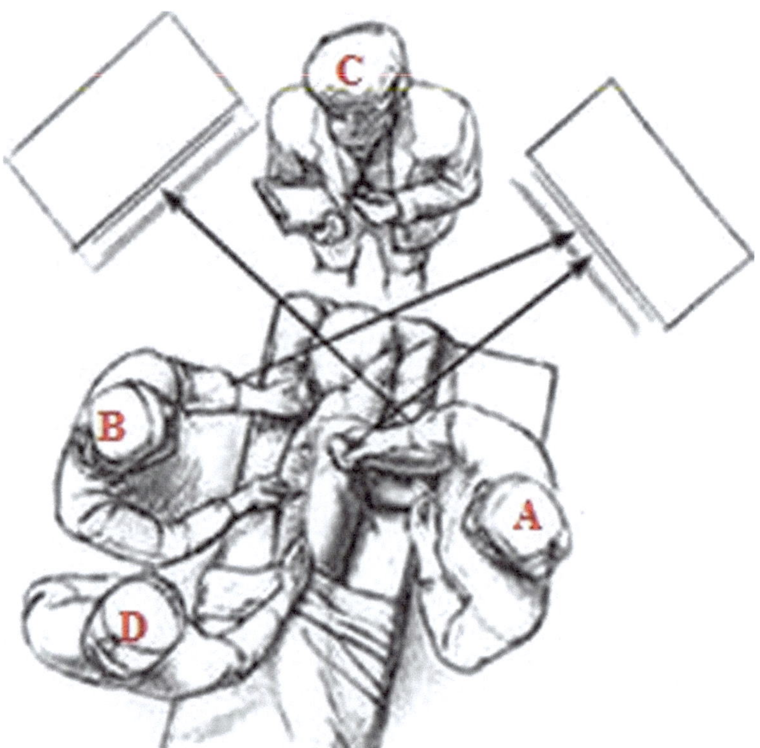

Fig. 7.19 (*A*) Operator, (*B*) assistant, (*C*) anesthetist, (*D*) nurse (However, medical thoracoscopy can also be done under local anesthesia with a single operator and a nurse in the room)

After this initial inspection, a film can be made, if indicated and if the equipment is available. Once this is performed, biopsies of suspicious lesions can be obtained using a rigid optical forceps through the same port.

7.4.2.4 Pleural Biopsy

We advise using a biopsy technique involving palpation and peeling. The initial biopsy should be performed over a hard surface, i.e., a rib – this avoids injury to the neurovascular bundle

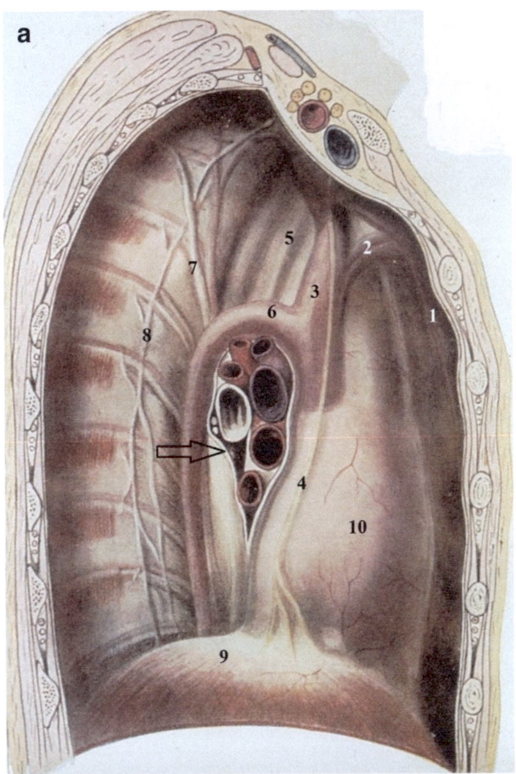

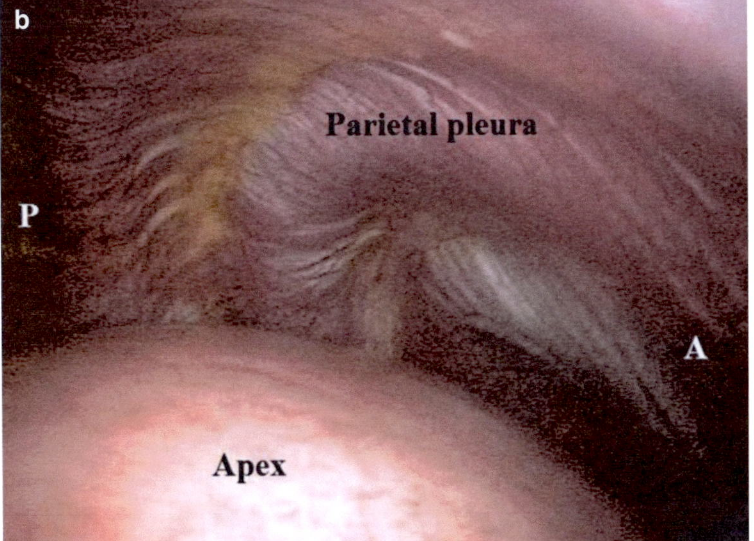

Fig. 7.20 (**a**) The right pleural cavity (*arrow*: hilum) – *1* internal mammary artery, *2* internal mammary vein, *3* superior vena cava, *4* phrenic nerve, *5* vagus nerve, *6* azygos arch, *7* intercostal venous trunk, *8* sympathetic trunk, *9* diaphragm, *10* heart. (**b**) *Right side – A* anterior parietal pleura. *P* posterior parietal pleura. (**c**) *Right side* – subclavian artery (*arrows*). Lung (●). (**d**) *Right side* – upper lobe (■). Middle lobe (●). Lower lobe (□). (**e**) *Right side* – fissures (*arrows*). Middle lobe (●). Lower lobe (■). (**f**) *Right side* – posterior parietal pleura. Intercostal space (●). Pleural fat (○). (**g**) *Right side* – posterior parietal pleura with pleural fat (*yellow*). Fissure (*arrow*)

Fig. 7.20 (continued)

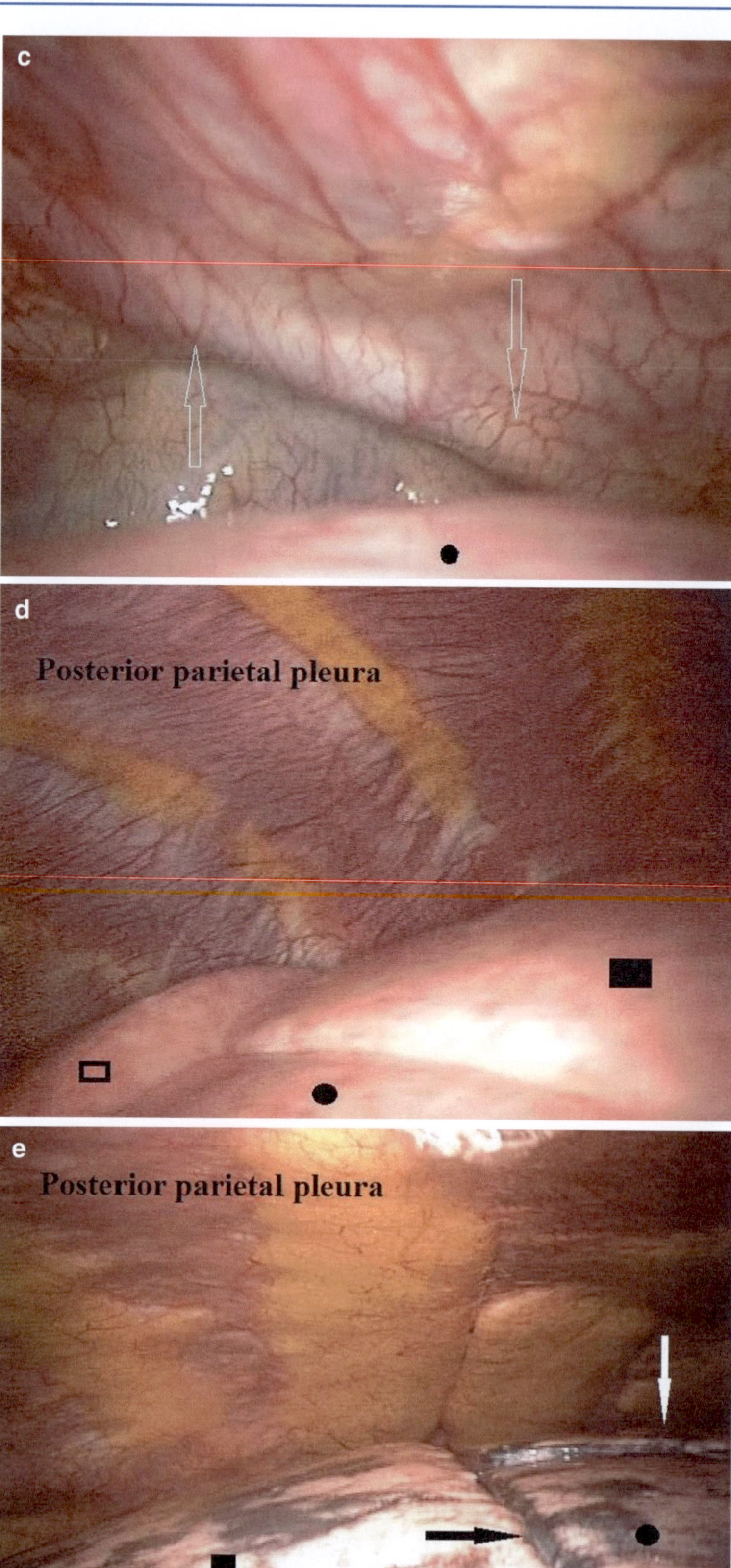

Fig. 7.20 (continued)

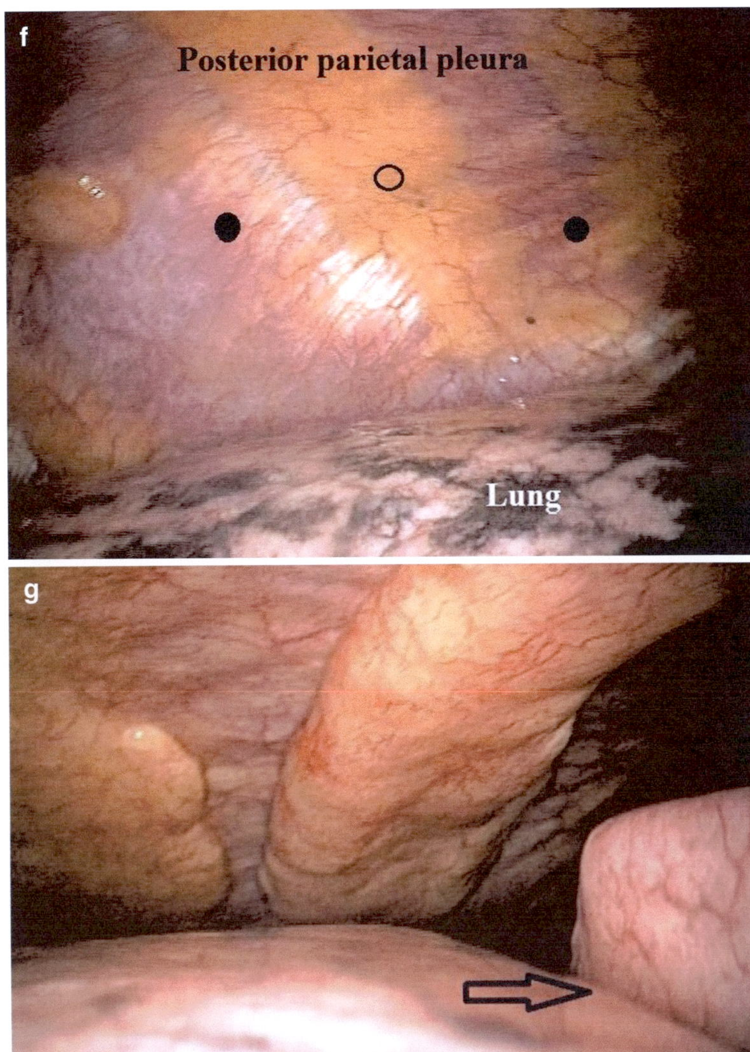

(Fig. 7.21d). Once a rib is confirmed by touching with the closed forceps, it is opened and the suspicious lesion is grasped. This is then peeled parallel to the chest wall. Once a small section is peeled, we return to the initial site of biopsy to ensure there is no excessive bleeding. The edge of the peel is then grasped and striped further (Fig. 7.22). This can be continued on a number of occasions to obtain a large biopsy sample. Multiple biopsies should be performed in this manner. In our practice we perform between 15 and 20 biopsies per case. This provides adequate sampling for pathology, immunohistochemistry, mutation analysis, and tumor markers – if indicated.

After biopsy, the cavity should be inspected again with the direct optical telescope to ensure that there is no excessive bleeding – if occurring, this may need additional treatment. If excessive bleeding occurs and coagulation is required, a second insulated port of entry must be placed in a suitable location to allow for this to be performed (Fig. 7.23).

If indicated, talc pleurodesis can be performed at this time through the single port or through an additional port of entry created with the Boutin needle. A second port allows visualization of the talcage during administration. However, in our opinion talcage can be performed safely through a single port with occasional revisualization of the cavity with the optic to ensure all surfaces are sufficiently coated. The goal is to obtain a light coating of talc on all pleural surfaces, both parietal and visceral (Fig. 7.24), using a dedicated device (Fig. 7.25) and avoid mass of talc which makes the procedure inefficient (Fig. 7.26). The pleura post talcage should resemble the first light fall of snow. In addition, in the setting of mesothelioma, a second port of entry may require

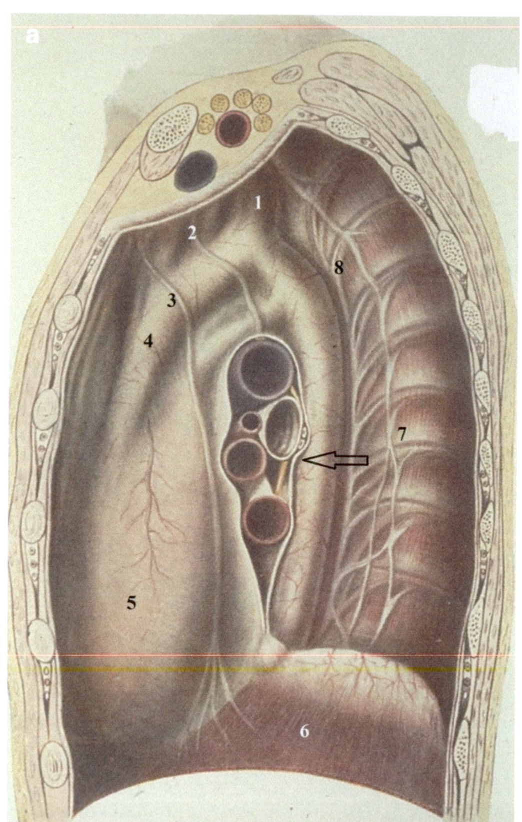

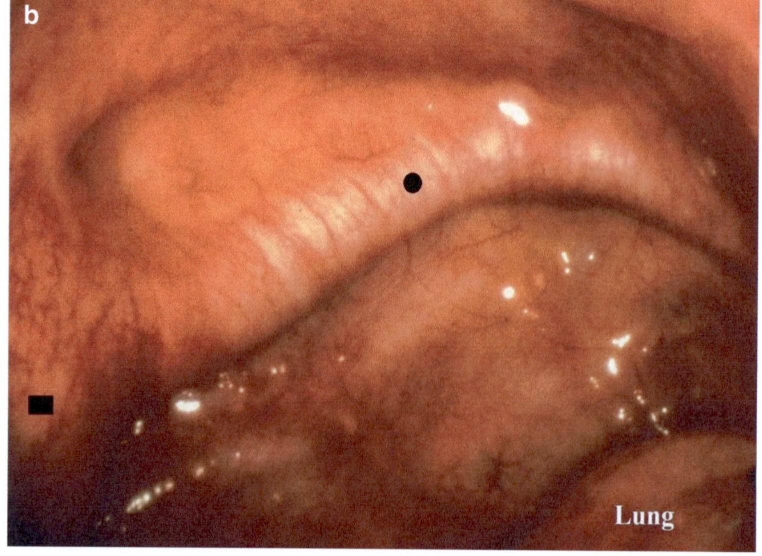

Fig. 7.21 (**a**) The left pleural cavity (*arrow*: hilum) – *1* subclavian artery, *2* vagus nerve, *3* phrenic nerve, *4* aortic arch, *5* heart, *6* diaphragm, *7* sympathetic trunk, *8* intercostal arteries and veins. (**b**) *Left side* – the subclavian artery (●) runs upwards through the upper half of the left pleural cavity. The aortic arch (■) is visible at the *left side* of the picture. (**c**) *Left side* – upper part of the pleural cavity with the upper lobe of the left lung; posterior parietal pleura (*white circle*) and apex (*white square*). (**d**) *Left side* – posterior parietal pleura with intercostal spaces (●), pleural fat (■), and the surface of the left lung (*star*). The intercostal vessels are clearly visible (*arrow*). When the pleura is thin, the biopsy should be performed against the ribs in order to eliminate the risk of bleeding. (**e**) *Left side* – costodiaphragmatic gutter with posterior parietal pleura where intercostal spaces and pleural fat are clearly visible (□). The diaphragm on the *right side* of the picture (○). Left lower lobe (*star*). (**f**) *Left side* – diaphragm with the costodiaphragmatic gutter (*star*). Fat deposits are visible at this level. Left lower lobe (○). Posterior parietal pleura (□). (**g**) *Left side* – anterior parietal pleura with internal mammary vessels (*arrow*). Surface of the lung (*star*). (**h**) *Left side* – fissure between the lower lobe (○) and the upper lobe (□). Fibrin deposits on the surface of the posterior parietal pleura are visible (*arrow*)

Fig. 7.21 (continued)

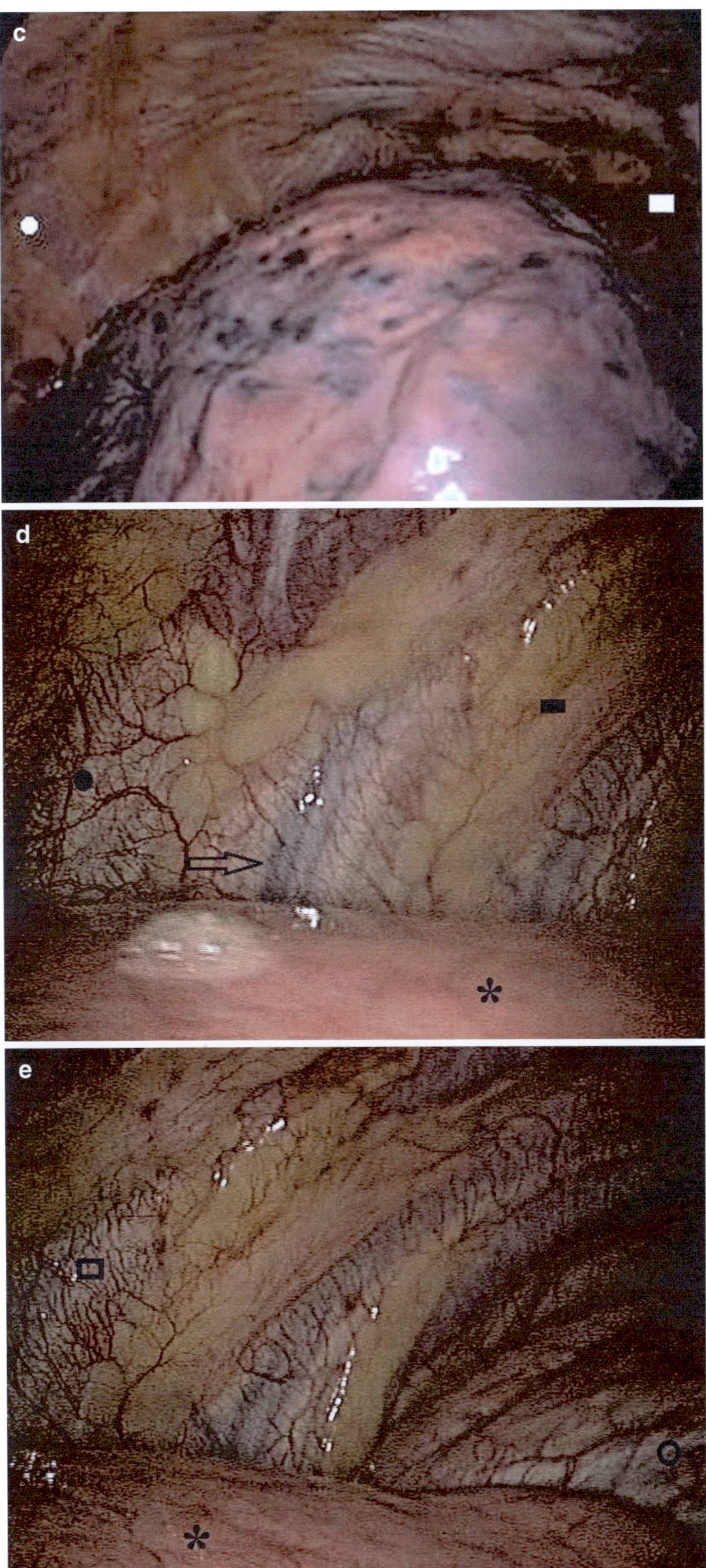

Fig. 7.21 (continued)

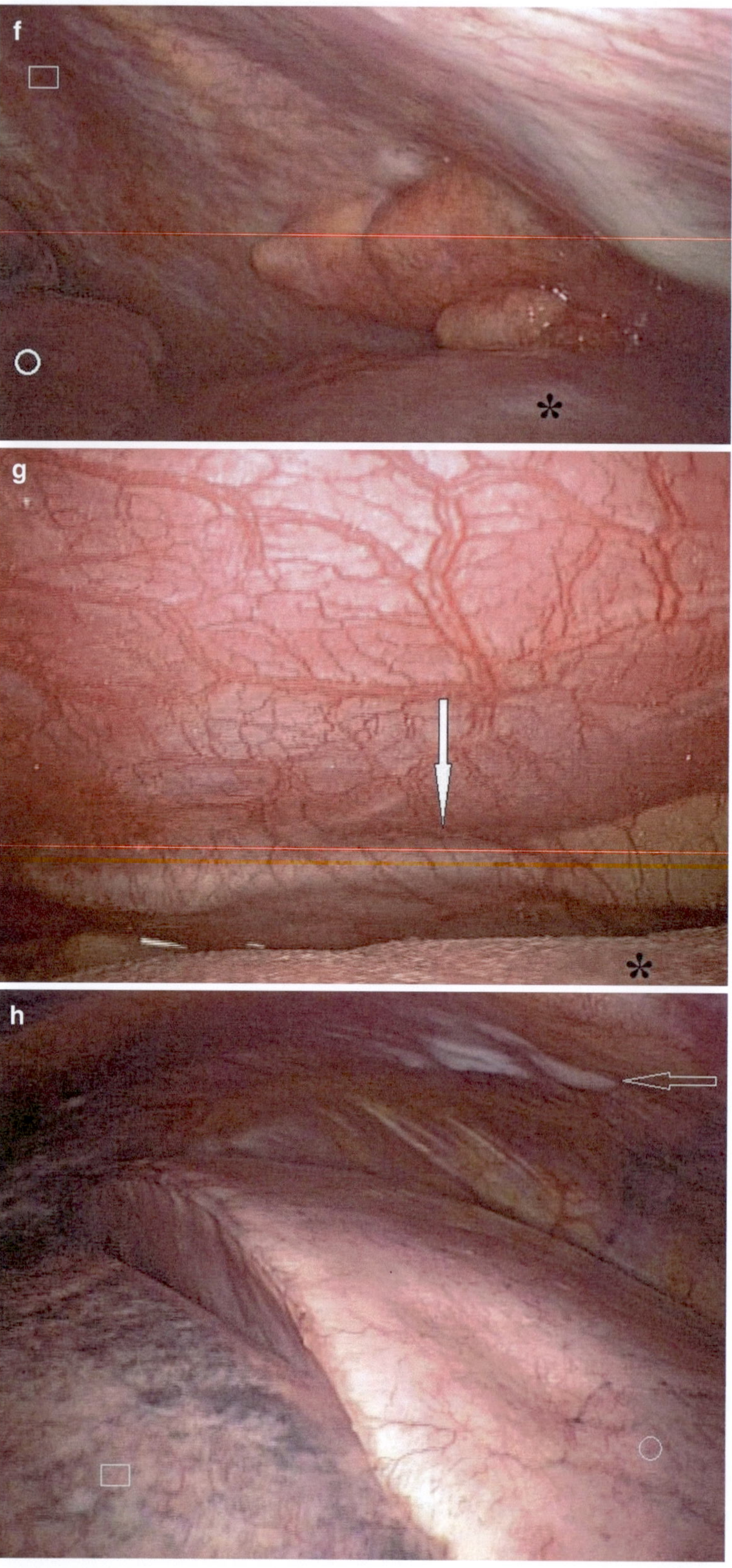

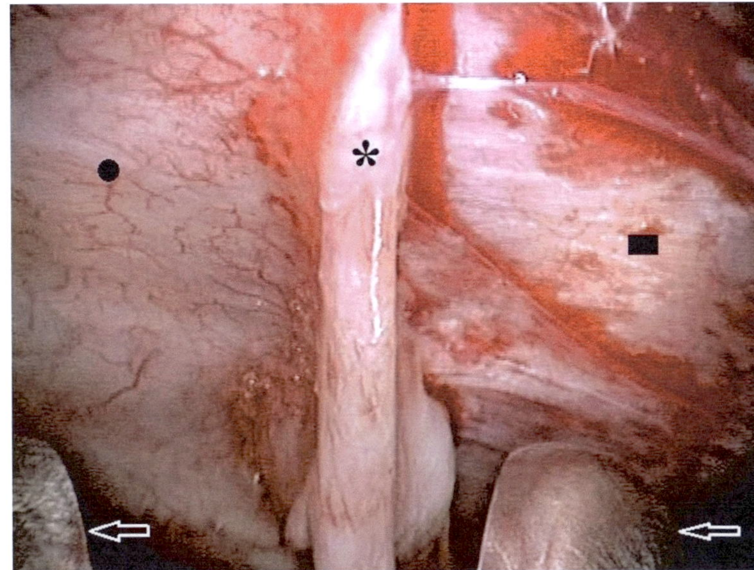

Fig. 7.22 Biopsy technique (peeled parietal pleura (*star*)). The pleural biopsies can be performed with a single point of entry (using an optical biopsy forceps) or through a second point of entry with jaws of the coagulating forceps (*arrow*). The biopsy should be taken against the rib when the pleura is thin so that the intercostal neurovascular bundle is not touched. On the view, the arrows and the star show the tip of the 5-mm double spoon forceps and the pleura specimen, respectively. (■): intercostal muscle is visible after deep peeling pleural biopsy. (●): posterior parietal pleura

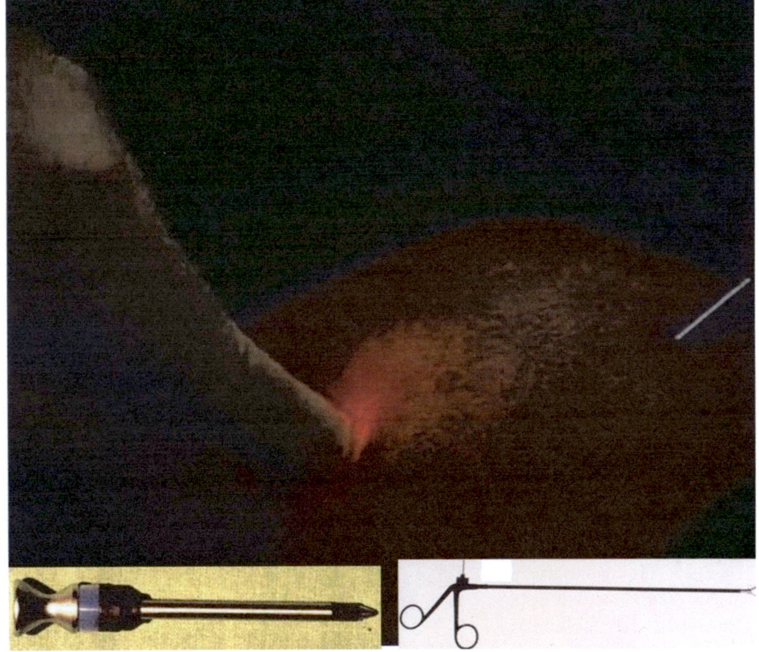

Fig. 7.23 A second point of entry must be done in a suitable location to allow the use of 5-mm insulated trocar (inserted picture, *bottom left*) for coagulating forceps (inserted picture, *bottom right*)

additional radiation therapy to minimize the occurrence of skin metastases.

7.4.2.5 End of Procedure

A drain should be inserted in every case at the end of the procedure. The optimal site and length for the chest drain is chosen under direct vision using the optic telescope. The drain is then directed blindly to that site at the end of the procedure and fixed to the skin with sutures. It is connected to an underwater seal and gentle step-by-step suction is applied until complete re-expansion of the lung has been achieved.

The duration of drainage depends on the procedure performed and on local policies. However, in our service, in patients who undergo diagnostic thoracoscopy alone, the drain can be removed on the table (Fig. 7.27). If pleurodesis is

Fig. 7.24 For a pleural symphysis, the goal is to obtain a light coating of dedicated talc on all pleural surfaces, both parietal and visceral

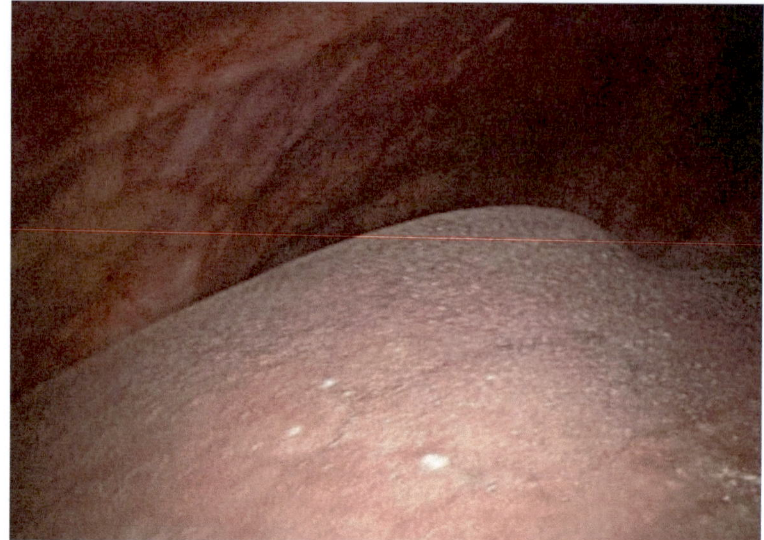

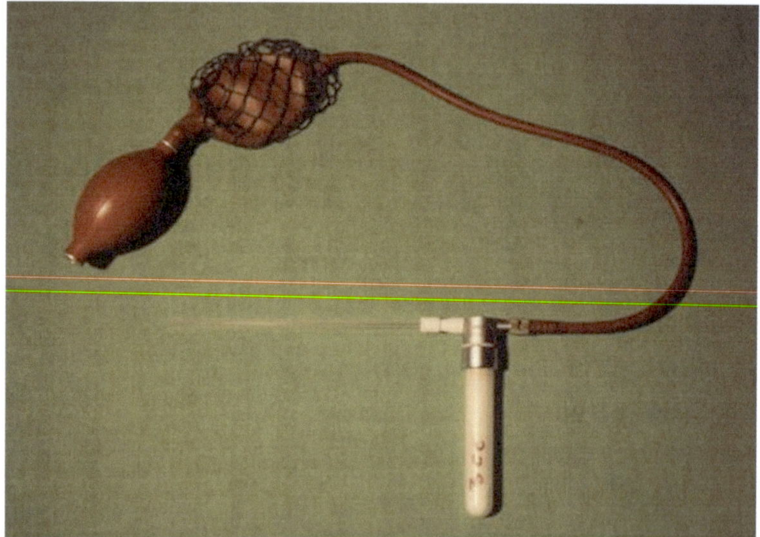

Fig. 7.25 For the treatment of chronic pleurisies (3–5 g) or spontaneous pneumothorax (1–2 g) is used. The talc should be sterile, free of asbestos and of a controlled granulometry (large particle size talc) preventing the talc from migrating and resulting in a systemic inflammatory reaction (Maskell 2004). A double- balloon atomizer (picture, *top*) or a disposable device (picture, *bottom* – Steritalc®, Novatech SA, France) can be used to insufflate the talc

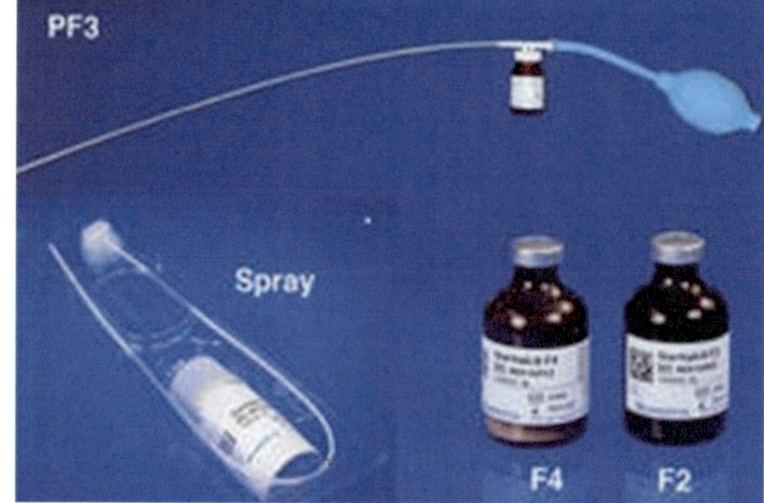

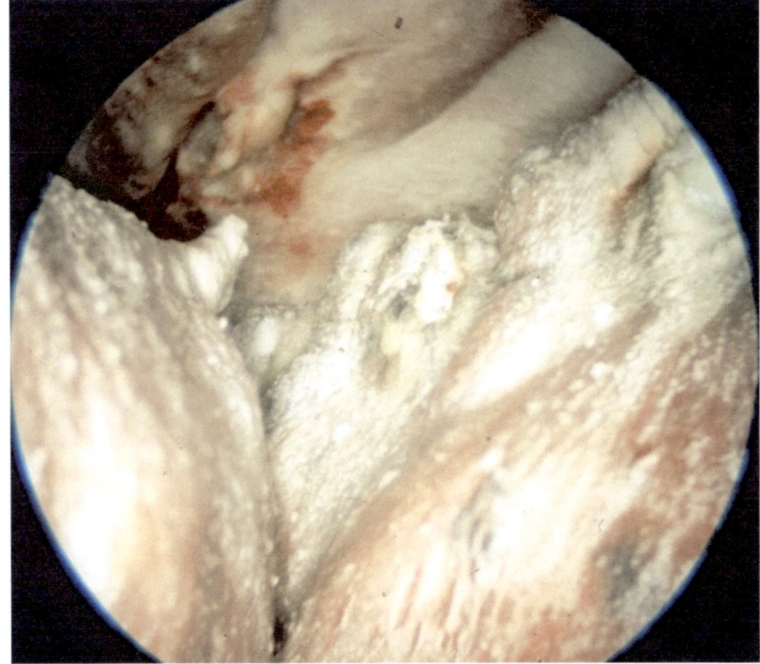

Fig. 7.26 In this case, the mass of talc has made the procedure inefficient. An attempted pleural symphysis will fail

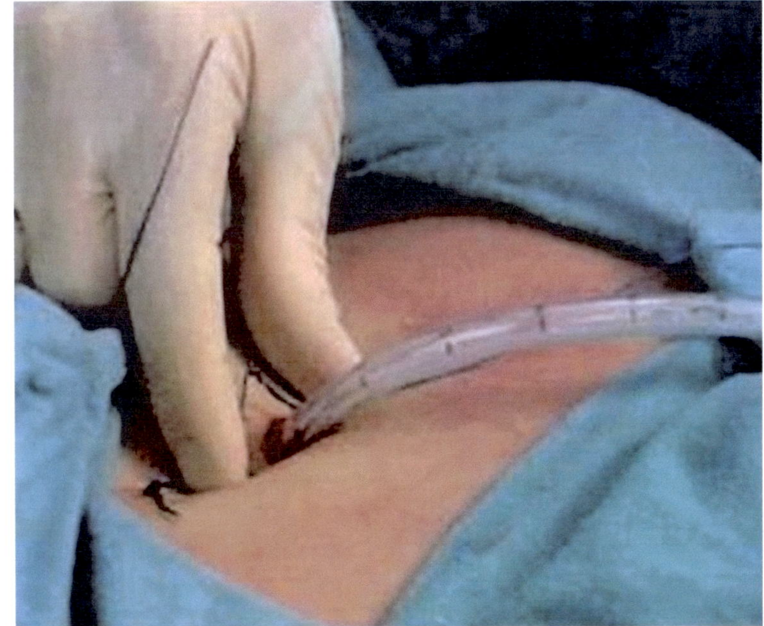

Fig. 7.27 At the end of the procedure, a chest tube is inserted through the point of entry and connected to a suction device. A gradual increase of the suction is applied (never > 50 cmH$_2$O) until full lung re-expansion has occurred. Ideally, the chest tube is directed posteriorly and pushed as close to the apex as possible. In case of pleurisy, fluid drainage can be improved by making one or two extra holes on the radiopaque side of the inferior part of the chest tube. When thoracoscopy is performed for diagnosis of a pleural effusion, the tube may be quickly removed as shown on the picture (Breen et al. 2009)

performed, the drain needs to remain in situ for a longer period depending on the etiology of the pleural effusion.

If the drain remains in situ, it is imperative that all staff are trained in the management of tube thoracostomy. Local policies should be implemented for effective analgesia for patients.

All patients should go to a recovery room post thoracoscopy where there is adequate cardiorespiratory monitoring available. Full resuscitation facilities are mandatory in the postoperative period.

Conclusion

Thoracoscopy is a safe and effective procedure in the assessment and management of pleural diseases. However, it is essential that patients are carefully selected and that their medical status is optimized prior to the intervention. Thoracoscopy is simple to perform, but all cases should be performed meticulously in a stepwise approach as outlined above. Physicians must be prepared for all eventualities, and, in particular, the chest drain and electrocautery should be available from the outset so that complications can be minimized.

References

Boutin C, Viallat JR, Cargnino P et al (1981a) La Thoracoscopie en 1980. Revue générale. Poumon Coeur 37:11–19

Boutin C, Viallat JR, Cargnino P et al (1981b) Thoracoscopy in malignant pleural effusions. Am Rev Respir Dis 124:588–592

Boutin C, Viallat JR, Cargnino P (1981c) Indications actuelles de la thoracoscopie. Compte rendu du Symposium de Marseille. Rev Fr Mal Respir 9:309–318

Breen D, Fraticelli A, Greillier L et al (2008) Redo medical thoracoscopy is feasible in patients with pleural disease: a series. Interact Cardiovasc Thorac Surg 8:330–338

Breen DP, Mallawathantri S, Fraticelli A (2009) Feasibility of short term drainage for diagnostic thoracoscopy. Monaldi Arch Chest Dis 71:54–58

Cruise F (1865) The utility of endoscope as an aid in the diagnosis and treatment of disease. Dublin Quarterly J Med Sci 39:329–363

Ishida A, Nakamura M, Miyazawa T, Astoul P (2011) Novel approach for talc pleurodesis by dedicated catheter through flexi-rigid thoracoscope under local anesthesia. Interact Cardiovasc Thorac Surg 12:667–670

Jacobaeus HC (1910) Über die Möglichkeit, die Zystoskopie bei Untersuchung seröser Höhlungen anzuwenden. Münch Med Wschr 40:2090–2092

Janssen JP, Boutin C (1992) Extended thoracoscopy: a biopsy method to be used in case of pleural adhesions. Eur Resp J 5:763–766

Maskell NA, Lee YC, Gleeson FV et al (2004) Randomized trials describing lung inflammation after pleurodesis with talc of varying particle size. Am J Respir Crit Care Med 170:377–382

Tassi GF, Marchetti GP, Pinelli V (2011) Minithoracoscopy: a complementary technique for medical thoracoscopy. Respiration 82:204–206

Part II

Thoracoscopy for the Beginners ('The Green Zone')

The Current Practice of Medical Thoracoscopy

8

Philippe Astoul, GianFranco Tassi, and Jean-Marie Tschopp

What do we mean by the green zone? Here we describe the classical indications for thoracoscopy that every pulmonologist interested in this technique should be able to practice easily after proper training. On one hand thoracoscopy is a diagnostic tool improving the diagnostic yield of malignant diseases or non-malignant pleural effusions such as tuberculosis in almost 100 % of the cases. On the other hand it is also an efficient therapeutic tool which allows control of pleural effusions responsible for breathlessness in patients with important such effusions and efficiently prevents further recurrence of pneumothorax by talc pleurodesis. As recently shown, talc if properly chosen and used is innocuous contrary to the talc used, for instance, in Brazil and North America. Talc pleurodesis under thoracoscopy is safe as recently shown in Europe by two large prospective studies in malignant pleural effusion and treatment of recurrence of spontaneous pneumothorax.

P. Astoul (✉)
Division of Thoracic Oncology, Pleural Diseases, and Interventional Pulmonology, Hôpital NORD, Marseille, France
e-mail: pastoul@ap-hm.fr

G. Tassi
Division of Pneumology,
Spedali Civili di Brescia, Brescia, Italy
e-mail: gf.tassi@tin.it

J.-M. Tschopp
Département de Médecine Interne
Centre valaisan de pneumologie,
CHCVs, Montana 3963, Switzerland
e-mail: jean-marie.tschopp@hopitalvs.ch

P. Astoul et al. (eds.), *Thoracoscopy for Pulmonologists*,
DOI 10.1007/978-3-642-38351-9_8, © Springer-Verlag Berlin Heidelberg 2014

Diagnostic Thoracoscopy: Malignant Pleural Effusion

9

Marios Froudarakis

9.1   Introduction

Malignant neoplasms are the second leading cause of death in the USA (Hoyert et al. 2006). Almost all neoplasms can metastasize to the pleura during their history, either as the initial presentation of cancer or during disease progression (Valdes et al. 1996). Every year, up to 150,000 cases of malignant pleural effusion are reported in the USA (Valdes et al. 1996). The optimal work-up for an undiagnosed pleural effusion remains a real problem for physicians (Froudarakis 2008). In developed countries, where the incidence of tuberculosis is low, a patient presenting with an undiagnosed pleural effusion has a significant likelihood of malignancy. Indeed, more than 50 % of the cases of undiagnosed pleural effusion are due to carcinomas; the second most common diagnosis (10 %) is tuberculosis (Valdes et al. 1996).

Carcinoma of the lung is the most common cause of malignant pleural effusion with 641 cases out of 1,783 patients (36 %) reported in a meta-analysis (Sahn 1998). All histological subtypes of bronchogenic carcinoma can result in a pleural effusion (Johnston 1985). The most frequent histology reported is adenocarcinoma – accounting for approximately 40 % of the cases – as it is more likely to occur in the lung periphery adjacent to the pleura, which may be directly invaded by the tumor. The second most common histological subtype is small-cell lung carcinoma, a highly invasive tumor, accounting for about 25 % of the cases (Johnston 1985). Breast carcinoma is the most common non-pulmonary cause of malignant pleural effusion ranging from 16 to 25 % of the cases (Sahn 1998). All neoplasms have been associated with pleural pathology, such as lymphomas (11 %), genitourinary (9.4 %) or gastrointestinal (7 %) carcinomas, while pleural carcinoma of unknown origin is reported in less than 8 % of cases (Table 9.1) (Johnston 1985; Antunes and Neville 2000).

Pleural effusion is usually diagnosed by a simple chest radiograph and/or computed tomography. In lung cancer, its presence is associated with advanced stage disease (M1a) and therefore with poor prognosis (Mountain 1997). However, in some cases, pleural effusion may be due to postobstructive pneumonia or atelectasis, venous obstruction by tumor compression, or lymphatic obstruction by mediastinal lymph nodes, and therefore it is not associated with direct pleural involvement (Antony et al. 2001). The confirmation of a benign pleural effusion in the setting of confirmed malignancy will have a major impact on treatment options and therefore prognosis. When pleural cytology is negative, thoracoscopy must be performed in order to evaluate the extent of the disease and confirm malignant infiltration of the pleura if present (Rodriguez Panadero 1995). Thoracoscopy also provides information about the extent of the disease especially in non-small-cell

M. Froudarakis
Department of Pulmonology,
University Hospital of Alexandroupolis,
Alexandroupolis, Greece
e-mail: mfroud@med.duth.gr

P. Astoul et al. (eds.), *Thoracoscopy for Pulmonologists*,
DOI 10.1007/978-3-642-38351-9_9, © Springer-Verlag Berlin Heidelberg 2014

Table 9.1 Primary carcinoma in patients with metastatic pleural effusion (Froudarakis 2008)

Lung carcinoma	37 %
Breast carcinoma	16.8 %
Lymphoma	11.5 %
Genitourinary carcinomas	9.4 %
Gastrointestinal carcinomas	6.9 %
Other carcinomas	7.3 %
Unknown primary	10.7 %

lung cancer (NSCLC) and mesothelioma. In NSCLC a positive thoracoscopy defines M1a disease, which excludes surgical resection and indicates a poor prognosis for the patient. In the case of a patient with NSCLC and pleural effusion, a negative thoracoscopy indicates a paramalignant effusion, and therefore the patient may be a candidate for radical surgery, with a presumed better prognosis. Thoracoscopy may have a role in early stage mesothelioma – the findings at the time of the procedure may suggest a role for multimodality treatments including extrapleural pneumonectomy. On the contrary, in a patient with known metastatic carcinoma or poor performance status (PS), establishing whether or not an effusion is malignant might not be necessary, since survival will be poor in either case.

9.2 Pathogenesis of Malignant Pleural Effusion

The occurrence of a pleural effusion in malignancy is usually secondary to obstruction of the lymphatic drainage from the pleural space, such as pleural thickening by widespread carcinomatosis, obstruction caused by infiltration of mediastinal lymph nodes, or obstruction caused by tumor emboli (Rodriguez-Panadero et al. 1989; Meyer 1966; Chernow and Sahn 1977). In addition a local inflammatory reaction to tumors next to the pleura might play an important role in the development of pleural effusions by increasing capillary permeability (Leff et al. 1978). These mechanisms explain the predominance of lymphocytes in malignant pleural effusion, although their role in the pathogenesis remains unclear. However, T lymphocytes might have an important role in host versus tumor local defense in malignant pleural effusions (Domagala et al. 1978).

The underlying mechanisms of pleural effusion due to neoplasms have been reported in postmortem studies (Rodriguez-Panadero et al. 1989; Meyer 1966). Most of the patients had both parietal and visceral pleura infiltration. It was shown that invasion of the parietal pleura is due to neoplastic spread across the pleural cavity from the visceral pleura along pleural adhesions which have been preformed or secondary to the malignant process. In addition, the parietal pleura is invaded by the attachment of exfoliated cells from the visceral pleura. The visceral pleura might be involved by direct pulmonary arterial invasion and embolization (Meyer 1966). When the tumor infiltrates blood vessels directly, and/or occludes venules, a bloody pleural effusion may occur. Another mechanism of hemorrhagic pleural effusion might be associated with capillary dilatation due to release of vasoactive substances (Meyer 1966; Chernow and Sahn 1977). Bilateral pleural metastases are due to hematogenous spread to the contralateral hemithorax (Meyer 1966).

Nonmalignant pleural effusions (paramalignant) may occur due to bronchial obstruction causing atelectasis or pneumonia with an associated parapneumonic effusion. In this situation the effusion is due to a mechanical obstruction without malignant cell infiltration of lymphatics or blood vessels. Lung carcinoma is also frequently associated with heart failure, as both bronchogenic carcinoma and heart disease have the same risk profiles. Thus, pleural effusion may be a transudate due to heart failure. The same finding may be observed in patients with bronchogenic carcinoma and hepatic insufficiency. In some patients there is an association between pulmonary embolism and pneumothorax (Kabnick et al. 1982) with bronchogenic carcinoma.

9.3 Clinical Presentation of Malignant Pleural Effusion

A pleural effusion in patients with neoplasm may present in two distinct clinical situations: as a presenting symptom, i.e., during the work-up a previously unknown carcinoma, or presenting as a pleural effusion during the evolution of a known carcinoma. The diagnostic approach, although basically the same, must be specific to each case as the patient's prognosis is dependent on it. In the former, the pleural effusion is discovered after the patient consults his physician for progressively worsening dyspnea, dry cough, lateral thoracic pain, or hemoptysis. General constitutional symptoms may also be present, such as fever, weight loss, loss of appetite, and impairment of activities of daily living (ADLs). Only 25 % of patients are totally asymptomatic despite the presence of a pleural effusion on imaging studies. Typically there is evidence of a pleural effusion on the physical examination which is confirmed by chest X-ray, which also demonstrates the extent of the pleural process (Hyde and Hyde 1974; Cohen 1974; Scagliotti 1995).

9.4 Imaging

Pleural effusions may be free-flowing or loculated (White et al. 1993). The chest X-ray may also demonstrate the likely cause of the pleural effusion, such as a peripheral lesion in contact with the thoracic wall or a central lesion with associated atelectasis or obstructive pneumonia. It may also provide useful information on associated findings, such as pericardial effusion, air in the pleural space, or mediastinal lymph node enlargement (White et al. 1993; Romney and Austin 1990; Woodring 1990). In 15 % of cases however, the chest X-ray is negative. A lateral chest X-ray may assist in these cases (White et al. 1993).

Pneumothorax is a rare manifestation of lung cancer and may be associated with pleural effusion. It was estimated that the occurrence of air in the pleural space is less than 1 % in patients with lung cancer (Kabnick 1982; Steinhausling and Cuttat 1985; Woodring 1990). Also, lung cancer is the cause of only 0.05 % of pneumothorax cases (Steinhausling and Cuttat 1985). A pneumothorax may develop as a complication of a bronchopleural fistula secondary to both pleural

and bronchial infiltration by the tumor, from a peripheral necrotizing tumor invading the pleura or from obstructive hyperinflation due to central obstruction (Steinhausling and Cuttat 1985; Woodring 1990). In most of the cases, pneumothorax occurs when lung cancer is already at an advanced stage (Woodring 1990).

The extension of the neoplasm to the pleura can also be assessed by chest computed tomography (Mountain 1997; Au and Thomas 2003). Chest computed tomography is sensitive in recognizing a pleural effusion, but cannot identify its possible malignant nature (McLoud 1998; Armstrong et al. 1995). However, some patterns may indicate malignancy, such as a pleural thickness over 1 cm indicating pleural carcinomatosis (Leung 1990). It is controversial whether computed tomography is more sensitive than the standard chest X-ray in recognizing associated findings such as a peripheral nodule and/or mass infiltrating the thoracic wall, the diaphragm, or the mediastinum (Armstrong et al. 1995; Glazer et al. 1989; Rato et al. 1991), as soft tissue swelling may be due to inflammation and/or fibrosis rather than direct infiltration of tumor (Pearlberg et al. 1987; Wang et al. 2004). Also, it appears that focal chest pain is more accurate than chest computed tomography in predicting chest wall invasion (Glazer et al. 1985). Computed tomography may also reveal mediastinal lymphadenopathy or associated pathology in the contralateral lung or pleura. The presence of these findings may be indicative of the malignant nature of the pleural effusion (Woodring 1990; Leung et al. 1990; Glazer et al. 1985).

Magnetic resonance imaging is less sensitive than computed tomography in diagnosing a pleural effusion (Au and Thomas 2003; McLoud 1998; Webb 1989). On T1-weighted images the signal from the fluid is very low and therefore may not be detected, although characteristic brightening on T2-weighted images allows detection (Au and Thomas 2003; Webb 1989; Templeton et al. 1990). In addition, magnetic resonance imaging has the same limitations as computed tomography in recognizing chest wall, mediastinal, pericardial, or diaphragmatic infiltration (Armstrong et al. 1995; Webb 1989; Templeton et al. 1990).

In malignant pleural disease, chest imaging with positron emission tomography (PET) using fluorine 18-labeled fluorodeoxyglucose (FDG) has a sensitivity ranging from 93 to 100 % and specificity from 67 to 89 %. The negative predictive value of the PET ranges from 94 to 100 % and its positive predictive value from 63 to 94 % (Duysinx et al. 2004; Erasmus et al. 2000; Schaffler et al. 2004). False-positive results occur in patients with any other inflammatory process such as parapneumonic effusions or pleurodesis after talc instillation (Wang et al. 2004; Kwek et al. 2004). When PF cytology is negative, a negative PET-FDG scan provides the most useful clinical information for ruling out a pleural effusion of malignant etiology (negative predictive value) (Wang et al. 2004).

Ultrasound is another noninvasive method for investigating the pleura (Herth 2004). Although its major indication is loculated pleural effusions usually due to infection, it may be also helpful in patients with a low performance status who are unsuitable for a more sophisticated examination, such as computed tomography of the thorax (O'Moore et al. 2004; Lipscomb et al. 1981). Ultrasound sensitivity in setting of pleural effusion is 92 % alone; combined with the standard chest radiograph, it is 98 % (Lipscomb et al. 1981; Henschke et al. 1989). It also assists in the recognition of associated findings such as pleural thickness, pleural or subpleural tumors, and parenchymal masses (Herth 2004; Yang et al. 1992).

9.5 Pleural Thoracentesis

The associated chemistry of pleural fluid in patients with malignancy has been the subject of many reports. There are no specific features of pleural fluid chemistry from patients with lung carcinoma when compared to those with extrapulmonary malignancy to the pleura (Sahn 1982; Sahn 1998). Thus, as in other malignant pleural effusions, we expect to find an exudate, with a protein concentration >3 g/dL levels (or pleural to serum protein ratio >0.5) and lactate dehydrogenase (LDH) >200 IU/L (or pleural to serum LDH ratio >0.6) (Light et al. 1972, 1973a).

Table 9.2 Pleural fluid tests in patients with exudative pleural effusion

Test of pleural fluid	Test value	Probability
pH	<7.30	In 30 % of malignant PE
Glucose	<0.6 g/dl	In 30 % of malignant PE
Red cells	>100,000/ml	High probability for malignancy
Lymphocytes	>50 %	Probable malignancy, do not rule out TB
Adenosine deaminase (ADA)	>40 U/L	High probability for TB (used in countries with high TB incidence)
Eosinophils	>10 %	Also present in malignancy
Cytology	>0	Malignant PE
Cytology	<0	Do not rule out malignancy
PCR for TB	<0	Rule out TB
Aneuploidy	>0	High probability for malignancy

PE pleural effusion, *TB* tuberculosis, *PCR* polymerase chain reaction

Some pleural fluid findings are useful in confirming the diagnosis (Table 9.2). In approximately 30 % of cases, the pH will be less than 7.30 and glucose levels less than 0.6 g/dL (or the ratio of pleural to serum glucose <0.5) (Light 1995; Light et al. 1973b; Berger and Maher 1971; Chavalittamrong et al. 1979; Good et al. 1985). Low pleural fluid pH (<7.20) may indicate trapped lung, a shorter expected survival, and a higher probability of a failed pleurodesis (Sanchez-Armengol and Rodriguez-Panadero 1993; Sahn 1998; Rodriguez-Panadero and Antony 1997). However, Aelony et al. reported that thoracoscopic talc poudrage was successful in 88 % of patients with malignant pleural effusion despite the low pH (Aelony et al. 1998). In malignant pleural effusions, when both low pH and glucose are present, there is an association with marked pleural thickening and inhibition of transfer between the pleural space and the systemic circulation (Rodriguez-Panadero and Lopez Mejias 1989). In rare occasions the pleural fluid is a transudate due to associated diseases such as congestive heart failure, atelectasis from bronchial obstruction, or hypoalbuminemia (Chernow and Sahn 1977; Sahn 1982). Tests to define whether the fluid is an exudate or transudate are not diagnostic, but provide a probability as to the likely nature of a pleural effusion (Heffner 1998).

Leukocytes in malignant pleural fluid are relatively low with mean values ranging from 2,000 to 2,500 cells/mL (Sahn 1998; Chernow and Sahn 1977). While the total amount of leukocytes is not helpful in the differential diagnosis, the type of cell is important. In malignant pleural effusions we may find the proportion of lymphocytes to be greater than 50 % (Chernow and Sahn 1977; Domagala et al. 1978). Neutrophils usually represent less than 25 % (Sahn 1998), while total eosinophils are low (7–10 %) (Kuhn et al. 1989; Rubins and Rubins 1996). Other nucleated cells may be found, such as macrophages and mesothelial cells. Erythrocytes (Table 9.2) average about 40,000–50,000 cells/mL, however, with a wide range dependent on the etiology, from none to hemothorax (Chernow and Sahn 1977).

Several tumor markers, such as carcinoembryonic antigen (CEA), CA-125, CA 19-9, CYFRA 21-1, and NSE, have been tested in patients with malignant pleural effusions (Cascinu et al. 1997; Alatas et al. 2001). Although results seem to be contradictory as to the usefulness of these markers in the differential diagnosis of pleural effusions even when comparing patients with malignant and nonmalignant effusions, some authors propose specific tumor markers for the diagnosis of pleural effusions due to bronchogenic carcinoma (Menard et al. 1993). A reasonable compromise may be that tests should be performed in a selected population of patients with negative cytology and a "suspect" clinical outcome (Falcone et al. 1996). Recently, a number of reports have emerged, studying various novel markers, such as oncogenes (Stoetzer et al. 1999), various cytokines involved in inflammation (Alexandrakis et al. 2000), or matrix metalloproteinases (Hurewitz et al. 1992) as predictive or prognostic indicators of malignant pleural effusions. Until now, none of these markers have proved their usefulness even in differentiating malignant from benign pleural effusions. Generally, biochemical or biological markers in the malignant pleural effusions, as well as in the serum, cannot replace the routine cytopathological examination in the diagnosis of the disease (Marel et al. 1995).

A diagnosis of malignant pleural effusion can be made only when cancer cells are found in the pleural fluid. The first step in the assessment is cytological examination of the pleural fluid obtained at the time of thoracentesis (Sahn 1998; Antony et al. 2001). Cytologists face two major problems: to prove malignancy by confirming the presence of malignant cells and, in addition, to establish the organ of origin of those malignant cells. The diagnostic accuracy of the cytological examination of the pleural fluid varies from series to series. It is very low for some authors ranging from 15 to 35 % (Storey et al. 1976; Salyer 1975), while very high for others ranging from 80 to 90 % (Johnston 1985; Light et al. 1973a). This yield is increased only slightly (approximately 20 %) if repeated cytology specimens are sent (Johnston 1985). The cytological yield is higher for adenocarcinoma and when smears and blocks are used (Johnston 1985). Variations in diagnostic yield are due to various factors including the stage of the disease and the origin of the primary malignancy (Antony et al. 2001).

9.6 Minimally Invasive Techniques

Blind pleural biopsy have similar results to pleural cytology (Salyer et al. 1975). However, the combination of both techniques seems to improve the diagnostic yield (Johnston 1985; Antony et al. 2001). The low diagnostic yield of closed pleural biopsy is explained by a number of factors including minimal pleural extension; localization of tumors in regions of the pleura unreachable by biopsy needle, including the visceral pleura (Canto et al. 1983); and the level of experience of the physician (Walshe et al. 1992). Furthermore, the diagnostic yield of blind biopsy increases with the number of specimens taken in malignant pleural effusion (Jimenez et al. 2002). At least four biopsy samples are needed for accurate diagnosis (Jimenez et al. 2002). Since malignant pleural invasion is preferentially located at the bases of the hemithorax, it is recommended the sample be taken from the lowest region of the costal pleura in order to achieve a higher diagnostic success (Canto et al. 1983; Rodriguez-Panadero et al. 1989). However, Prakash reported that only 20 out of 281 patients (7 %) with malignant pleural effusion and initially negative fluid cytology had a closed biopsy which confirmed the disease (Prakash and Reiman 1985). Therefore, this result argues against performing concurrent thoracentesis and closed biopsy as an initial step, when a malignant origin for the pleural effusion is suspected. In cases with initial negative cytology and an indeterminate exudative pleural effusion, it may then be reasonable to repeat the thoracentesis with a pleural biopsy. However, negative pleural cytology and closed biopsy do not rule out a malignant origin for the pleural effusion. On the contrary, both techniques are indicated as the initial approach when considering a tuberculous pleural effusion as the diagnostic yield from the biopsy is consistently higher than that found in malignant disease (Prakash and Reiman 1985; Loddenkemper et al. 1978).

When pleural thoracentesis and/or biopsy does/do not show malignant cells, and lung carcinoma is highly suspected, it is reasonable to perform a fiber-optic bronchoscopy, since it may help in obtaining a diagnosis (Vergnon and Froudarakis 1999). Pleural effusions of unknown origin after the initial work-up are associated with bronchogenic carcinoma in about 30 % of the cases (Vergnon and Froudarakis 1999; Poe et al. 1994). In addition, fiber-optic bronchoscopy is important in assessing the extent of the disease in the tracheobronchial tree, which may be important for the patient's treatment and prognosis (Vergnon and Froudarakis 1999).

9.7 Thoracoscopy in the Diagnosis of Malignant Pleural Effusion

Thoracoscopy is the "gold standard" in the diagnosis of pleural effusion, and it is indicated when less invasive tests have failed (Maskell and Butland 2003; Colt 1999; Mathur et al. 1995; Boutin and Astoul 1998). Thoracoscopy is a simple and safe method and should be the procedure of choice in the diagnosis of an exudative pleural effusion (Mathur et al. 1995; Boutin and Astoul 1998). This minimally invasive method can be performed by a pulmonologist under local anesthesia in the endoscopy suite, thus sparing the patient more invasive techniques such as video-assisted thoracic surgery (VATS) or open thoracotomy as performed by the thoracic surgeons under general anesthesia with selective ventilation in an operating theater (Mathur and Loddenkemper 1995). Before performing a thoracoscopy and to minimize complications, the performance status and expected benefit in terms of patient's overall survival should be considered. Other relative contraindications such as coagulation disorders, with or without anticoagulant therapy; thrombocytopenia; severe respiratory insufficiency with hypercapnea; and unstable cardiac status must also be ruled out and if possible corrected prior to undertaking the thoracoscopy (Froudarakis 2008; Rodriguez-Panadero et al. 2006).

The sensitivity of thoracoscopy ranges from 92 to 97 % (Boutin et al. 1981, 1993a), and its specificity is 99–100 % (Boutin et al. 1981, 1993 b; Roeslin et al. 1992) for patients with a malignant pleural effusion (Table 9.3). The diagnostic sensitivity of thoracoscopy does not alter according to the origin of the malignant pleural effusion: it is 96 % for lung carcinomas, 92 % for mesotheliomas, and 96 % for extrathoracic metastatic malignancies (Antony et al. 2001). Biopsies may be taken not only from the parietal, but also from the visceral and diaphragmatic pleuras, since during thoracoscopy the whole pleural cavity is inspected under direct vision (Boutin et al. 1981; Loddenkemper 1998). In addition, there is the possibility to perform lysis of adhesions which may have limited the access to the pleural cavity (Antony et al. 2001; Rodriguez-Panadero et al. 2006). It appears that the recently developed semirigid (or semiflexible, or flex-rigid) thoracoscope has the same diagnostic accuracy as the classical rigid one (Ernst et al. 2002; Lee 2007). However, problems exist as biopsies are usually of a smaller size than those done with the rigid scope, as it utilizes a flexible forceps (same as

Table 9.3 Diagnostic accuracy of thoracoscopy for malignant pleural effusion

Series	Patients (*n*)	Thoracoscopy (*n*)	Malignancy with thoracoscopy/total pleural malignancies (%)	True benign disease (*n*)	Idiopathic pleuritis (*n*)
De Camp et al (1973)	126	121	47/50 (94 %)	32	44
Canto et al (1977)	208	172	129/137 (94 %)	12	59
Weissberg et al (1980)	127	73	69/69 (100 %)	–	–
Boutin et al (1980)	233	195	131/150 (88 %)	25	40
Boutin et al (1981)	215	215	131/150 (87 %)	25	40
Page et al (1989)	121	107	90/91 (99 %)	15	15
Wu et al (1989)	152	152	71/74 (96 %)	63	15
Hucker et al (1991)	102	102	61/76 (80 %)	5	21
Menzie et al (1991)	102	91	42/44 (96 %)	31	22
Ohri et al 1992	56	56	37/38 (97 %)	11	7
Harris et al. (1995)	182	124	70/73 (96 %)	25	26
Colt (1995)	52	28	12/12 (100 %)	14	2
Hansen et al (1998)	147	147	91/103 (88 %)	11	33
Janssen et al (2004)	709	709	318/349 (91 %)	183	177
Ferrer et al (2005)	93	93	50/56 (89 %)	26	11
Sakuraba et al (2006)	138	138	37/39 (95 %)	40	58
Simpson (2007)	89	89	73/77 (94.5 %)	–	–
Fletcher et al (2007)	50	50	40/42 (95 %)	3	4
Lee et al (2007) (flex-rigid)	51	51	34/36 (94 %)	13	2

flexible bronchoscopy) (Lee and Colt 2005a). This is especially an issue in patients suspected of malignant mesothelioma, where large biopsies are needed for accurate histological subtyping (Froudarakis 2008). The role of thoracoscopy with autofluorescence in undiagnosed pleural effusions is still under investigation. Primary results showed a high sensitivity (100 %) but low specificity (75 %) for malignant pleural effusion due to false-positive fluorescence of nonspecific pleuritis (Chrysanthidis and Janssen 2005).

Macroscopically, the lesions seen during thoracoscopy may vary from polypoid tumors, masses, "candle wax drops" (Fig. 9.1), nodules, and/or pleural thickening – diffuse or localized, with associated islands of metastatic invasion from uninvolved pleura (Colt 1999; Mathur et al. 1995; Boutin and Astoul 1998; Rodriguez-Panadero et al. 2006). Also, nonspecific inflammation, localized or diffuse, may be observed, which has to be biopsied (Canto et al. 1983). Biopsies of the parietal pleura should be performed over a rib so as to avoid the neurovascular bundle. The closed forceps should be first used to probe the rib in order to feel the hard

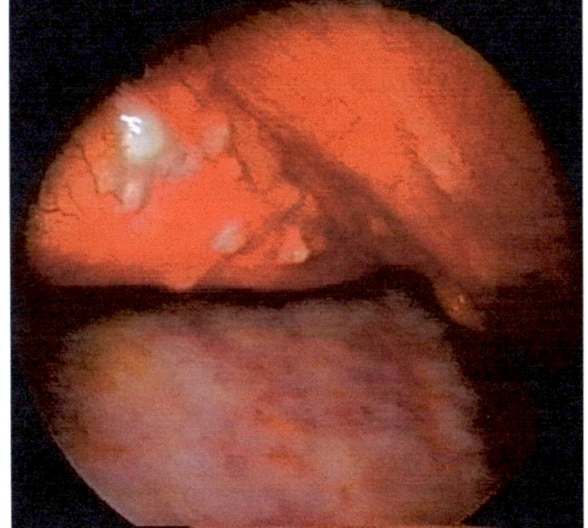

Fig. 9.1 Candle wax metastatic nodules on the pericardium of a 70-year-old patient with a pleural effusion from breast adenocarcinoma. Note the diffuse invasion of the parietal pleura

undersurface; this is followed by the grasping of the parietal pleura overlying it and removing the pleura with a long tearing motion ("peeling"), rather than a "grab and pull" (Lee and Colt 2007). Multiple biopsies have to be taken (>10)

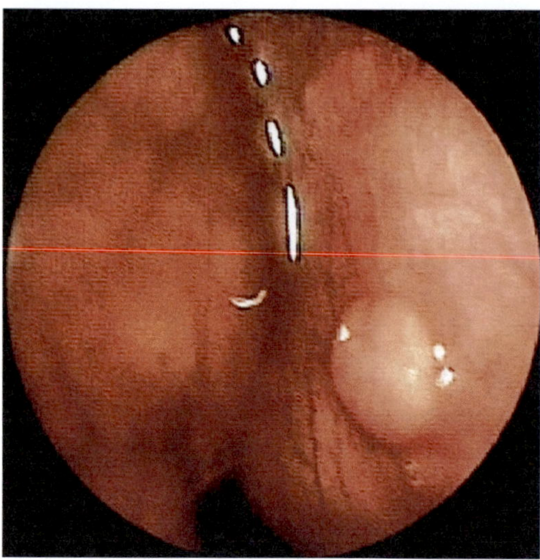

Fig. 9.2 Invasion of the parietal pleura from Hodgkin's lymphoma as discovered during thoracoscopy in a 39-year-old patient with a pleural effusion. In addition to the nodule, there is diffuse invasion of the parietal pleura as well as a mass within the mediastinum

of the abnormal areas as well as additional "bites" of the same area (deep biopsy) to obtain tissue of sufficient depth for accurate diagnosis (Rodriguez-Panadero et al. 2006; Lee and Colt 2007).

Survival of patients with malignant pleural effusion is very much related to the primary tumor, with ovarian tumors having the longest survival and lung tumors the shortest (Lee and Colt 2007; Froudarakis 2009). The biopsies taken must be of significant number and size in order to identify tumor invading the pleura and to perform additional investigations such as hormonal receptors in the case of breast carcinoma (Schwarz et al. 2004). Lymphoma is also difficult to diagnose by thoracentesis and closed biopsy, and thoracoscopy should be performed if this tumor is suspected, and initial investigations are negative (Alifano et al. 1997; Celikoglu et al. 1992). Lymphomatous pleural effusion usually results from impaired lymphatic drainage of the pleural space as well as from direct pleural involvement (Steiropoulos et al. 2009). Large and numerous biopsy specimens are necessary for immunohistochemistry/molecular techniques to identify and subclassify lymphomas (Fig. 9.2) (Celikoglu

et al. 1992; Alifano et al. 1997; Steiropoulos et al. 2009).

Some authors have attempted to identify features which would give a high pretest probability of malignancy. Martensson performed logistic analysis using seven variables (the patient's sex, age, smoking habits, asbestos exposure, size of effusion, pleural fluid color, and eosinophils) to discriminate malignant from nonmalignant disease in 334 patients with undiagnosed pleural effusion, in order to better select patients for diagnostic thoracoscopy (Martensson 1989). His predictions were correct in 79 % of the effusions; the strongest variable for malignancy was the presence of a bloody effusion. On the contrary, the variables with the strongest negative predictive value for malignancy were the presence of eosinophils (>30 %) in the pleural fluid as well as patient age younger than 50 years (Martensson 1989). Harris has published a series of 182 patients with undiagnosed pleural effusion who underwent thoracoscopy for diagnosis. He observed that a previous history of malignancy and an age older than 50 years were statistically significant as positive predictors for identifying malignancy by thoracoscopy. The combination of high pleural LDH, lymphocytosis, and hemorrhagic fluid was associated with intrapleural malignancy, and therefore, patients with those characteristics should undergo diagnostic thoracoscopy. In the same study, patient management was directly affected by thoracoscopy in 85 % of patients (Harris et al. 1995).

In undiagnosed pleural effusions in developed countries, thoracoscopy has an absolute indication since the patient has a significant likelihood of malignancy (Light 2006). Indeed, in developed countries, where the incidence of tuberculosis is low, more than 50 % of the cases of undiagnosed pleural effusion are due to carcinomas, the second most common diagnosis being tuberculosis (10 %) (Boutin et al. 1981; Kendall et al. 1992; Harris et al. 1995). Post thoracoscopy, less than 10 % of the cases, will have a diagnosis of nonspecific (idiopathic) pleuritis (Boutin et al. 1981; Harris et al. 1995). During the follow-up period of these patients, 4–8 % of patients will later present with a malignancy.

Most of the cases (about 80 %) follow a true benign course with spontaneous resolution, while few cases are "idiopathic" (Janssen et al. 2004; Venekamp et al. 2005).

Janssen and associates have followed their 208 patients with inconclusive thoracoscopy out of a total of 709 subjects who underwent thoracoscopy for investigation of an undiagnosed pleural effusion; 391 cases (55 %) had malignant pleural disease and 183 (26 %) a true benign pleural effusion. A final diagnosis of malignancy was achieved in 31 patients out of the 208 patients who underwent long-term follow-up (4.3 %) (Janssen et al. 2004). The overall mean interval between initial diagnostic thoracoscopy and the final diagnosis was 4.4 months (range 4 days–24 months). For mesothelioma, this mean interval was 8.7 months. Therefore, after long-term follow-up the sensitivity of diagnostic thoracoscopy was 91 % and the specificity 100 %. The positive predictive value was 100 %, the negative predictive value 92 %. False-negative results were associated with pleural adhesions and a fibrinous layer on the pleura. They suggested a wait-and-see approach, in such a patient population, unless repeated thoracocentesis suggests a progressive pleural process (Janssen et al. 2004). A recent study published by Venekamp and colleagues reported results from 60 evaluable patients with pleural effusion who remained undiagnosed after the initial thoracoscopy with a histological diagnosis of nonspecific pleuritis. The majority of those patients (92 %) followed a course of benign pleuritis, with only 8 % of the subjects proved to have a malignancy during a 3-year follow-up period. However, in some (25 %) of the patients with true benign evolution, no cause was identified and idiopathic pleuritis remained the final diagnosis (Venekamp et al. 2005).

These findings suggest that a histological diagnosis of nonspecific pleuritis does not necessarily mean a benign pleural process. Therefore, we can conclude that when nonspecific pleuritis is diagnosed histologically, after initial thoracoscopy for pleural effusion, a follow-up must be undertaken as a proportion of patients will manifest malignancy at a later date. If there are any doubts at any moment during this follow-up period, a repeat thoracoscopy or another more invasive procedure should be undertaken for diagnosis.

9.8 Thoracoscopy in Patients with Lung Cancer and Pleural Effusion

Lung cancer remains the most common fatal malignancy. Carcinoma of the lung is the most common cause of a malignant pleural effusion. The incidence of pleural effusion in patients with lung carcinoma ranges between 7 % (280 out of 4,000 cases) and 23 % (5,888 out of 25,464 cases) (Froudarakis 2009). Thoracoscopy is an important tool in the assessment of the extent of lung carcinoma within the pleural cavity (Canto et al. 1985; Roeslin and Kessler 1992; Rodriguez Panadero et al. 1995; Froudarakis 2009) (Fig. 9.3). If thoracocentesis is negative, thoracoscopy can be performed to further assess the cavity and to detect localized or diffuse pleural infiltration and in so doing determine – in cases of non-small-cell lung carcinoma (NSCLC) – the unresectable character of the tumor (M1a)

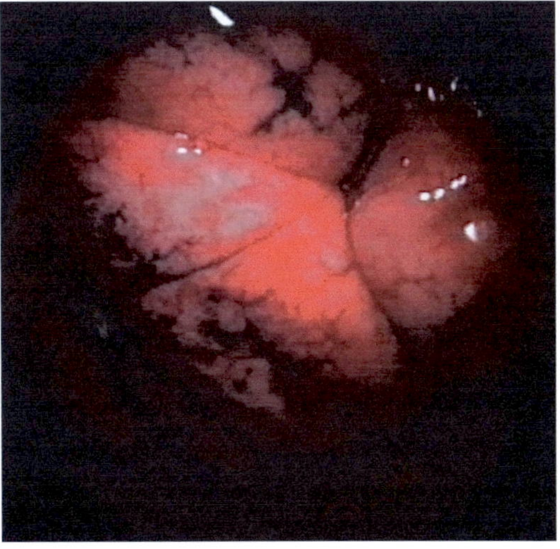

Fig. 9.3 A peripheral lung adenocarcinoma in a 46-year-old male, nonsmoker, presenting as an "undiagnosed" pleural effusion. Note the satellite nodule on the visceral pleura and the invasion of the parietal pleura

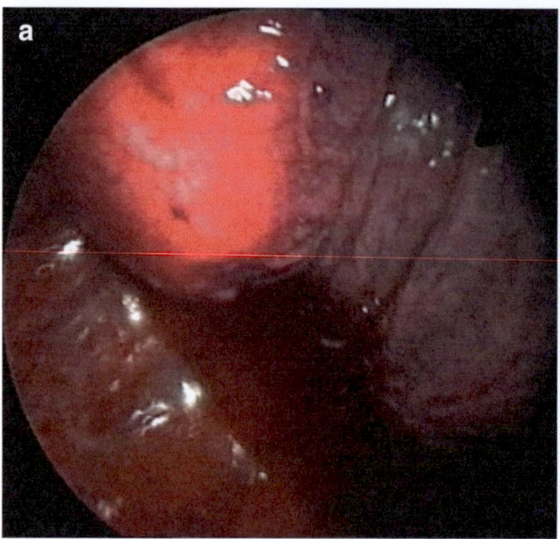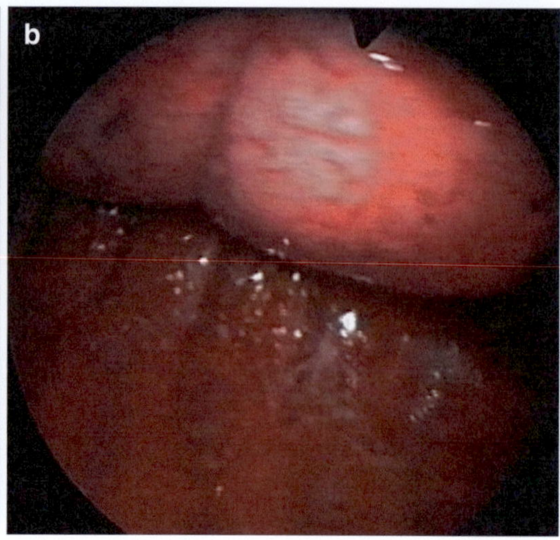

Fig. 9.4 (**a**) Segmental atelectasis of the left lower lobe caused by a central epidermoid carcinoma in a 65-year-old smoker male, presenting with a negative pleural effusion by cytology. (**b**) Paramalignant origin of the pleural effusion was confirmed by revealing extensive invasion of the parietal pleura, thus staging the patient as locally advanced NSCLC (T4 disease- IIIB) at that time. This is now defined as M1a, stage IV disease

(Fig. 9.4) (Rodriguez-Panadero et al. 1989; Colt 1995). Several series have been published in the last decades, showing the utility of thoracoscopy in staging NSCLC. Generally these series confirm the low rate of resectability, ranging from 0 to 36 %, and hence the poor prognosis, in patients with lung cancer and pleural effusion (Le Roux 1968; Rodriguez Panadero 1995). Many lung cancers, even in the setting of paramalignant pleural effusions, may be unresectable, due to the extent of the intrathoracic tumor. Limitations of thoracoscopy in recognizing the intrapleural extent of the disease exist, for example, localized disease may be missed and areas such as costo-diaphragmatic angles and/or mediastinal pleura may be difficult to explore (Colt 1995).

Patients with NSCLC and confirmed malignant pleural effusion are now classified as IV-M1a, unresectable disease, according to the Mountain revised classification (Mountain CF *AJCC TNM Staging*, 7th edition), although it was already known since 1974 that NSCLC patients with malignant pleural effusion represented a group of patients with a particularly poor prognosis (Carr and Mountain 1974; Mountain et al. 1974). Malignant pleural effusion was previously classified as IIIB-T4 disease; however, the poor prognosis associated with this manifestation is now accepted with a change in staging from T4 to M1a.

Sugiura and collaborators compared the survival of 197 patients with stage IIIB disease without pleural effusion, stage IIIB with pleural effusion, and stage IV disease as previously characterized by the 6th AJCC TNM classification. They found that the median survival of the three groups was 15.3, 7.5, and 5.5 months, respectively. Survival curves for stage IIIB patients with effusion were significantly worse than those for stage IIIB patients without effusion, but not significantly different from stage IV patients. In addition, they found no significant difference in survival whether pleural fluid cytology was positive or negative; or the effusion was negative but exudative and/or bloody; and clinically judged malignant. Recently, the IASLC Lung Cancer Staging Project has reviewed the T and M stage of 18198 NSCLC patients (Rami-Porta et al. 2007; Postmus et al. 2007). Patients with pleural dissemination and classified as T4 according to the previous Mountain classification were 471. Five-year and median survival for those patients was 2 % and 8 months, respectively, versus 14 % and 13 months for defined T4 disease other than due to pleural effusion ($p < 0.0001$). Based on these observations it is more appropriate to classify patients with malignant pleural effusion due to NSCLC as having M1a, stage IV rather than T4, and stage IIIB disease, since both prognosis and management for these patients are similar to that for other stage IV disease (Goldstraw et al. 2007; Groome et al. 2007).

In small-cell lung carcinoma (SCLC), disease-free and overall survival of patients with ipsilateral malignant pleural effusion appears to be worse than in patients with limited stage disease (LD) without pleural effusion, but better than those with extensive stage disease (ED) (Livingston et al. 1982; Shepherd et al. 1993; Perng et al. 2007). It has been suggested however that these patients should benefit from the same treatment as LD (Livingston et al. 1982).

Shepherd and colleagues have reviewed the data from the SCLC database. Information concerning the presence or absence of pleural effusion or other distant sites was available for 1,258 patients with otherwise defined LD disease (1,113 of whom were without pleural effusion, 145 with pleural effusion) and 4,500 patients with ED with other defined metastatic sites. Of the 145 cases of limited disease with pleural effusion, 81 were actually designated as ED without any other metastatic sites. These 81 were assumed to have LD with pleural effusion. Surgically managed cases were excluded. The survival of patients with LD with effusion (median survival 12 months) is intermediate between those of patients with LD without effusion (median survival 18 months) and patients with ED (median survival 7 months) ($p = 0.0001$) The result of cytological examination of the pleural effusion was available for only 68 patients in the database. The survival of patients with LD and effusion, whether cytologically negative (median survival 13 months) or positive (median survival 12 months), remained intermediate between those of patients with LD without effusion (median survival 18 months) and patients with ED (median survival 7 months) ($p = 0.0001$) (Shepherd et al. 2007).

Their analysis showed that patients who have pleural effusion without extrathoracic metastases (M1a) have a survival that is intermediate between that of stage I–III without effusion and stage IV. Perng et al. reported a similar observation in a series of patients treated in Taiwan. Therefore, they recommended that pleural effusion should be a stratification parameter in clinical trials for both LD and ED SCLC. Having even a small proportion of patients with pleural effusion in LD trials could affect outcome significantly if they are not well divided between studied groups. The authors did not make a clear statement concerning cytology-positive or negative effusions since they did not have enough patients in their analysis (Perng et al. 2007).

9.9 Thoracoscopy in Malignant Pleural Mesothelioma

Malignant pleural mesothelioma (MPM) is a neoplasm with an increasing incidence and poor prognosis, since median survival is 12 months, with death resulting from respiratory failure. In the United States MPM occurs in about 2,500 individuals every year, while 72,000 cases are expected to occur in the next 20 years. In Western Europe 5,000 patients die of the disease each year (Robinson and Lake 2005; Robinson et al. 2005). Malignant pleural mesothelioma is also the most difficult pleural malignancy to diagnose by cytology and closed biopsy (Ryan et al. 1981; Scherpereel 2007). Thoracoscopy is the method of choice to obtain the diagnosis of malignant pleural mesothelioma (MPM) when suspected on clinical or radiological grounds (Scherpereel et al. 2007). The diagnostic yield of thoracoscopy in MPM is >90 %. Boutin and Rey prospectively analyzed the records of 188 patients with malignant pleural mesothelioma in order to compare the diagnostic value of thoracoscopic biopsy, fluid cytology, and closed needle biopsy. They achieved a diagnosis by fluid cytology in 26 %, needle biopsy in 21 %, combined fluid cytology and needle biopsy in 39 %, and thoracoscopy in 98 %. Thoracoscopy reduces the need for thoracotomy as it provides equal quantity and quality pleural biopsies for diagnosis (Boutin and Rey 1993). In addition, fibrohyaline or calcified,

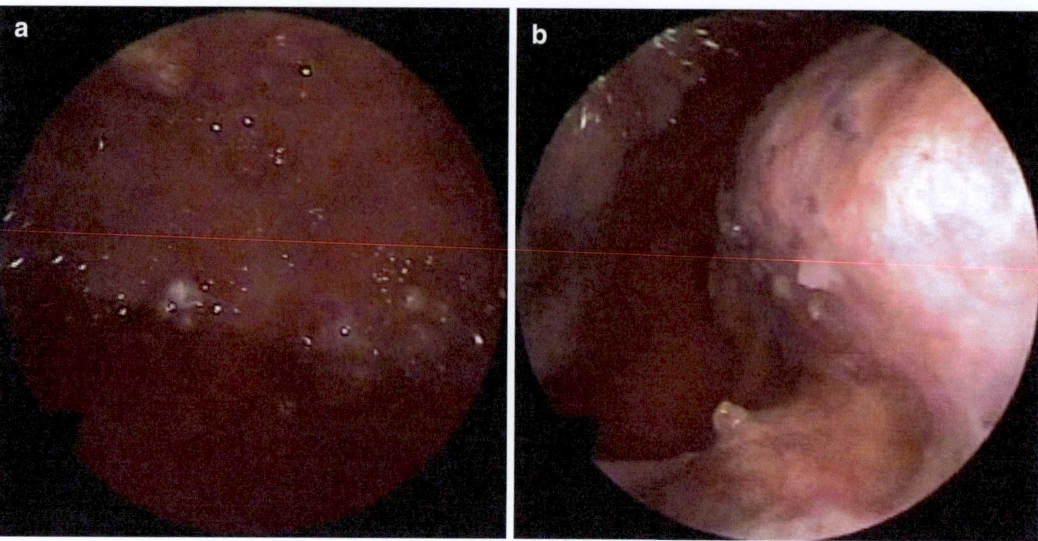

Fig. 9.5 (**a**) Multiple masses of the parietal pleura in a patient with pleural effusion secondary to mesothelioma. (**b**) Note the minimal involvement of the visceral pleura, comparing to the parietal pleura (**a**). In addition there is homogenous mesothelial thickening of the visceral pleura strangling the lung parenchyma (trapping)

thick, pearly white pleural plaques may be found, diagnosing benign asbestos pleural effusion (BAPE) and excluding mesothelioma or malignancies (Boutin and Astoul 1998). However, in case of macroscopically nonspecific pleural lesions, biopsies should be performed on the parietal pleura around the fibrohyaline plaques and in pleural zones marked by anthracosis (Boutin et al. 1996; Boutin and Astoul 1998).

The appearance of malignant mesotheliomas is that of a firm, grayish tumor coalescing on the visceral and parietal pleural surfaces into discrete plaques and nodules (Fig. 9.5a) (Boutin and Astoul 1998). The lung may be completely "strangled" by the tumor. Adjacent structures are involved at an advanced stage, with invasion of the chest wall, pericardium, diaphragm, and interlobar fissures. However, these endoscopic features depend on the stage of the disease. Lesions of MPM observed during thoracoscopy present macroscopically as nodules and masses associated with parietal pleural thickening (Boutin and Rey 1993). In some early stage patients, the presence of nonspecific lesions is noted. Pleural lymphangitis might also be present, especially in the posterior and inferior regions of the parietal pleura, where lymphatic

vessels are most numerous, and this may be associated with irregular thickening. An important diagnostic finding is involvement of the visceral pleura and lung (Boutin et al. 1993b). These structures can be easily visualized during thoracoscopy. The visceral pleura is always involved to a lesser degree than the parietal pleura, with the nodules less numerous and smaller (Fig. 9.5b). In many cases, the visceral pleura appears macroscopically normal, but routine biopsy should be performed to assess further (Astoul 1999).

An important point to consider in patients with MPM is that trocar introduction for thoracoscopy (Boutin et al. 1995) but also pleural thoracentesis, closed pleural biopsy, and thoracotomy (Agarwal et al. 2006) may induce tumor seeding in the thoracic wall (Fig. 9.6). The incidence of this complication is 5–22 % for percutaneous imaging-guided needle biopsy (Metintas et al. 1995; Agarwal et al. 2006) and 16–40 % for thoracoscopy (Boutin et al. 1995; Agarwal et al. 2006), while thoracotomy has an incidence of 24 % (Agarwal et al. 2006). These subcutaneous nodules are extremely painful, often impairing the patients' quality of life. To prevent track seeding in those patients, early local external radiation therapy of 21 Gys is proposed on the site of

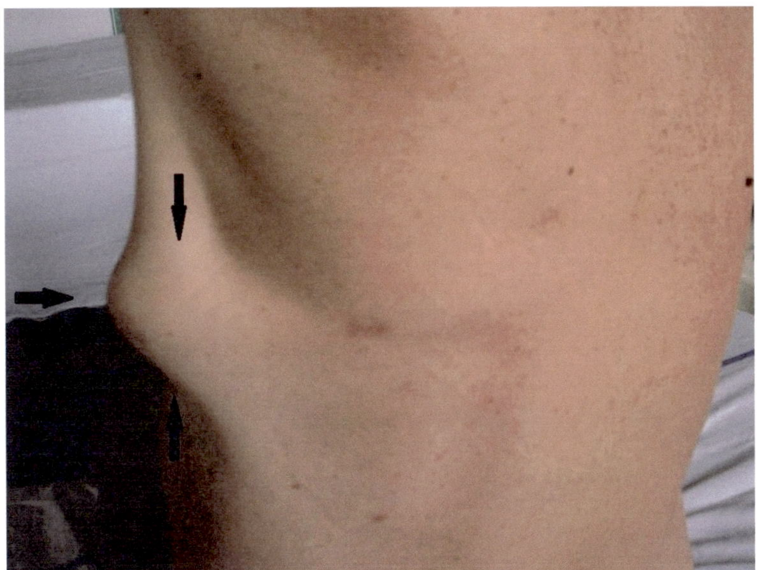

Fig. 9.6 A subcutaneous malignant nodule which has developed at the site of trocar insertion for a previous medical thoracoscopy in a patients with a malignant pleural mesothelioma *(Courtesy Ph Astoul, Marseille, France)*

the trocar introduction 10–15 days after thoracoscopy, with excellent results (Boutin et al. 1995).

Important prognostic factors in MPM are the histological type of the tumor with epithelial tumors having the better prognosis, sarcomatous the worst, and mixed tumors intermediate (Robinson and Lake 2005; Robinson et al. 2005). Thus the need for well-documented pleural histology of the MPM is mandatory (Scherpereel 2007). Most of the clinical trials measuring efficacy of different agents and survival of patients are based on biopsies taken transthoracically under thoracic imaging guidance (Vogelzang et al. 2003; van Meerbeeck et al. 2005). Closed biopsies from the pleural tumor may be diagnostic under the guidance of chest computed tomography or chest ultrasound (Adams et al. 2001; Herth 2004; Metintas et al. 1995; Rahman and Gleeson 2008). Both methods have comparable diagnostic yield in pleural mesothelioma, while their yield is poorer in extrathoracic pleural metastatic disease (Macha et al. 1993; Adams et al. 2001; Rahman and Gleeson 2008). Rates of complications such as pneumothorax or bleeding are rare (<10 %), and costs are lower for chest ultrasound comparing to CT (Adams et al. 2001; Herth 2004; Metintas et al. 1995; Rahman and Gleeson 2008). However, in MPM the situation is more complicated: different histological

mesothelioma subtypes may coexist in the same patient's pleura (van Gelder et al. 1991; Greillier et al. 2007b), and this significantly affects the prognosis even after extrapleural pneumonectomy for early stage disease (Boutin et al. 1993a, b; Greillier et al. 2007a).

Staging patients with mesothelioma, before inclusion in therapeutic trials, is based on imaging. Imaging may underestimate or miss mesothelioma tumor localized to the visceral, diaphragmatic, or mediastinal pleura, as well as pericardial and lymph node invasion (Webb 1989; Leung et al. 1990; Boutin et al. 1993b; McLoud 1998; Au and Thomas 2003; Wang et al. 2004). Thoracoscopy is therefore necessary in all patients with suspected mesothelioma for accurate histological diagnosis, staging, and prognosis as well as therapeutic management of the effusion (Boutin et al. 1993b; Tassi et al. 1997; Astoul 1999, 2005; Greillier et al. 2007b). All patients should undergo thoracoscopy before being included in therapeutic trials since response rates and survival depend very much on thoracoscopic parameters. Improvement in response rates and survival benefits as reported in clinical trials in patients with MPM should be interpreted with caution especially when only percutaneous biopsy confirmation and/or clinico-radiological staging of the disease was performed (Karpathiou et al. 2007).

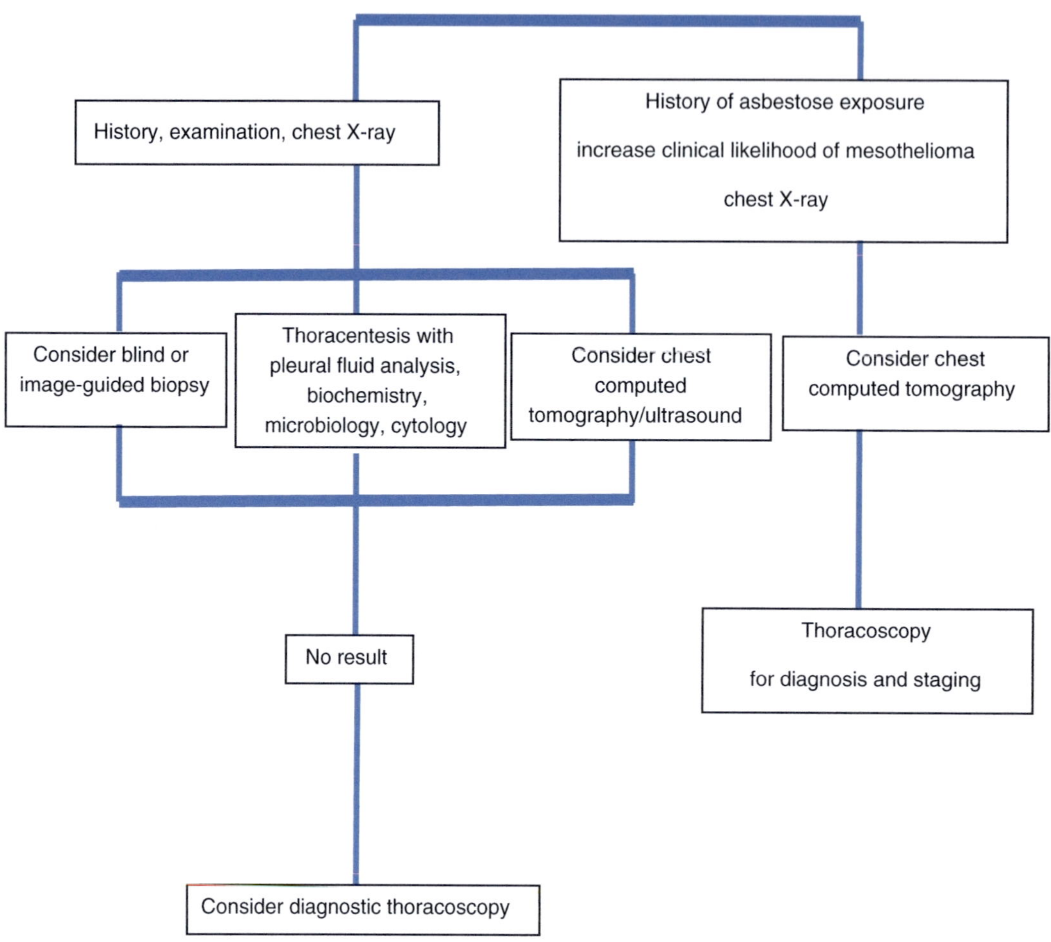

Table 9.4 Place of thoracoscopy in the work-up of a suspect malignant pleural effusion

Conclusion

Thoracoscopy in patients with undiagnosed pleural effusion is an important diagnostic tool, since noninvasive techniques have a low diagnostic yield (Table 9.4). More than 50 % of those patients will be diagnosed as having a malignancy if resident in countries with a low incidence of tuberculosis. Histological diagnosis of primary tumor in patients with pleural effusion and good performance status is important, since patients' treatment and prognosis relies on it. In addition, in patients with NSCLC and pleural effusion, thoracoscopy differentiates malignant from paramalignant etiologies which would result in totally different therapeutic approaches. Finally, in patients with mesothelioma, other than the prognostic importance associated with a precise histological type, the mapping of the intracavitary lesions of the tumor at thoracoscopy helps with the accurate staging of the patient and subsequent management.

References

Adams RF, Gray W, Davies RJ et al (2001) Percutaneous image-guided cutting needle biopsy of the pleura in the diagnosis of malignant mesothelioma. Chest 120:1798–1802

Aelony Y, King RR, Boutin C (1998) Thoracoscopic talc poudrage in malignant pleural effusions: effective pleurodesis despite low pleural pH. Chest 113:1007–1012

Agarwal PP, Seely JM, Matzinger FR et al (2006) Pleural mesothelioma: sensitivity and incidence of needle track seeding after image-guided biopsy versus surgical biopsy. Radiology 241:589–594

Alatas F, Alatas O, Metintas M et al (2001) Diagnostic value of CEA, CA 15-3, CA 19-9, CYFRA 21-1, NSE and TSA assay in pleural effusions. Lung Cancer 31:9–16

Alexandrakis MG, Coulocheri SA, Bouros D et al (2000) Evaluation of inflammatory cytokines in malignant and benign pleural effusions. Oncol Rep 7:1327–1332

Alifano M, Guggino G, Gentile M et al (1997) Management of concurrent pleural effusion in patients with lymphoma: thoracoscopy a useful tool in diagnosis and treatment. Monaldi Arch Chest Dis 52:330–334

Antony VB, Loddenkemper R, Astoul P et al (2001) Management of malignant pleural effusions. Eur Respir J 18:402–419

Antunes G, Neville E (2000) Management of malignant pleural effusions. Thorax 55:981–983

Armstrong P, Reznek RH, Phillips RR (1995) Diagnostic imaging of lung cancer. Eur Respir Mon 1:137–187

Astoul P (1999) Pleural mesothelioma. Curr Opin Pulm Med 5:259–268

Astoul P (2005) Diagnostic clinique et endoscopique du mésothéliome pleural. In: Astoul P (ed) Mésothéliome pleural. Elsevier, Paris, pp 77–88

Au VW, Thomas M (2003) Radiological manifestations of malignant pleural mesothelioma. Australas Radiol 47:111–116

Berger HW, Maher G (1971) Decreased glucose concentration in malignant pleural effusions. Am Rev Respir Dis 103:427–429

Boutin C, Cargnino P, Viallat JR (1980) Thoracoscopy in the early diagnosis of malignant pleural effusions. Endoscopy 12:155–160

Boutin C, Astoul P (1998) Diagnostic thoracoscopy. Clin Chest Med 19:295–309

Boutin C, Rey F (1993) Thoracoscopy in pleural malignant mesothelioma: a prospective study of 188 consecutive patients. Part 1: diagnosis. Cancer 72:389–393

Boutin C, Viallat JR, Cargnino P et al (1981) Thoracoscopy in malignant pleural effusions. Am Rev Respir Dis 124:588–592

Boutin C, Loddenkemper R, Astoul P (1993a) Diagnostic and therapeutic thoracoscopy: techniques and indications in pulmonary medicine. Tuber Lung Dis 74:225–239

Boutin C, Rey F, Gouvernet J et al (1993b) Thoracoscopy in pleural malignant mesothelioma: a prospective study of 188 consecutive patients. Part 2: prognosis and staging. Cancer 72:394–404

Boutin C, Rey F, Viallat JR (1995) Prevention of malignant seeding after invasive diagnostic procedures in patients with pleural mesothelioma. A randomized trial of local radiotherapy. Chest 108:754–758

Boutin C, Dumortier P, Rey F et al (1996) Black spots concentrate oncogenic asbestos fibers in the parietal pleura. Thoracoscopic and mineralogic study. Am J Respir Crit Care Med 153:444–449

Cantó A, Blasco E, Casillas M et al (1977) Thoracoscopy in the diagnosis of pleural effusion. Thorax 32:550–554

Canto A, Rivas J, Saumench J et al (1983) Points to consider when choosing a biopsy method in cases of pleurisy of unknown origin. Chest 84:176–179

Canto A, Ferrer G, Romagosa V et al (1985) Lung cancer and pleural effusion. Clinical significance and study of pleural metastatic locations. Chest 87:649–652

Carr DT, Mountain CF (1974) The staging of lung cancer. Semin Oncol 1:229–234

Cascinu S, Del Ferro E, Barbanti I et al (1997) Tumor markers in the diagnosis of malignant serous effusions. Am J Clin Oncol 20:247–250

Celikoglu F, Teirstein AS, Krellenstein DJ et al (1992) Pleural effusion in non-Hodgkin's lymphoma. Chest 101:1357–1360

Chavalittamrong B, Angsusingha K, Tuchinda M et al (1979) Diagnostic significance of pH, lactic acid dehydrogenase, lactate and glucose in pleural fluid. Respiration 38:112–120

Chernow B, Sahn SA (1977) Carcinomatous involvement of the pleura: an analysis of 96 patients. Am J Med 63: 695–702

Chrysanthidis MG, Janssen JP (2005) Autofluorescence videothoracoscopy in exudative pleural effusions: preliminary results. Eur Respir J 26:989–992

Cohen MH (1974) Signs and symptoms of bronchogenic carcinoma. Semin Oncol 1:183–189

Colt HG (1995) Thoracoscopic management of malignant pleural effusions. Clin Chest Med 16:505–518

Colt HG (1999) Thoracoscopy: window to the pleural space. Chest 116:1409–1415

De Camp PT, Moseley PW, Scott ML et al (1973) Diagnostic thoracoscopy. Ann Thorac Surg 16:79–84

Domagala W, Emeson E, Kass LG (1978) Distribution of T-lymphocytes and B-lymphocytes in peripheral blood and effusions in patients with cancer. J Natl Cancer Inst 61:295–301

Duysinx B, Nguyen D, Louis R et al (2004) Evaluation of pleural disease with 18-fluorodeoxyglucose positron emission tomography imaging. Chest 125: 489–493

Erasmus JJ, McAdams HP, Rossi SE (2000) FDG PET of pleural effusions in patients with non-small cell lung cancer. AJR Am J Roentgenol 175:245–249

Ernst A, Hersh CP, Herth F et al (2002) A novel instrument for the evaluation of the pleural space: an experience in 34 patients. Chest 122:1530–1534

Falcone F, Marinelli M, Minguzzi L et al (1996) Tumor markers and lung cancer: guidelines in a cost-limited medical organization. Int J Biol Markers 11:61–66

Ferrer J, Roldán J, Teixidor J et al (2005) Predictors of pleural malignancy in patients with pleural effusion undergoing thoracoscopy. Chest 127:1017–1022

Fletcher SV, Clark RJ (2007) The Portsmouth thoracoscopy experience, an evaluation of service by retrospective case note analysis. Respir Med 101:1021–1025

Froudarakis ME (2008) Diagnostic work-up of pleural effusions. Respiration 75:4–13

Froudarakis ME (2009) Diagnosis and management of pleural effusion in lung cancer. In: Bouros D (ed) Pleural diseases. Marcel Dekker, New York

Glazer HS, Duncan-Meyer J, Aronberg DJ et al (1985) Pleural and chest wall invasion in bronchogenic carcinoma: CT evaluation. Radiology 157:191–194

Glazer HS, Kaiser LR, Anderson DJ et al (1989) Indeterminate mediastinal invasion in bronchogenic carcinoma: CT evaluation. Radiology 173:37–42

Goldstraw P, Crowley J, Chansky K et al (2007) The IASLC Lung Cancer Staging Project: proposals for the revision of the TNM stage groupings in the forthcoming (seventh) edition of the TNM Classification of malignant tumours. J Thorac Oncol 2:706–714

Good JT Jr, Taryle DA, Sahn SA (1985) The pathogenesis of low glucose, low pH malignant effusions. Am Rev Respir Dis 131:737–741

Greillier L, Cavailles A, Fraticelli A et al (2007a) Accuracy of pleural biopsy using thoracoscopy for the diagnosis of histologic subtype in patients with malignant pleural mesothelioma. Cancer 110:2248–2252

Greillier L, Scherpereel A, Astoul P (2007b) Pleural mesothelioma: impact of the staging for the therapeutic strategy. Rev Mal Respir 24:6S146–6S156

Groome PA, Bolejack V, Crowley J et al (2007) The IASLC Lung Cancer Staging Project: validation of the proposals for the revision of the TNM stage groupings in the forthcoming (seventh) edition of the TNM Classification of malignant tumours. J Thorac Oncol 2:694–705

Hansen M, Faurschou P, Clementsen P (1998) Medical thoracoscopy, results and complications in 146 patients: a retrospective study. Respir Med 92:228–232

Harris RJ, Kavuru MS, Rice TW et al (1995) The diagnostic and therapeutic utility of thoracoscopy: a review. Chest 108:828–841

Heffner JE (1998) Evaluating diagnostic tests in the pleural space. Clin Chest Med 19:277–293

Henschke CI, Davis SD, Romano PM et al (1989) Pleural effusions: pathogenesis, radiologic evaluation and therapy. J Thorac Imaging 4:49–60

Herth F (2004) Diagnosis and staging of mesothelioma transthoracic ultrasound. Lung Cancer 45(Suppl 1):S63–S67

Hoyert DL, Heron MP, Murphy SL et al (2006) Deaths: final data for 2003. Natl Vital Stat Rep 54:1–120

Hucker J, Bhatnagar NK, al-Jilaihawi AN (1991) Thoracoscopy in the diagnosis and management of recurrent pleural effusions. Ann Thorac Surg 52:1145–1147

Hurewitz AN, Zucker S, Mancuso P et al (1992) Human pleural effusions are rich in matrix metalloproteinases. Chest 102:1808–1814

Hyde L, Hyde CI (1974) Clinical manifestations of lung cancer. Chest 65:299–306

Janssen JP, Ramlal S, Mravunac M (2004) The long term follow-up of exudative pleural effusion after non-diagnostic thoracoscopy. J Bronchol 11:169–174

Jimenez D, Perez-Rodriguez E, Diaz G et al (2002) Determining the optimal number of specimens to obtain with needle biopsy of the pleura. Respir Med 96:14–17

Johnston WW (1985) The malignant pleural effusion: a review of cytopathologic diagnosis of 584 specimens from 472 consecutive patients. Cancer 56:905–909

Kabnick EM, Sobo S, Steinbaum S et al (1982) Spontaneous pneumothorax from bronchogenic carcinoma. J Natl Med Assoc 74:478–479

Karpathiou G, Argiana E, Koutsopoulos A et al (2007) Response of a patient with pleural and peritoneal mesothelioma after second-line chemotherapy with lipoplatin and gemcitabine. Oncology 73:426–429

Kendall SW, Bryan AJ, Large SR et al (1992) Pleural effusions: is thoracoscopy a reliable investigation? A retrospective review. Respir Med 86:437–440

Kuhn M, Fitting JW, Leuenberger P (1989) Probability of malignancy in pleural fluid eosinophilia. Chest 96:992–994

Kwek BH, Aquino SL, Fischman AJ (2004) Fluorodeoxyglucose positron emission tomography and CT after talc pleurodesis. Chest 125:2356–2360

Le Roux BT (1968) Bronchial carcinoma. E&S Livingstone, London

Lee P, Colt HG (2005a) Flex-rigid pleuroscopy step-by-step. CMPMedica, Singapore

Lee P, Colt HG (2005b) Rigid and semirigid pleuroscopy: the future is bright. Respirology 10:418–425

Lee P, Colt HG (2007) State of the Art: pleuroscopy. J Thorac Oncol 2:663–670

Lee P, Hsu A, Lo C et al (2007) Prospective evaluation of flex-rigid pleuroscopy for indeterminate pleural effusion: accuracy, safety and outcome. Respirology 12:881–886

Leff A, Hopewell PC, Costello J (1978) Pleural effusion from malignancy. Ann Intern Med 88:532–537

Leung AN, Müller NL, Miller RR (1990) CT in differential diagnosis of diffuse pleura disease. AJR Am J Roentgenol 154:487–492

Light RW (1995) Approach to the patient. In: Light RW (ed) Pleural disease, 3rd edn. Williams & Wilkinson, Baltimore, pp 75–82

Light RW (2006) The undiagnosed pleural effusion. Clin Chest Med 27:309–319

Light RW, Macgregor MI, Luchsinger PC et al (1972) Pleural effusions: the diagnostic separation of transudates and exudates. Ann Intern Med 77:507–513

Light RW, Erozan YS, Ball WC (1973a) Cells in pleural fluid. Their value in differential diagnosis. Arch Intern Med 132:854–860

Light RW, MacGregor MI, Ball WC Jr et al (1973b) Diagnostic significance of pleural fluid pH and PCO2. Chest 64:591–596

Lipscomb DJ, Flower CD, Hadfield JW (1981) Ultrasound of the pleural: an assessment of its clinical value. Clin Radiol 32:289–290

Livingston RB, McCracken JD, Trauth CJ et al (1982) Isolated pleural effusion in small cell lung carcinoma: favorable prognosis. A review of the Southwest Oncology Group experience. Chest 81:208–211

Loddenkemper R (1998) Thoracoscopy: state of the art. Eur Respir J 11:213–221

Loddenkemper R, Mai J, Scheffler N et al (1978) Prospective individual comparison of blind needle biopsy and of thoracoscopy in the diagnosis and differential diagnosis of tuberculous pleurisy. Scand J Respir Dis Suppl 102:196–198

Macha HN, Reichle G, von Zwehl D et al (1993) The role of ultrasound assisted thoracoscopy in the diagnosis of pleural disease. Clinical experience in 687 cases. Eur J Cardiothorac Surg 7:19–22

Marel M, Stastny B, Melinova L et al (1995) Diagnosis of pleural effusions. Experience with clinical studies, 1986 to 1990. Chest 107:1598–1603

Martensson G (1989) Prediction of the diagnostic utility of thoracoscopy in pleural effusion. Pneumologie 43:72–75

Maskell NA, Butland RJA (2003) BTS guidelines for the investigation of a unilateral pleural effusion in adults. Thorax 58(Suppl II):ii8–ii17

Mathur PN, Loddenkemper R (1995) Medical thoracoscopy. Role in pleural and lung diseases. Clin Chest Med 16:487–496

Mathur PN, Astoul P, Boutin C (1995) Medical thoracoscopy: technical details. Clin Chest Med 16:479–486

McLoud TC (1998) CT and MRI in pleural space. Clin Chest Med 19:261–276

Menard O, Dousset B, Jacob C et al (1993) Improvement of the diagnosis of the cause of pleural effusion in patients with lung cancer by simultaneous quantification of carcinoembryonic antigen (CEA) and neuron-specific enolase (NSE) pleural levels. Eur J Cancer 13:1806–1809

Metintas M, Ozdemir N, Isiksoy S et al (1995) CT-guided pleural needle biopsy in the diagnosis of malignant mesothelioma. J Comput Assist Tomogr 19:370–374

Meyer PC (1966) Metastatic carcinoma of the pleura. Thorax 21:437–443

Mountain CF (1997) Revisions for the international system for staging lung cancer. Chest 111:1710–1717

Mountain CF, Carr DT, Anderson WA (1974) A system for the clinical staging of lung cancer. Am J Roentgenol Radium Ther Nucl Med 120:130–138

Ohri SK, Oswal SK, Townsend ER (1992) Early and late outcome after diagnostic thoracoscopy and talc pleurodesis. Ann Thorac Surg 53:1038–1041

O'Moore PV, Mueller PR, Simeone JF et al (2004) Sonographic guidance in diagnostic and therapeutic interventions in the pleural space. AJR Am J Roentgenol 149:1–5

Page RD, Jeffrey RR, Donnelly RJ (1989) Thoracoscopy: a review of 121 consecutive surgical procedures. Ann Thorac Surg 48:66–68

Pearlberg JL, Sandler MA, Beute GH (1987) Limitations of CT in evaluation of neoplasms involving chest wall. J Comput Assist Tomogr 11:290–293

Perng RP, Chen CY, Chang GC et al (2007) Revisit of 1997 TNM staging system–survival analysis of 1112 lung cancer patients in Taiwan. Jpn J Clin Oncol 37:9–15

Poe RH, Levy PC, Israel RH et al (1994) Use of fiberoptic bronchoscopy in the diagnosis of bronchogenic carcinoma. A study in patients with idiopathic pleural effusions. Chest 105:1663–1667

Postmus PE, Brambilla E, Chansky K et al (2007) The IASLC Lung Cancer Staging Project: proposals for the

revision of the M descriptors in the forthcoming (seventh) edition of the TNM classification of lung cancer. J Thorac Oncol 2:686–693

Prakash UB, Reiman HM (1985) Comparison of needle biopsy with cytologic analysis for the evaluation of pleural effusion: analysis of 414 cases. Mayo Clin Proc 60:158–164

Rahman NM, Gleeson FV (2008) Image-guided pleural biopsy. Curr Opin Pulm Med 14:331–336

Rami-Porta R, Ball D, Crowley J et al (2007) The IASLC Lung Cancer Staging Project: proposals for the revision of the T descriptors in the forthcoming (seventh) edition of the TNM classification for lung cancer. J Thorac Oncol 2:593–602

Rato GB, Piacenza G, Frola C et al (1991) Chest wall involvement by lung cancer: computed tomography detection and results of operation. Ann Thorac Surg 51:182–188

Robinson BW, Lake RA (2005) Advances in malignant mesothelioma. N Engl J Med 353:1591–1603

Robinson BWS, Musk AW, Lake RA (2005) Malignant mesothelioma. Lancet 366:397–408

Rodriguez Panadero F (1995) Lung cancer and ipsilateral pleural effusion. Ann Oncol 6:S25–S27

Rodriguez-Panadero F, Antony VB (1997) Pleurodesis: state of the art. Eur Respir J 10:1648–1654

Rodriguez-Panadero F, Lopez Mejias J (1989) Low glucose and pH levels in malignant pleural effusions. Diagnostic significance and prognostic value in respect to pleurodesis. Am Rev Respir Dis 139: 663–667

Rodriguez-Panadero F, Borderas Naranjo F, Lopez Mejias J et al (1989) Pleural metastatic tumours and effusions. Frequency and pathogenic mechanisms in a post-mortem series. Eur Respir J 2:366–369

Rodriguez-Panadero F, Janssen JP, Astoul P (2006) Thoracoscopy: general overview and place in the diagnosis and management of pleural effusion. Eur Respir J 28:409–421

Roeslin N, Kessler R (1992) Quelle est la place de la thoracoscopie dans le bilan d'extension pré-opératoire du cancer bronchique non à petites cellules? Rev Mal Respir 9:R247–R251

Romney BM, Austin JH (1990) Plain film evaluation of carcinoma of the lung. Seminars in roentgenology 5:45–63

Rubins JB, Rubins HB (1996) Etiology and prognostic significance of eosinophilic pleural effusions. A prospective study. Chest 110:1271–1274

Ryan CJ, Rodgers RF, Unni KK et al (1981) The outcome of patients with pleural effusion of indeterminate cause at thoracotomy. Mayo Clin Proc 56:145–149

Sahn SA (1982) Pleural effusion in lung cancer. Clin Chest Med 3:443–452

Sahn SA (1998) Malignancy metastatic to the pleura. Clin Chest Med 19:351–361

Sakuraba M, Masuda K, Hebisawa A et al (2006) Diagnostic value of thoracoscopic pleural biopsy for pleurisy under local anaesthesia. ANZ J Surg 76: 722–724

Salyer WA, Eggleston JC, Erozan YS (1975) Efficacy of pleural needle biopsy and pleural fluid cytopathology in the diagnosis of malignant neoplasm involving the pleura. Chest 67:536–538

Sanchez-Armengol A, Rodriguez-Panadero F (1993) Survival and talc pleurodesis in metastatic pleural carcinoma, revisited. Report of 125 cases. Chest 104: 1482–1485

Scagliotti GV (1995) Symptoms and signs and staging of lung cancer. Eur Respir Mon 1:91–136

Schaffler GJ, Wolf G, Schoellnast H et al (2004) Non-small cell lung cancer: evaluation of pleural abnormalities on CT scans with 18F FDG PET. Radiology 231:858–865

Scherpereel A (2007) Guidelines of the French Speaking Society for Chest Medicine for management of malignant pleural mesothelioma. Respir Med 101:1265–1276

Schwarz C, Lubbert H, Rahn W et al (2004) Medical thoracoscopy: hormone receptor content in pleural metastases due to breast cancer. Eur Respir J 24:728–730

Shepherd FA, Ginsberg RJ, Haddad R et al (1993) Importance of clinical staging in limited small-cell lung cancer: a valuable system to separate prognostic subgroups. The University of Toronto Lung Oncology Group. J Clin Oncol 11:1592–1597

Shepherd FA, Crowley J, Van Houtte P et al (2007) The IASLC Lung Cancer Staging Project: proposals regarding the clinical staging of small cell lung cancer in the forthcoming (seventh) edition of the TNM Classification for lung cancer. J Thorac Oncol 2:1067–1077

Simpson G (2007) Medical thoracoscopy in an Australian regional hospital. Intern Med J 37:267–269

Steinhausling CA, Cuttat JF (1985) Spontaneous pneumothorax a complication of lung cancer? Chest 88: 709–713

Steiropoulos P, Kouliatsis G, Karpathiou G et al (2009) Rare cases of primary pleural Hodgkin and non-Hodgkin lymphomas. Respiration 77:459–463

Stoetzer OJ, Munker R, Darsow M et al (1999) P53-immunoreactive cells in benign and malignant effusions: diagnostic value using a panel of monoclonal antibodies and comparison with CEA- staining. Oncol Rep 6:455–458

Storey DD, Dines DE, Coles DT (1976) Pleural effusion: a diagnostic dilemma. JAMA 236:2183–2186

Tassi GF, Marchetti GP, Fattibene F et al (1997) Thoracoscopy in pleural malignant mesothelioma diagnosis. Diagn Ther Endosc 3:147–151

Templeton PA, Caskey CI, Zerhouni EA (1990) Current uses of CT and MR imaging in the staging of lung cancer. Radiol Clin North Am 28:631–646

Valdes L, Alvarez D, Valle JM et al (1996) The etiology of pleural effusions in an area with high incidence of tuberculosis. Chest 109:158–162

Van Gelder T, Hoogsteden HC, Vandenbroucke JP (1991) The influence of the diagnostic technique on the histopathological diagnosis in malignant mesothelioma. Virchows Arch A Pathol Anat Histopathol 418: 315–317

Van Meerbeeck JP, Gaafar R, Manegold C et al (2005) Randomized phase III study of cisplatin with or without raltitrexed in patients with malignant pleural mesothelioma: an intergroup study of the European Organisation for Research and Treatment of Cancer Lung Cancer Group and the National Cancer Institute of Canada. J Clin Oncol 23:6881–6889

Venekamp LN, Velkeniers B, Noppen M (2005) Does 'Idiopathic Pleuritis' exist? Natural history of non-specific pleuritis diagnosed after thoracoscopy. Respiration 72:74–78

Vergnon JM, Froudarakis M (1999) Bronchoscopy. In: Grassi C (ed) Pulmonary diseases. McGraw-Hill International, London, pp 39–43

Vogelzang NJ, Rusthoven JJ, Symanowski J et al (2003) Phase III study of pemetrexed in combination with cisplatin versus cisplatin alone in patients with malignant pleural mesothelioma. J Clin Oncol 21: 2636–2644

Walshe AD, Douglas JG, Kerr KM et al (1992) An audit of the clinical investigation of pleural effusion. Thorax 47:734–737

Wang ZJ, Reddy GP, Gotway MB et al (2004) Malignant pleural mesothelioma: evaluation with CT, MR imaging, and PET. Radiographics 24:105–119

Webb WR (1989) The role of magnetic resonance imaging in the assessment of patients with lung cancer. A comparison with computed tomography. J Thorac Imaging 4:65–75

Weissberg D, Kaufmann M (1980) Diagnostic and therapeutic pleuroscopy. Experience with 127 patients. Chest 78:732–735

White CS, Templeton PA, Belani CP (1993) Imaging in lung cancer. Semin Oncol 20:142–152

Woodring JH (1990) Unusual radiographic manifestations of lung cancer. Radiol Clin North Am 28: 599–618

Wu MH, Hsiue RH, Tseng KH (1989) Thoracoscopy in the diagnosis of pleural effusions. Jpn J Clin Oncol 19:116–119

Yang PC, Luh KT, Chang DB et al (1992) Value of sonography in determining the nature of pleural effusion: analysis of 320 cases. AJR Am J Roentgenol 159:29–33

Philippe Astoul

- Metastatic pleural malignancies
- Malignant pleural mesothelioma

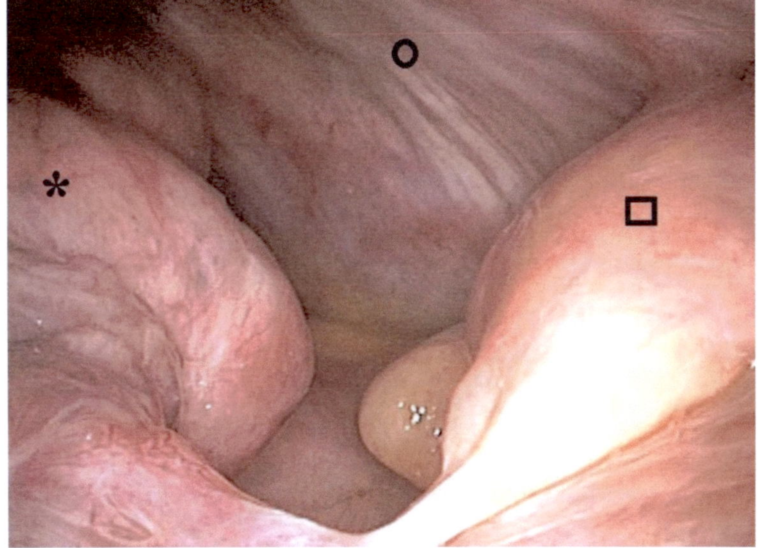

Fig. 10.1 Trapped lung (left lower lobe in this case – *star*) is not a contraindication to medical thoracoscopy in case with high clinical suspicion of neoplastic disease. In this case, a diagnosis of pleural adenocarcinoma was obtained after multiple biopsies of the posterior parietal pleura which had demonstrated non-specific white lymphangitis (O). Pleural fat is visible on the diaphragm (□)

P. Astoul
Division of Thoracic Oncology, Pleural Diseases, and Interventional Pulmonology, Hôpital NORD, Marseille, France
e-mail: pastoul@ap-hm.fr

P. Astoul et al. (eds.), *Thoracoscopy for Pulmonologists*,
DOI 10.1007/978-3-642-38351-9_10, © Springer-Verlag Berlin Heidelberg 2014

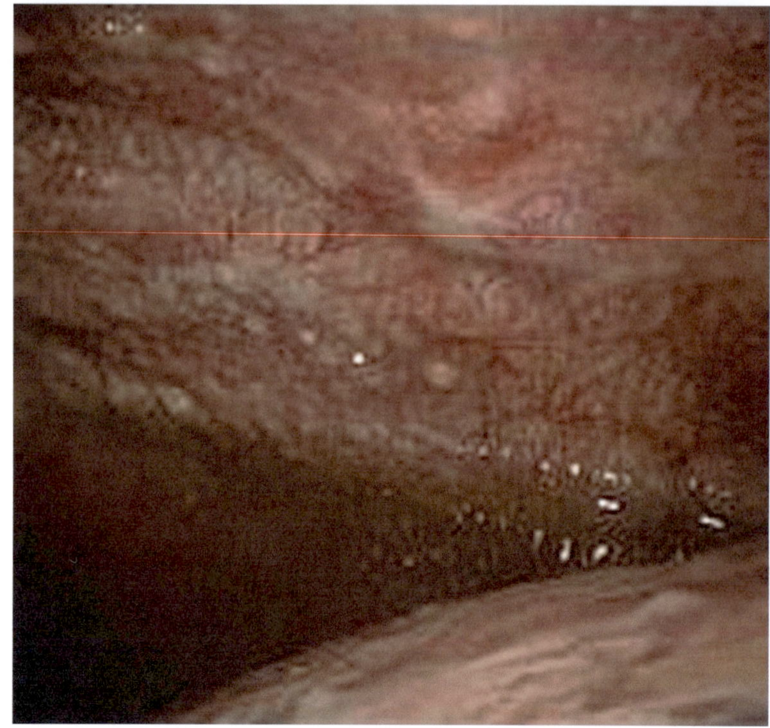

Fig. 10.2 Left side. Typical features of metastatic pleural effusion. Nodules are clearly visible on the posterior parietal pleura with hypertrophic lymphatic vessels (*white bundles*). The diaphragm is also invaded with nodules on the surface. After removal of the fluid, the costodiaphragmatic gutter will be carefully examined

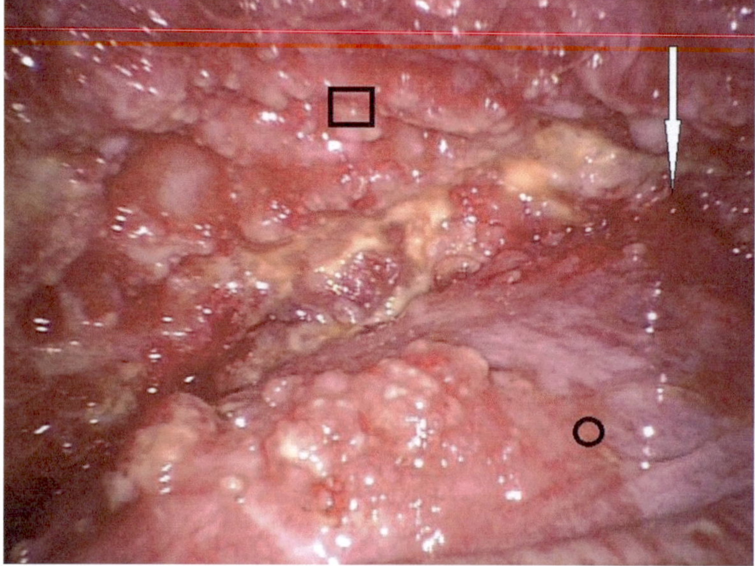

Fig. 10.3 Advanced malignant pleural effusion from a cancer of unknown origin. Disseminated pleural carcinomatosis is seen invading the posterior parietal pleura (□) and the lung (○)

Fig. 10.4 Metastatic pleural cancer. The view of the upper part of the right pleural cavity. Huge nodules and neoplastic lymphangitis are visible on the parietal pleura (O). Nodules are also present on the surface of the lung (*star*)

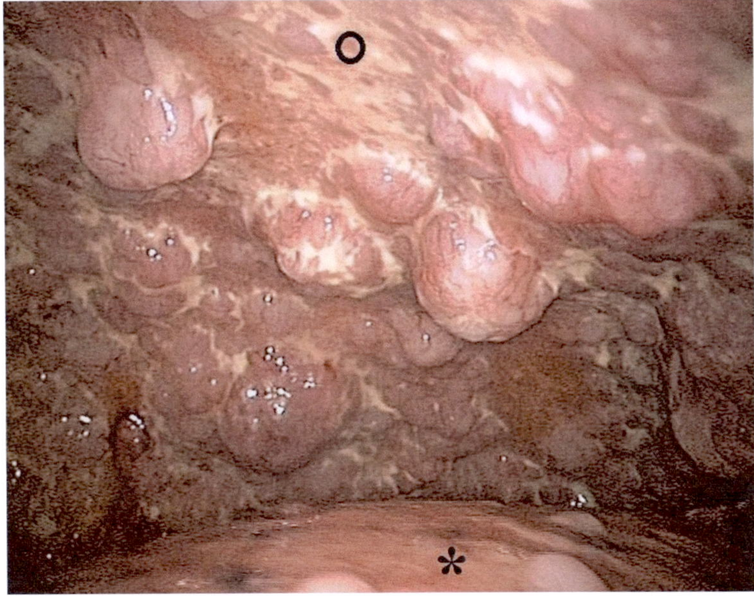

Fig. 10.5 Metastatic pleural cancer (same patient). Posterior parietal pleura (*star*). Upper lobe (O). Lower lobe (□). Fissure (*white arrow*)

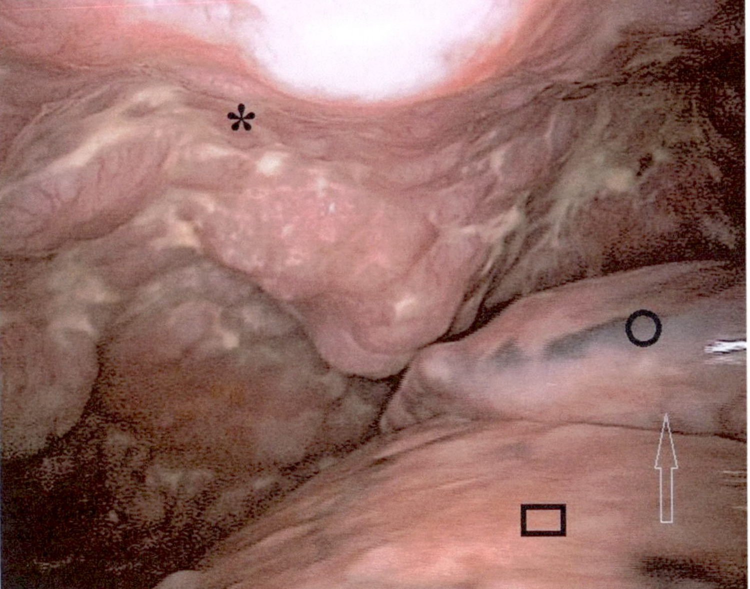

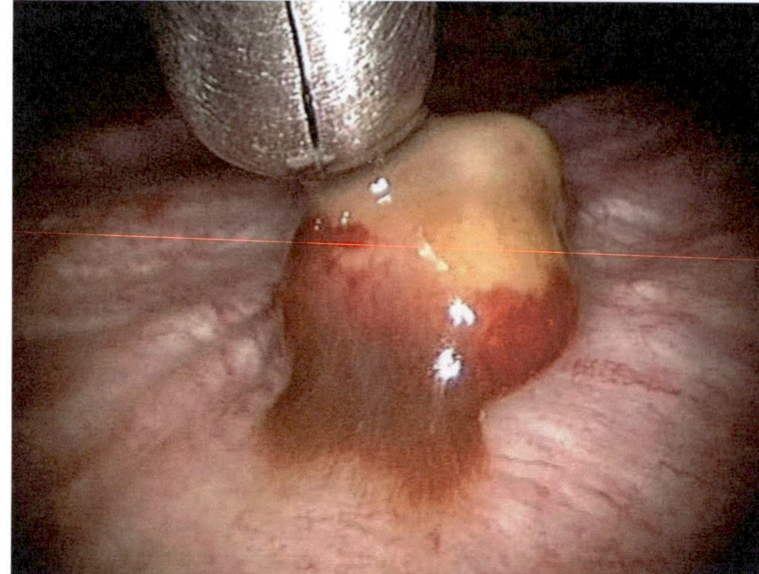

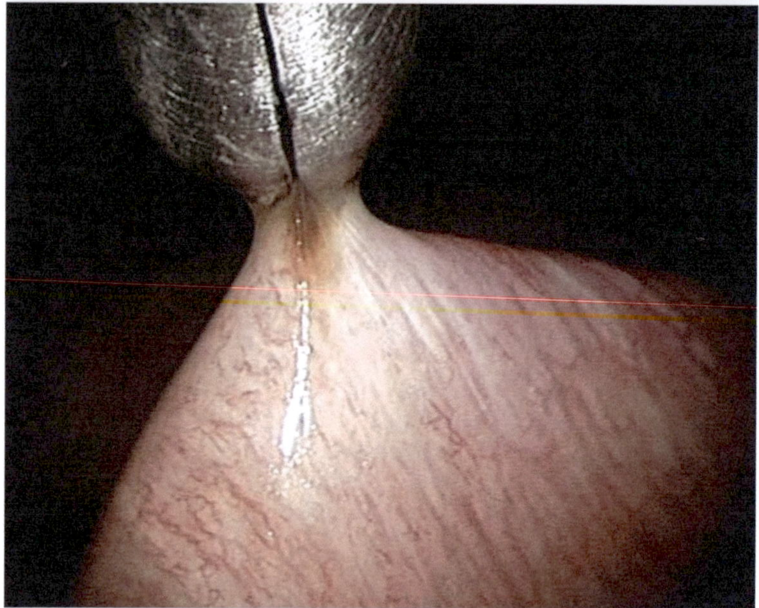

Fig. 10.6 After aspiration of the fluid, a single nodule can be seen. In this case, using an optical biopsy forceps, the nodule located on the diaphragm is removed (adenocarcinoma from primary lung cancer). To perform the procedure with absolute safety, the tip (5 mm) of the forceps has to be visible at all times without any blind periods

Fig. 10.7 A malignant nodule on the parietal pleura

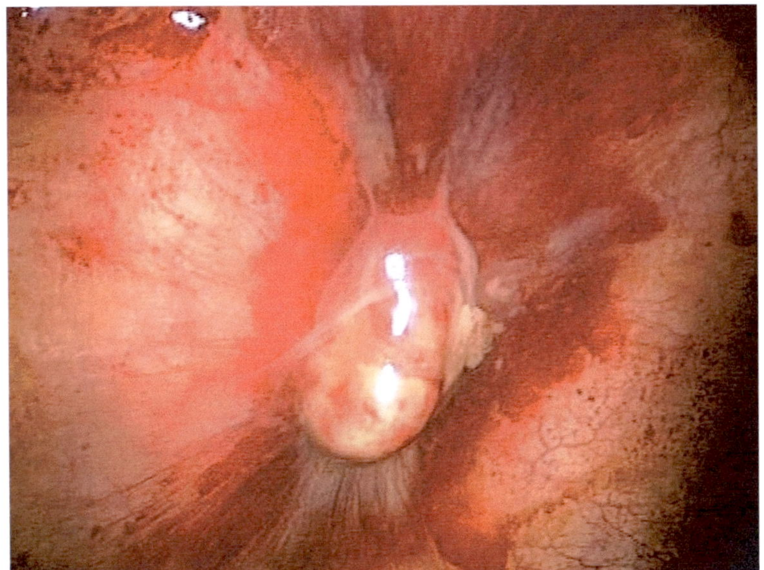

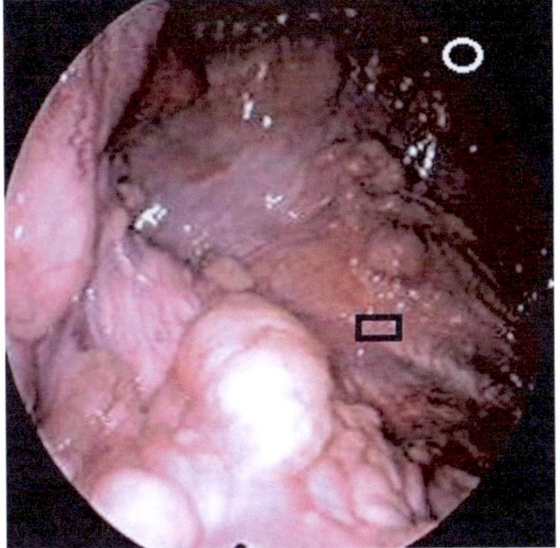

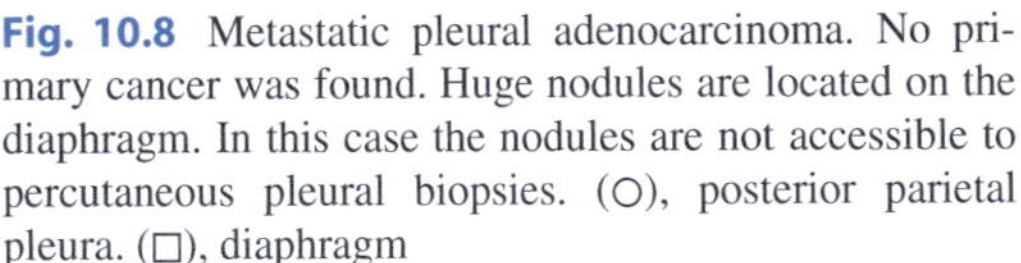

Fig. 10.8 Metastatic pleural adenocarcinoma. No primary cancer was found. Huge nodules are located on the diaphragm. In this case the nodules are not accessible to percutaneous pleural biopsies. (O), posterior parietal pleura. (□), diaphragm

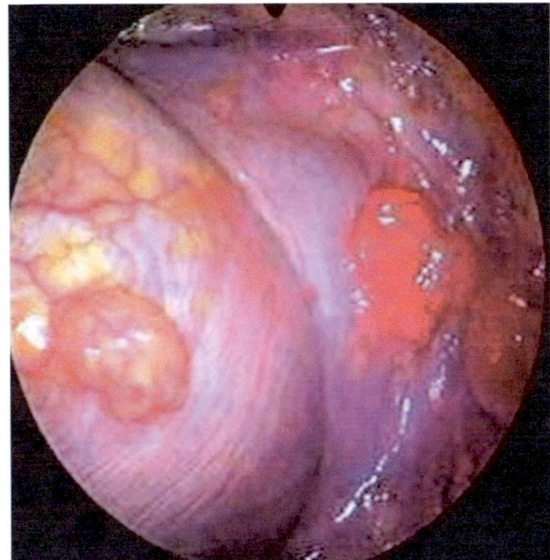

Fig. 10.9 Malignant nodules on the diaphragm. The costal pleura was not invaded by the disease. Previous percutaneous procedures failed to obtain a diagnosis

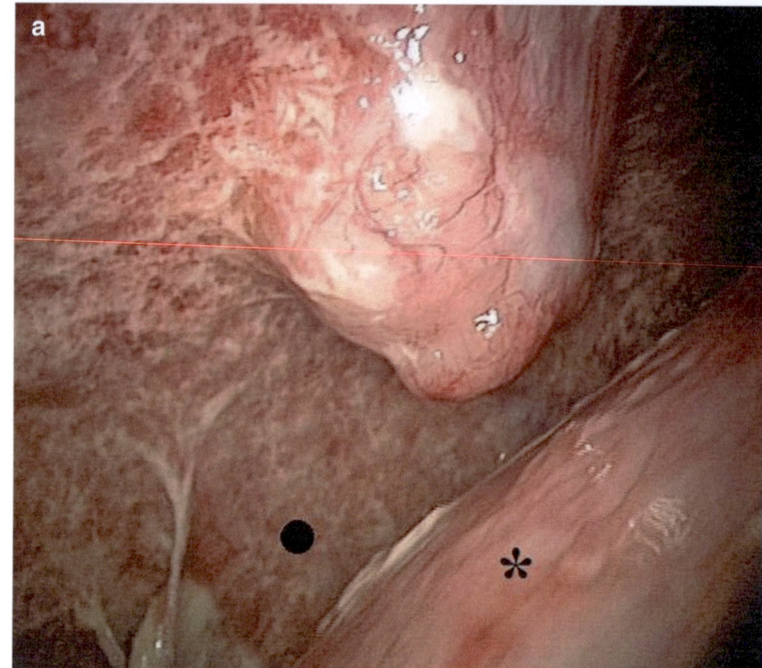
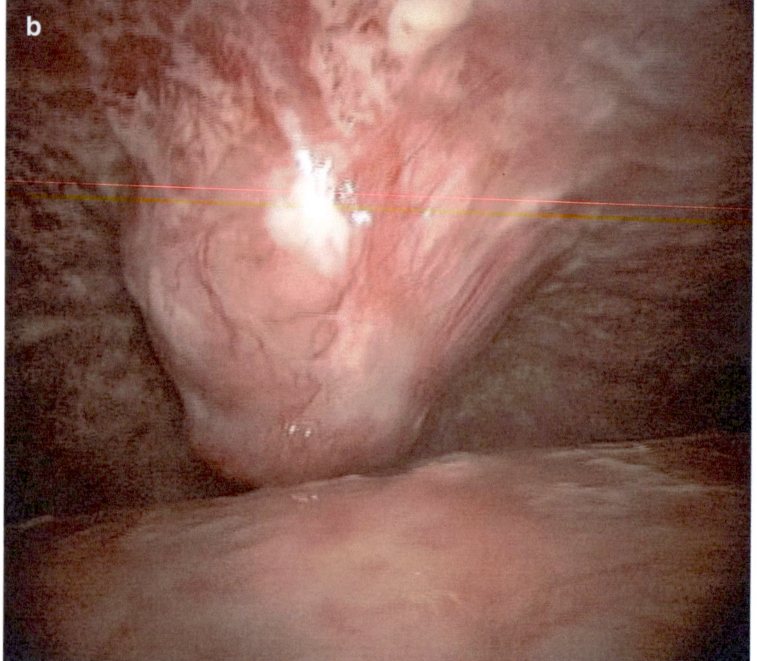

Fig. 10.10 'A kissing nodule'. Panel (**a**): A malignant nodule on the parietal pleura at the level of the left costodiaphragmatic gutter (●). Vessels are visible on the surface of the nodule. In addition, there is malignant pleural lymphangitis. (*star*), diaphragm. Panel (**b**): The procedure is performed in spontaneous breathing, and during the respiratory cycle, the nodule can be seen to be in contact with the diaphragm

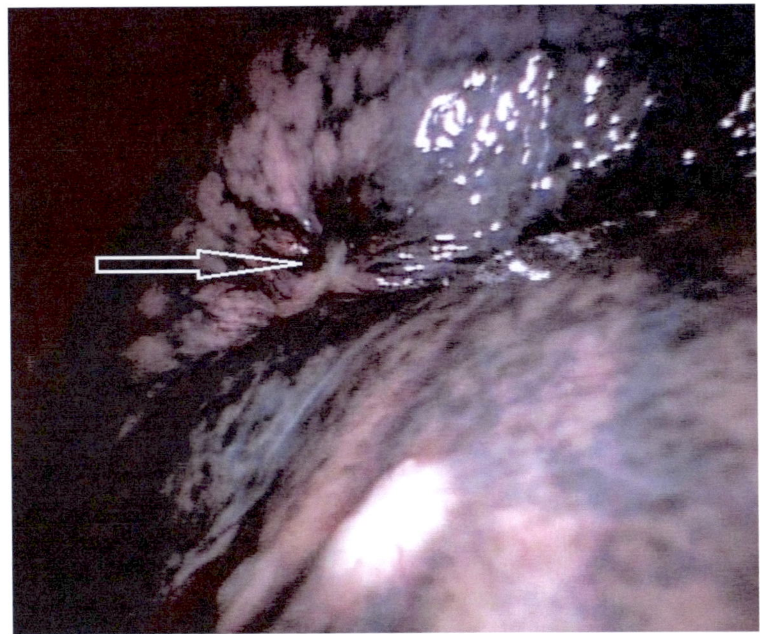

Fig. 10.11 Lung nodule with umbilication (*arrow*) close to the fissure

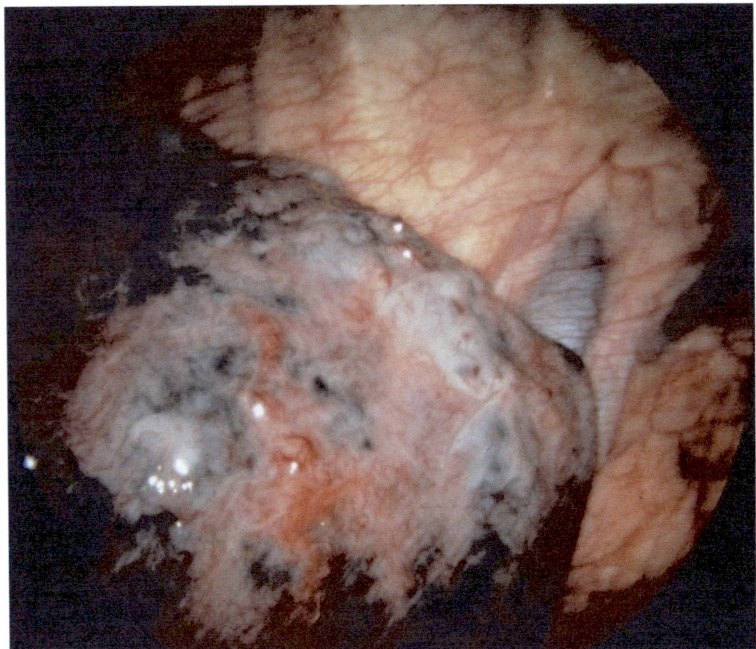

Fig. 10.12 An atelectatic left lower lobe with nodule on the surface

Fig. 10.13 Multiple lung
metastases visible on the
surface of this trapped lung

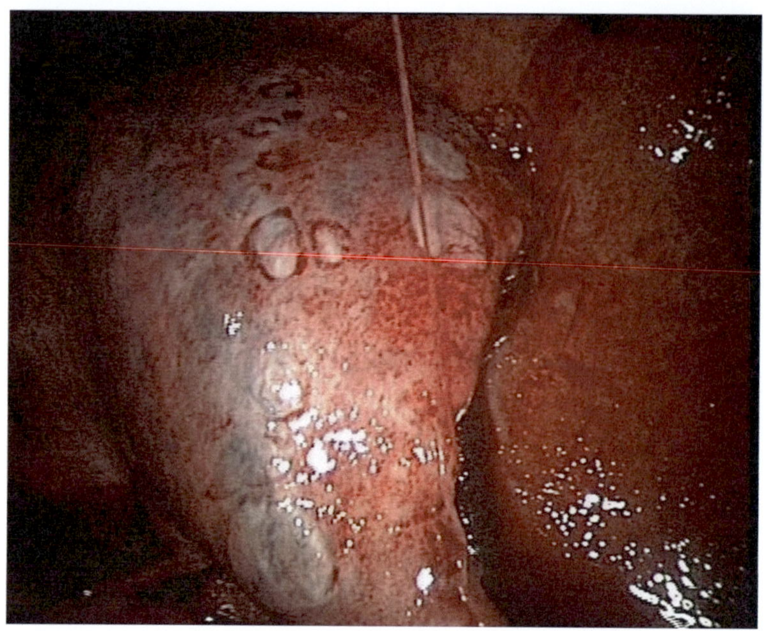

Fig. 10.14 A lung tumour of
the left lower lobe. Fibrotic
inflammation (*white inflammation*) is visible on the
visceral pleura and parietal
pleura (*star*)

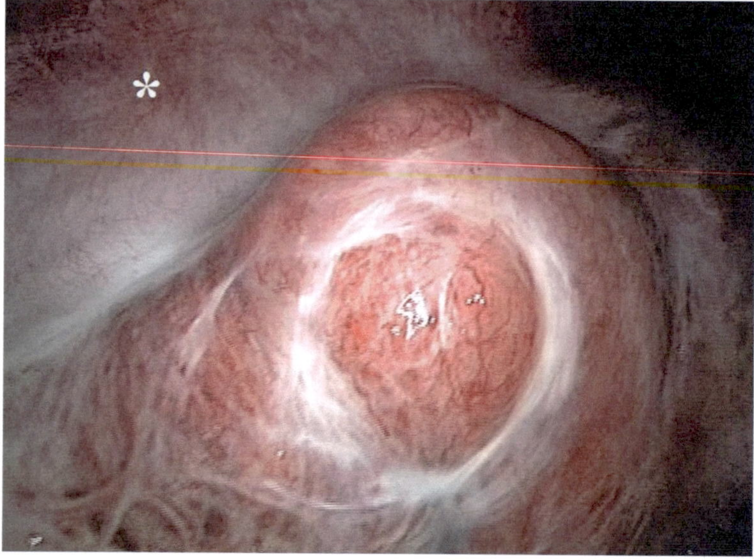

Fig. 10.15 Metastatic small cell lung cancer. Multiple nodules are visible on the surface of the lung at the level of the fissure. There are pleural adhesions between anterior parietal pleura and left upper lobe. The left lower lobe is on the right side of the figure

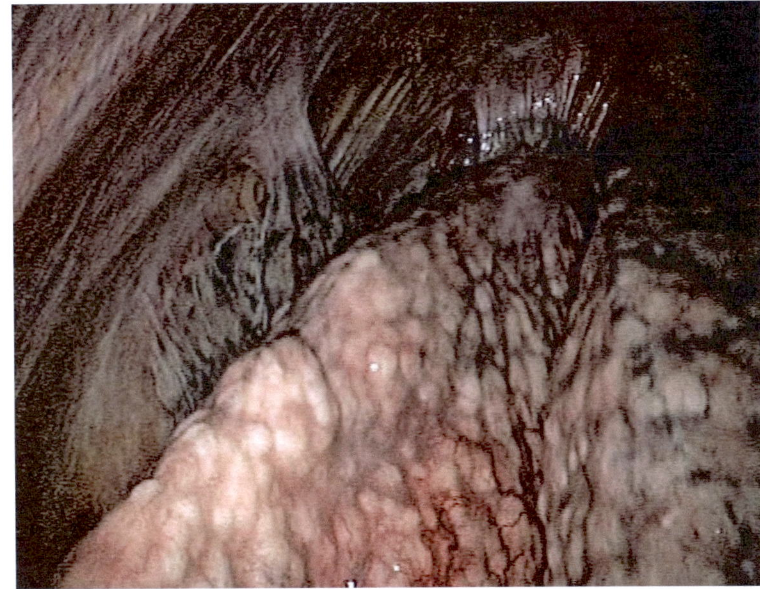

Fig. 10.16 Flat malignant pleural lesions in breast cancer. The parietal pleura (□) and the diaphragm (O) are invaded. The lung (*star*) is free of disease

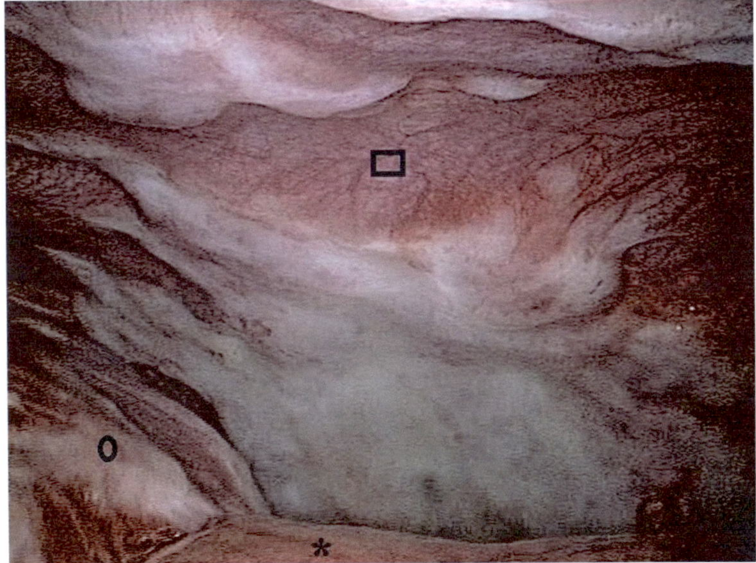

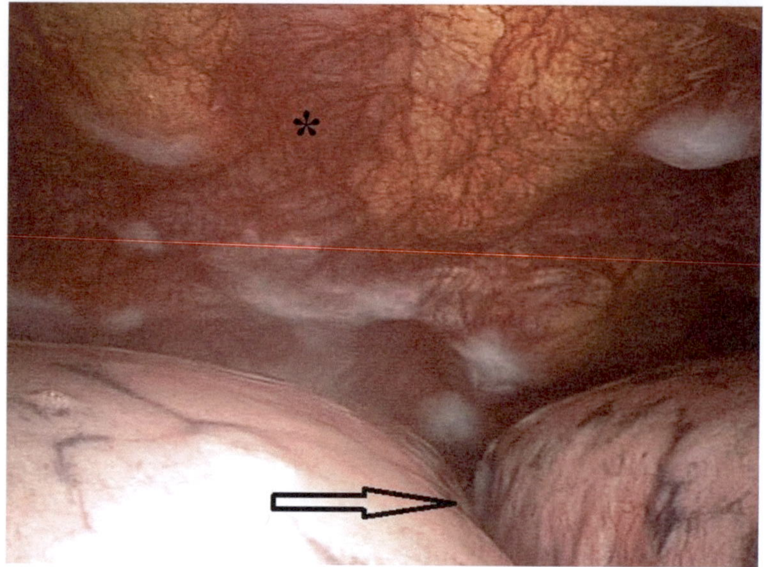

Fig. 10.17 Left side. Metastasis on the posterior parietal pleura (*star*) in woman with breast cancer. The surface of the two lobes of the left lung separated by the fissure (*arrow*) is normal with few anthracotic deposits

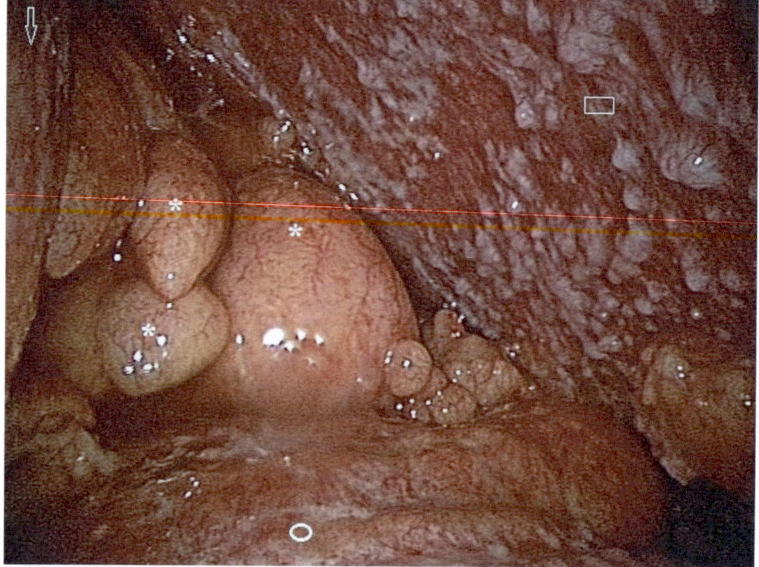

Fig. 10.18 The costodiaphragmatic gutter on the left side in a patient with a metastatic ovarian cancer. Multiple nodules are disseminated on the parietal pleura (□), the diaphragm (○), and the pericardial fat (*star*). Lower lobe (*arrow*)

Fig. 10.19 Non-specific lymphangitis on the posterior parietal pleura. Pleural biopsies demonstrated pleural lymphoma

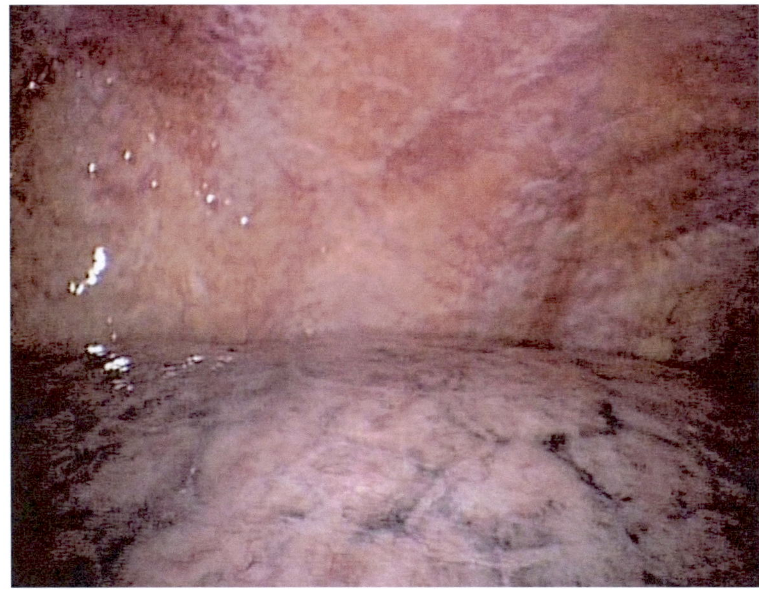

Fig. 10.20 Huge nodules in a patient with a malignant pleural effusion from metastatic sarcoma

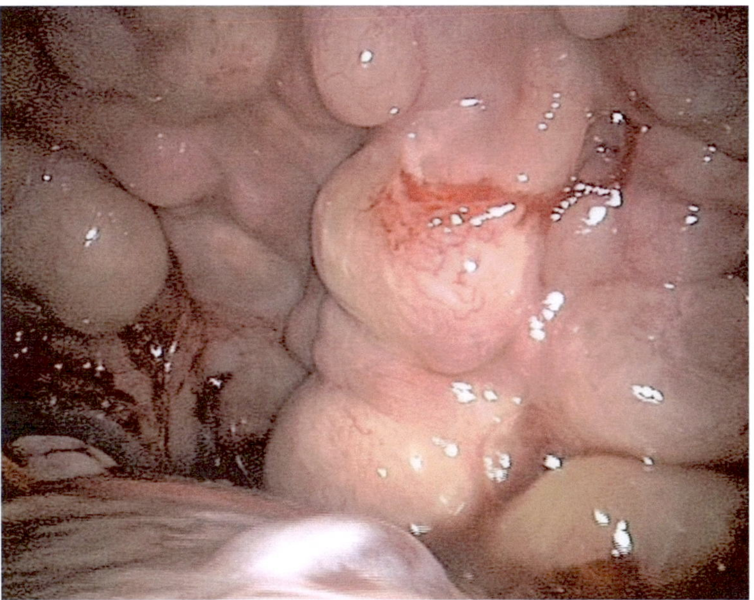

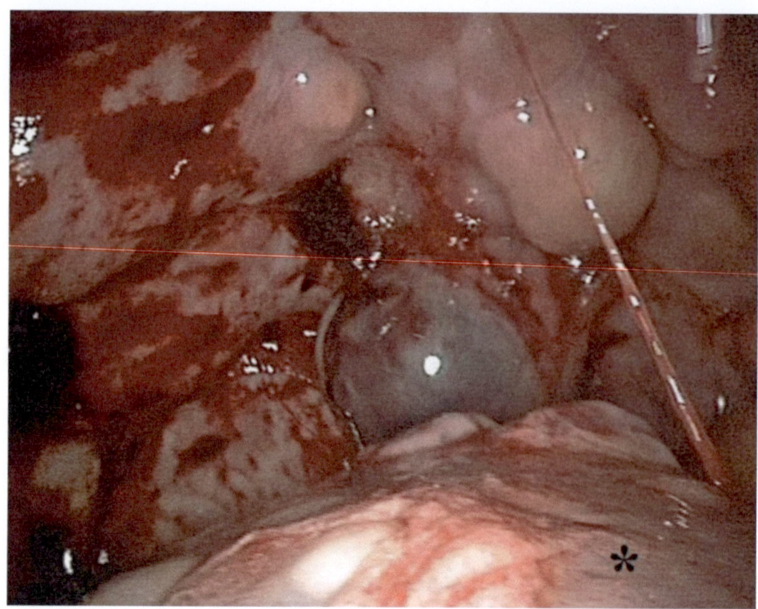

Fig. 10.21 Right side. Pleural sarcoma with invasion of the apex of the lung (*star*)

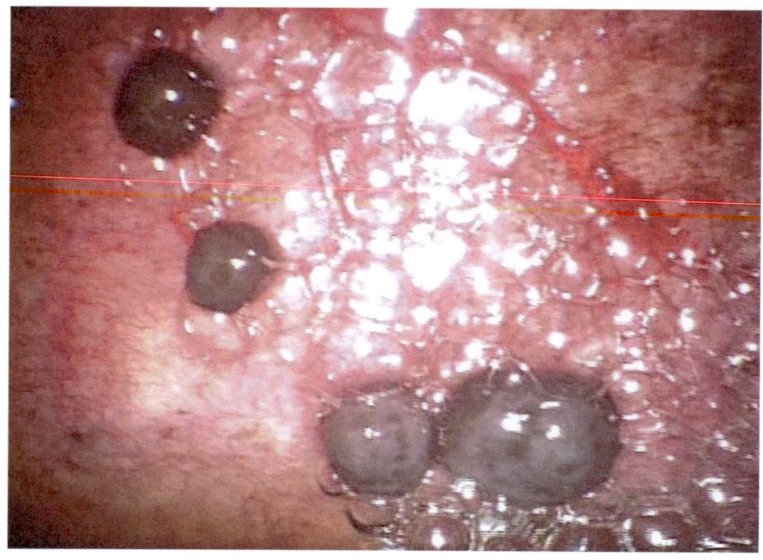

Fig. 10.22 Metastatic pleural nodules on the parietal pleura in a patient with malignant melanoma

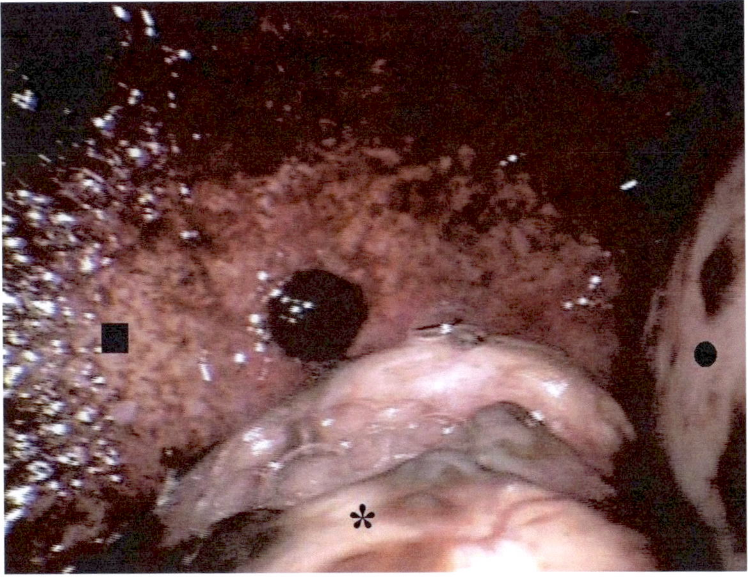

Fig. 10.23 Metastatic nodules from malignant melanoma on the parietal pleura (■), diaphragm (●), and on the surface of the lung (*star*)

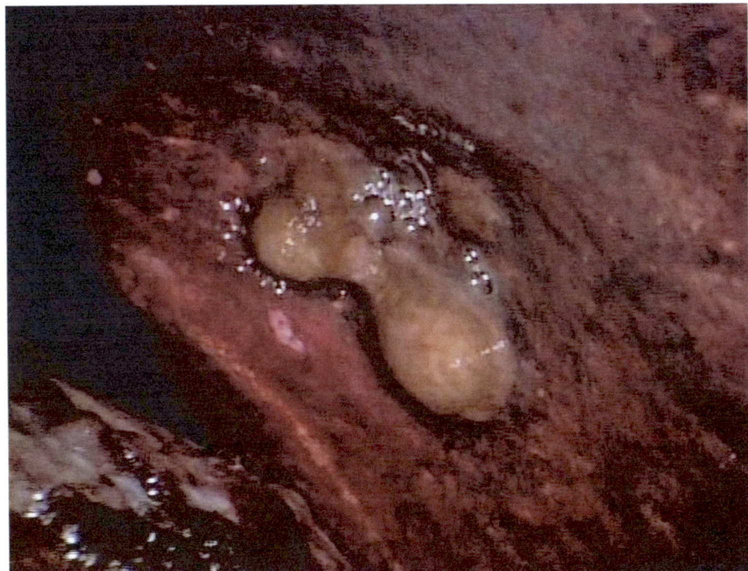

Fig. 10.24 Pleural metastasis of malignant melanoma may be amelanocytic

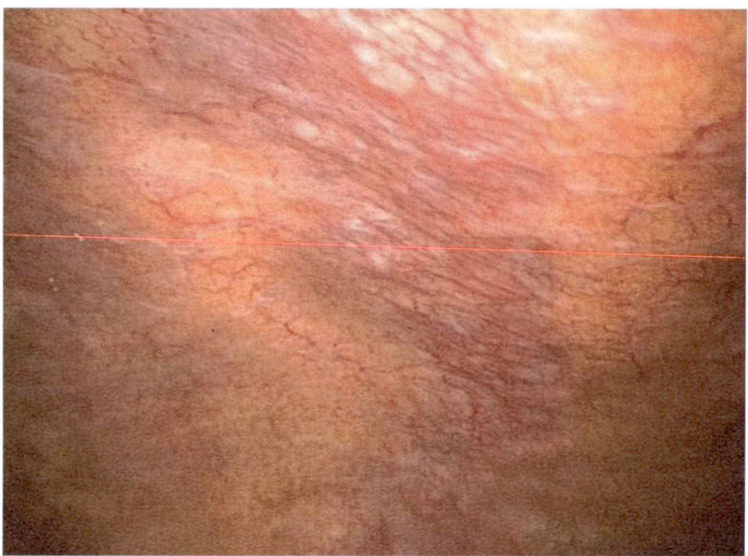

Fig. 10.25 Malignant pleural mesothelioma (epithelial type). Early-stage disease with a few flat nodules and non-specific parietal pleural lymphangitis

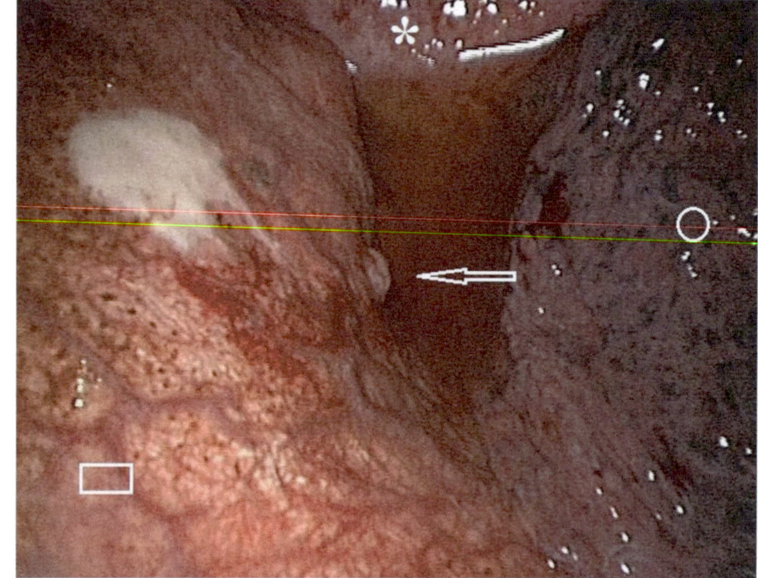

Fig. 10.26 Early-stage epithelial malignant pleural mesothelioma. A nodule is visible (*white arrow*) on the diaphragm (□) close to a pleural plaque. The right lower lobe is atelectatic (○). There is residual fluid in the costodiaphragmatic gutter and non- specific inflammation of the parietal pleura (*star*)

Fig. 10.27 Malignant pleural mesothelioma (epithelial type) in an asbestos- exposed patient. *1*- Typical pleural plaques on the anterior parietal pleura. *2*- Parietal pleura with small nodules and neoplastic lymphangitis. *3*- Fissure. *4*- Pleural fluid. Lung (*white square*)

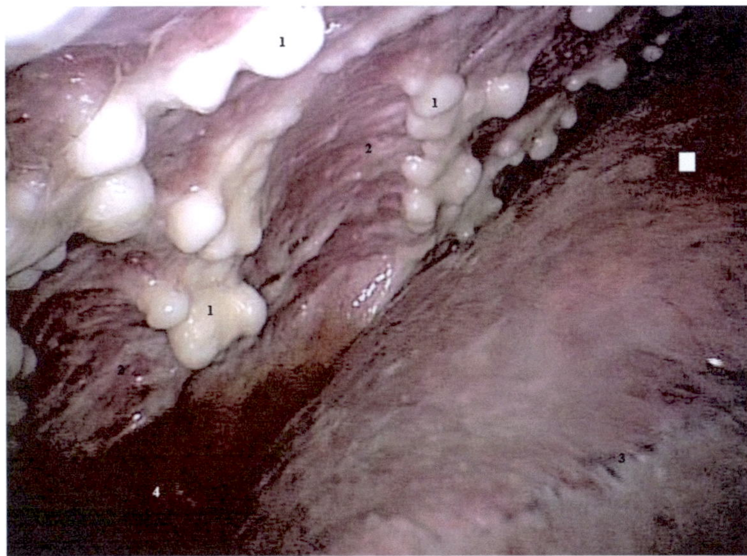

Fig. 10.28 Malignant pleural mesothelioma (sarcomatoid type). Pleural plaque (*black arrow*). Neoplastic lymphangitis (*white arrow*). Lung (*star*)

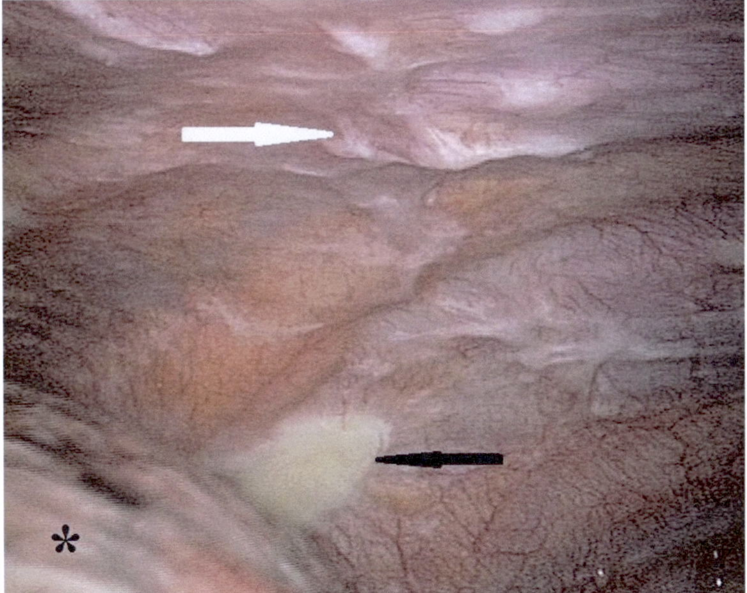

Diagnostic Thoracoscopy: Nonmalignant Pleural Effusion

Wolfgang Frank and Nicolas Schönfeld

11.1 Introduction

Nonmalignant effusion is a term that covers a broad spectrum of both inflammatory and noninflammatory conditions, including pleural involvement by cardiac and hepatic disease (transudative hydrothorax). Cardiac disease accounts for about 90 % of all transudative effusions, and effusions of varying extent are present in 58–73 % of all unselected hospitalized cardiac patients (Weiss and Spodick 1984). Indeed, since there is usually no pleural pathology in transudative effusion, such patients rarely, if ever, need thoracoscopic exploration. As there is a high prevalence of cardiac disease, it is therefore extremely important to establish whether an effusion is transudative or exudative in nature. Traditionally, this is best achieved by means of simple *thoracocentesis* using the classical Light's criteria (protein and LDH levels). An overall discriminatory accuracy of 90 % can be achieved with the expanded *triple test* using well-established cutoff values and including additional cholesterol determinations in pleural fluid and serum (Table 11.1) (Heffner

et al. 1997). Very recently, the determination of the marker NT-proBNP (a precursor of B-type natriuretic peptide) has been shown to be equally successful in identifying effusions secondary to cardiogenic hydrothorax, having an overall accuracy of 92 % (Kolditz et al. 2006). On the basis of these criteria and current epidemiology, the pretest odds relationship of transudative vs exudative etiologies in unselected patients with pleural effusion will be about 0.4/0.6.

In the diagnosis of exudative etiologies, apart from its classical role in malignancy, thoracoscopy is also an excellent tool for the diagnosis of various benign diseases. The etiologic spectrum and relative frequency of benign exudative effusion, i.e., mostly inflammatory pleural disease, are summarized in Table 11.2 ,in which bacterial pleurisy (parapneumonic effusion and empyema) is clearly the main cause (Light 1995a). Tuberculous pleurisy has become rare in Western populations but remains a crucial issue in light of globalization and in developing countries, particularly in the context of the HIV epidemic. Nonspecific pleurisy is caused by different conditions such as thromboembolism and rheumatological disease that are often clinically underestimated and also by a variety of difficult-to-diagnose inflammatory conditions, which may have anecdotic importance only, for example, benign asbestos. Nevertheless, thoracoscopy may also play an important role in some of these conditions. The diagnostic value and overall role of thoracoscopy in the management of various benign pleural effusions will be discussed in this chapter.

W. Frank (✉)
Department of Pulmonology Deseases,
Lungenklinik, AmseeWaren, Müritz, Germany
e-mail: wfrank@klinikamsee.de

N. Schönfeld
Department of Pulmonology,
Lungenklinik Heckeshorn,
HELIOS Klinikum Emil von Behring,
Berlin, Germany
e-mail: nicolas.schoenfeld@helios-kliniken.de

P. Astoul et al. (eds.), *Thoracoscopy for Pulmonologists*,
DOI 10.1007/978-3-642-38351-9_11, © Springer-Verlag Berlin Heidelberg 2014

Table 11.1 Commonly used parameters and recommended cutoff values for distinguishing transudates and exudates

Parameter	Cutoff	Cutoff
	Absolute values	PF/S[a] – Ratio
	Transudate↓	*Transudate↓*
	Exudate↑	*Exudate↑*
Protein	3 g/dl	0.5
Lactic dehydrogenase (LDH)	200 IU/dl[b]	0.6
Cholesterol	60 mg/dl[c]	

Light 1972; Heffner et al. 1997
[a]Pleural effusion/serum
[b]3.3 µmol/l
[c]1.5 mmol/l

Table 11.2 Etiologic spectrum and causes of exudative pleural effusion and their relative incidence

Etiology	Incidence (%)
Pneumonia	50.9
Pleural malignancies	25.5
Thromboembolism	18.0
Gastrointestinal disease	4.0
Rheumatic-autoimmunologic disease	0.8
Tuberculosis	0.55
Benign asbestos pleuritis	0.25

Analysis of one year incidence of 785,000 exudative effusions, USA (1991) – adapted from Light (1995a)

Table 11.3 Differentiation between empyema and lung abscess on a (contrast) CT scan

Signs favoring empyema
Signs of lung compression
Smooth margins of membranes
Dissection of the thickened visceral parietal pleura
Blunt angle with the chest wall
Signs favoring abscess
Spherical shape with irregular and thicker wall structures
Absence of lung compression
Sharp angle with the chest wall
Visible airway connection
Demonstration of vasculature around abscess (definite proof)

11.2 Parapneumonic Effusion and Empyema

11.2.1 Clinical Background

Parapneumonic effusion and empyema are inter-related, overlapping manifestations of bacterial pleurisy. The most common cause, pneumonia, is present in about 55 % of cases, while bacterial pleurisy complicates pneumonia in 20–57 % of cases. Thus in the majority of cases, the condition presents as *pleuropneumonia* (Alfageme et al. 1993). Bacterial pleurisy is estimated to account for 20–30 % of all cases of pleural effusion. Serious and debilitating predisposing conditions are observed in up to 82 % of cases, of which compromised immunity due to alcoholism is the single biggest risk factor (Alfageme et al. 1993). The effusion is unilateral in 80 % of cases and may be profuse or sometimes even lead to intra-thoracic displacement and compression. The most important differential diagnosis relevant to local treatment is *lung abscess*, which, however, will not usually require thoracostomy. Contrast-enhanced CT is helpful for making this distinction using the criteria presented in Table 11.3.

11.2.2 Prethoracoscopic Investigations

The diagnosis of parapneumonic effusion may be straightforward in situations where the clinical background is compatible and the culture is positive, foul smelling turbid effusion has been recovered, or frank empyema is found at thoracocentesis. In the presence of serous clear pleural fluid and negative microbiological findings, further investigations are needed to establish a diagnosis of bacterial pleurisy. Light's criteria, including pH, glucose content, and LDH, are then commonly recommended for subclassification of

Table 11.4 Classification of parapneumonic effusion (bacterial pleurisy) and derived indications to tube drainage

Empyema/complicated parapneumonic effusion **ACCP category IV&III**	Intermediate effusion - quality **ACCP category II?**	Uncomplicated parapneumonic effusion **ACCP category I–II**
. frank empyema . bacterial culture + . any effusion amount . mono-/multilocular- . Light criteria glucose < 40 mg/dl LDH > 1000 IU/dl pH < 7.00 leucocyte count > 15/nl . air leaks	**serial pleurocentesis + clinical follow-up** ? ?	. clear-serous effusion . bacterial effusion - . effusion < ca. 1000 ml . monolocular . Light criteria glucose > 40 mg/dl LDH < 1000 IU/dl pH > 7.00 leucocyte count < 10/nl
TUBE DRAINAGE REQUIRED	← →	**CHEST TUBE NOT REQUIRED**

bacterial pleurisy into *uncomplicated* and *complicated parapneumonic effusions*. Previously, these overlapping conditions were referred to as *exudative or fibrinopurulent* pleurisy and *organizing or chronic* empyema. As shown in Table 11.4, empyema and complicated parapneumonic effusion, which are classical high-dependency indications for thoracostomy and drainage, are characterized by low pH (<7.0) and glucose (<2.2 mmol/l (40 mg/dl)) and elevated lactate dehydrogenase (LDH) levels (>10,000 IU/l) and WBC count ($>15 \times 10^9$/l), with a bacterial culture which is usually positive (Heffner et al. 1995; Maskell and Davies 2003). While uncomplicated effusion warranting noninvasive management is well defined, on the other hand, these criteria may leave a predictive gap for poorly defined intermediate effusions, as is also shown in Table 11.4. Based on the key parameter, pH, and a comprehensive body of evidence from individual studies and meta-analyses, current recommendations of the American College of Chest Physicians (ACCP) propose a more stringent differentiation into four risk and outcome categories (Davies et al. 2003; Antunes et al. 2003):

- Category I – minimal free-flowing effusion, culture and pH unknown
- Category II – small to moderate free-flowing effusion, negative culture, and pH>7.2
- Category III – large free-flowing effusion, loculations and membranes, pH<7.2
- Category IV – category III plus evidence of frank pus

In broad practical terms, taking into account the clinical presentation and fluid characteristics, thoracostomy with tube drainage is therefore vitally important in one or more of the following conditions:

- Frank empyema at thoracocentesis – ACCP category IV
- Ongoing sepsis
- Profuse effusion (>2 l), particularly where it causes displacement
- Presence of air in the pleural space suggesting a bronchopleural fistula
- Biochemical fluid parameters as defined in ACCP category III (usually termed "complicated parapneumonic effusion")

11.2.3 The Role of Thoracoscopy

Any invasive approach that focuses on chest drainage clearly addresses and highlights the use of thoracoscopy (Colice et al. 2000; Loddenkemper and Frank 2006). The rationale of thoracoscopy in empyema and complicated parapneumonic effusion is mainly management related. The diagnostic value of biopsies taken under direct vision in neutrophilic inflammation of bacterial pleurisy is usually negligible – unless differential diagnoses such as tuberculosis or other specific etiologies are being considered.

The role of medical thoracoscopy in the management of empyema and parapneumonic effusion has long been under debate; this indication is only reluctantly accepted by pulmonologists as there is a paucity of evidence-based data and competitive surgical treatment options. Video-assisted thoracic surgery (VATS), in particular, has become a gold standard. For many years, experienced pulmonologists in Western Europe have routinely performed thoracoscopy in the setting of bacterial pleurisy and this has created a body of expertise. However, it remains largely on the evidence level of expert opinion. The "inventor" of medical thoracoscopy himself (Jacobaeus) was the first to report an extensive experience in 100 cases as early as 1925 (Jacobaeus 1925). Boutin and colleagues describe their good results in the preceding edition of this book (Boutin et al. 1991). In Israel, Weissberg successfully performed thoracoscopy in empyema in the early 1970s, using a mediastinoscope (Weissberg 1980). More recently, in a large retrospective series of 127 patients from various hospitals in Switzerland and Italy, all of whom presented with multiloculated empyema, medical thoracoscopy as the first-line intervention under local anesthesia was successful in 91 % of cases, with 94 % of patients being cured by nonsurgical means (Brutsche et al. 2005). In another series of 16 consecutive cases in whom medical thoracoscopy was performed after tube drainage had failed, clinical improvement was achieved in all cases and definitive cure in 12, thus only four cases required surgical debridement (Solèr et al. 1997). In America, Landreneau and colleagues also reported similarly successful use of thoracoscopy in 63 out of 99 patients (Landreneau et al. 1995). In pediatric cases, medical thoracoscopy performed under local anesthesia does not appear to be feasible, and thus video-assisted thoracic surgery (VATS) is considered the intervention of choice and given clear preference over formal thoracostomy (Colice et al. 2000; Davies

et al. 2003; Antunes et al. 2003). Medical thoracoscopy is now also becoming increasingly accepted in English-speaking countries and has been adopted as a treatment option by many scientific societies. Surgical thoracoscopy (VATS) for the treatment of bacterial pleurisy is now firmly incorporated into the current guidelines and consensus statements of both the ACCP and the British Thoracic Society (BTS). According to the BTS guidelines, fibrinolysis, VATS, and formal surgery are equally acceptable interventions in empyema, but VATS is preferred to fibrinolysis (evidence level C) (Colice et al. 2000; Davies et al. 2003; Antunes et al. 2003). In this setting, medical thoracoscopy introduces the intriguing additional option of using a combined thoracoscopy/fibrinolysis approach which has the advantage of being only moderately invasive and more cost-effective. This concept is currently under investigation in a European multicenter project.

11.2.4 Procedure

The technical approach to performing a *thoracoscopy* in empyema is basically the same as that used for other types of effusion but, importantly, must specifically take into account loculations and membranes, which are typical for and frequently occur in empyema. A careful evaluation with CT and ultrasound, to define safe entry points, is mandatory prior to the thoracoscopy (Figs. 11.1 and 11.2) (Hersh et al. 2003). This is particularly important when sharp obturators are employed, in order to avoid injury to the lung. To define a safe entry compartment in a loculated effusion, an accessible liquid compartment must be firstly identified by fluid aspiration. In our opinion, this should be confirmed by fluoroscopy using gas insufflation (air or better CO_2) to demonstrate gas deposition and thus lung detachment at the intended point of entry. Following entry into the pleural cavity, exploration may reveal widely varying inflammatory patterns.

- One typical macroscopic finding is the presence of an abundant, viscous accumulation of pus (of up to several liters) often in a monolocular cavity; the intensely inflamed parietal and visceral

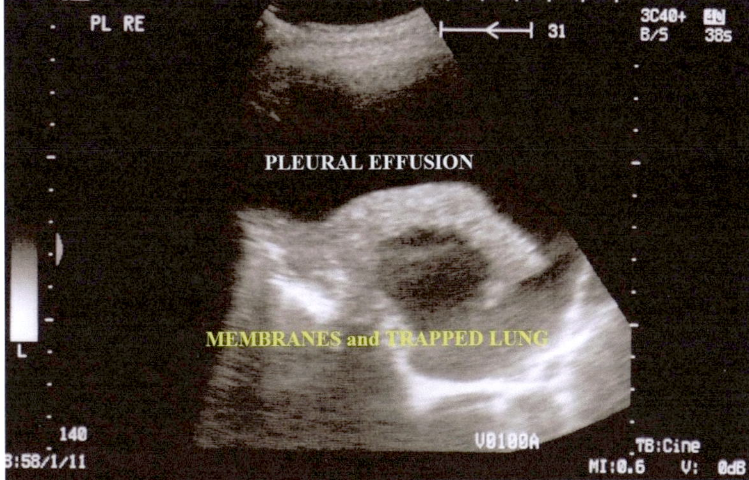

Fig. 11.1 Ultrasound to detect inflammatory visceral membranes and therefore a trapped lung secondary to empyema

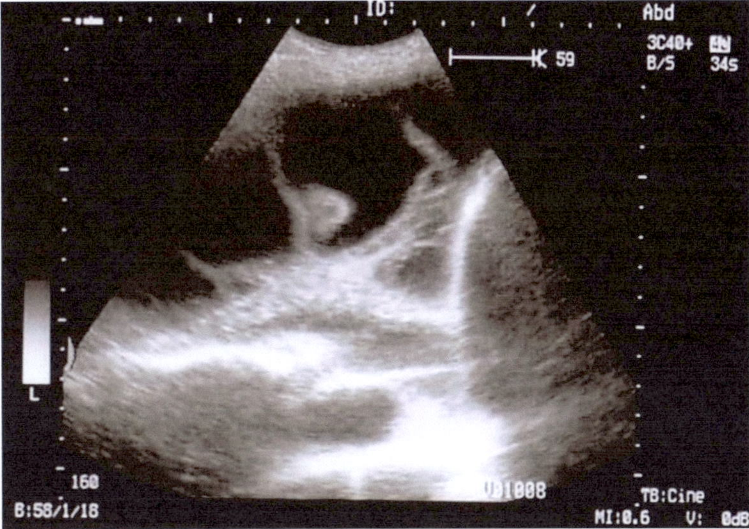

Fig. 11.2 Ultrasound detection of a multiple loculated empyema

pleura is associated with purulent adherent membranes and hemorrhage, which may occur spontaneously. An example of such changes, which used to be referred to as the *fibrinopurulent stage* of empyema, is shown in Fig. 11.3.

- More often, as is typically seen in complicated parapneumonic effusions, the endoscopic finding is of multiple fibrinous loculations. The operator often visualizes adhesions and sponge-like chambers following the introduction of the telescope (Fig. 11.4). The investigation may then be expanded to include mechanical separation of compartments and blunt dissection of membranes and adhesions in order to create a large monolocular cavity which will subsequently be easier to treat. This procedure can also include peeling of thick visceral membranes, making it possible to free and re-expand a trapped lung. With these dissection procedures, particular care must be taken to spare adhesions that are already organized and vascularized. This may occur in cases where the clinical course is prolonged and in the setting of chronic empyema. A typical sequence is shown in Fig. 11.5, with initial visualization of extensive loculations which are then broken down (debridement) to reveal the originally entrapped lung.

Fig. 11.3 Typical features of a single cavity secondary to empyema (parietal pleura, fibropurulent stage). Male, 48 years, purulent peels (**a**) including spontaneous hemorrhage (**b**) and biopsy lesion (to exclude TB) (**c**)

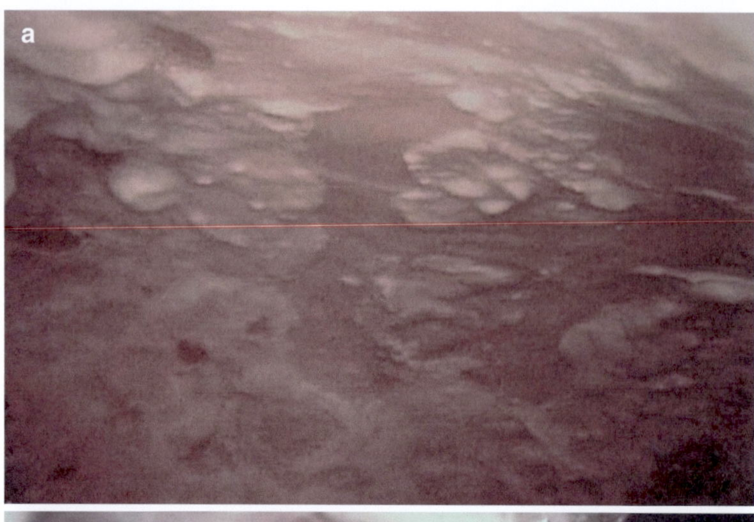

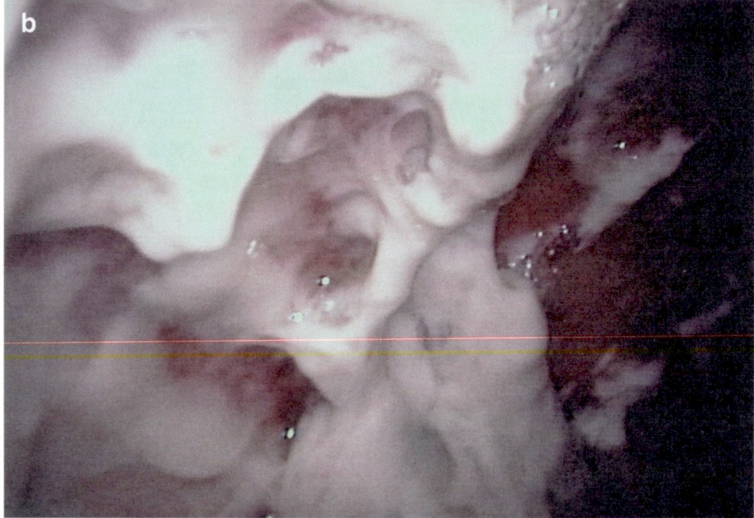

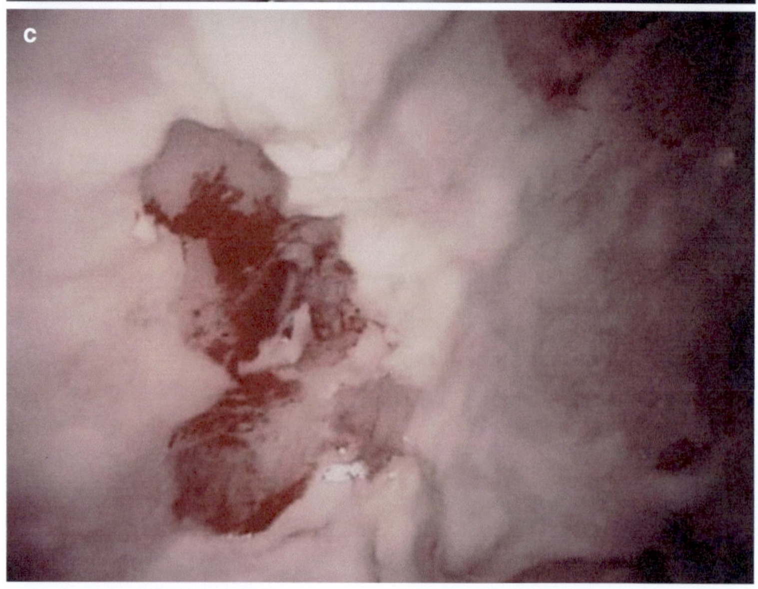

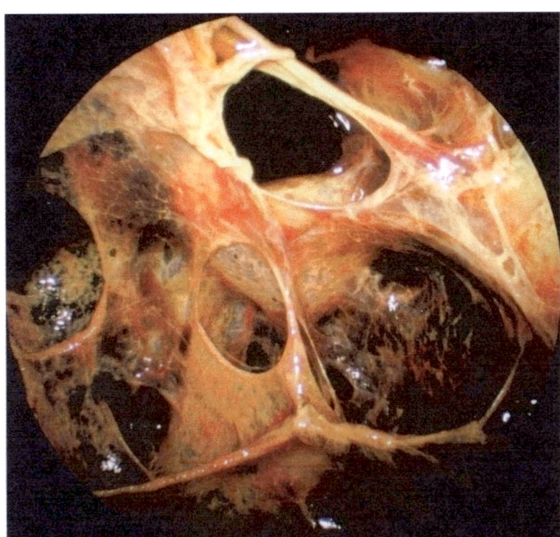

Fig. 11.4 The benefit of pleuroscopy in tube drainage management: recognition and elimination of multiloculation in empyema

11.2.5 Combined Treatment Modalities

Drain insertion is a vital procedure which is carried out in the acute phase of empyema, but it is also crucial for optimal long-term results. Another important advantage of thoracoscopy is that it allows visual control and thus also optimal drain placement. Drainage is performed not only to remove fluid but should also usually include irrigation with or without instillation of fibrinolytics. The drainage specifications should therefore give preference to large-bore, double-lumen catheters ($\geq$24 F) to ensure clearance of thick secretions and initiation of closed circuit irrigation. If fibrinolysis is considered, streptokinase and urokinase are equally effective agents. According to several guidelines, the instillation of fibrinolytics is indicated in the presence of:

- Thick pus with apparent or suspected retention of the secretion
- Membranes and loculations
- Trapped lung. (Davies et al. 2003; Antunes et al. 2003; Colice et al. 2000)

Fibrinolysis enhances the effects of interventional thoracoscopy and may obviate the need for two or more drains in multiloculated empyema. There will be a transient increase in

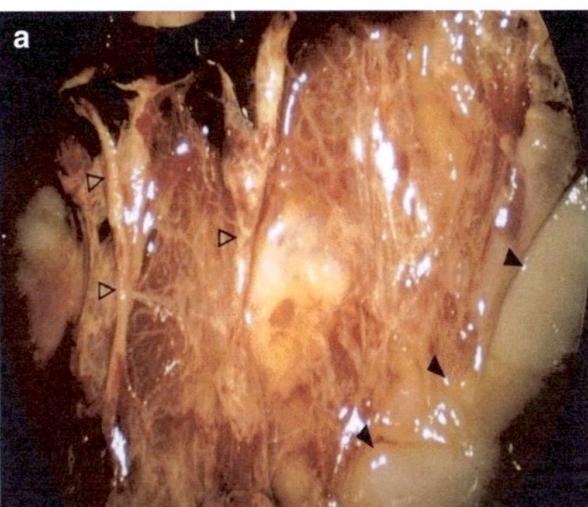

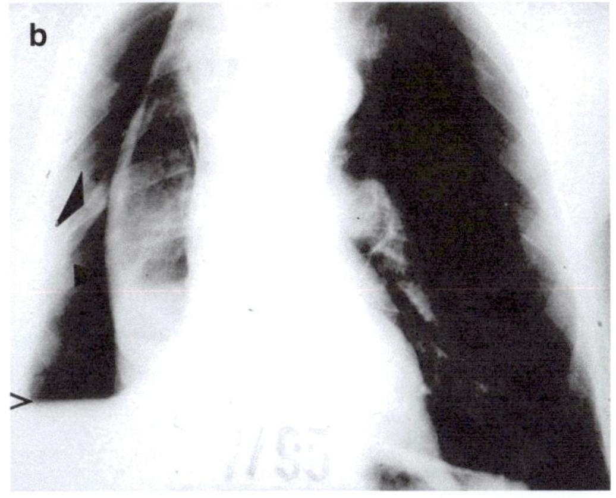

Fig. 11.5 The benefit of pleuroscopy in tube drainage management in empyema: same case as Fig. 11.4. Pleuroscopic features of the visceral membrane after dissection of the inflammatory adhesions. *Black arrowheads* pus deposits, *white arrowheads* visceral membrane (**a**). The visceral peel with indwelling chest tube preventing re-expansion of the trapped lung post pleuroscopy. *Black arrowheads* visceral peel (**b**). The lung subsequently expanded after fibrinolysis

fluid production due to the resolution and liquidation of pus and membranes. With irrigation and fibrinolysis protocols, the output of mostly turbid fluid will initially exceed the irrigation input. Irrigation is continued until a clear sterile fluid is obtained and the net fluid production falls below 50 ml/day. Our protocol has been well tried and proven in practice and uses a combination of streptokinase and streptodornase (DNAse) (see Table 11.5). The value of the streptodornase component has not yet been firmly established clinically; however, experimental data strongly suggest that the

Table 11.5 Combined irrigation/instillation protocol for fibrinolytic chest tube management of empyema (own protocol)

A: *Interventional approach*
1. Ultrasound-guided thoracentesis
2. Double-lumen irrigation/suction drainage (20–24 F, 40 cm), ultrasound guided pleuroscopy guided
3. Empyema evacuation (standard suction: 20 cm H_2O)
4. Imaging control (X-ray/fluoroscopy/sonography)
5. Irrigation using isotonic saline solution with aseptic additives (polyvidone iodine 2 %) until recovery of clear irrigation fluid (before and after fibrinolysis)
6. Fibrinolytic agent instillation: Varidase® (1 ampule = 100,000 IE streptokinase + 25,000 IE streptodornase) with a 2–4 h clamping period
B: *Empiric and subsequent targeted antibiotic therapy*

effectiveness of fibrinolysis can be improved by decreasing the DNA-dependent viscosity of the pus (Simpson et al. 2000). The only relevant contraindication to the use of streptokinase is suspected allergy. However, fibrinolytics may also be cautiously applied in the presence of bronchopleural fistula to avoid spilling and contamination of the ipsilateral and contralateral bronchial systems. Adverse effects of both streptokinase and urokinase may include fever >38.5 °C and pain (both up to 7 % of cases). Pleural fibrinolysis is safe as regards systemic effects, and there is no evidence that systemic fibrinolysis occurs at cumulative doses of up to six times the therapeutic level (Davies et al. 1998). A review of the evidence based on fibrinolysis from multicenter studies and meta-analyses reveals that 200,000–250,000 IU streptokinase was equally as effective as 50,000–100,000 IU urokinase (Bouros et al. 1997). Fibrinolysis was significantly more effective than pure irrigation as assessed on the basis of some secondary endpoints such as time to clearance of empyema and radiological resolution (Diacon et al. 2004; Maskell et al. 2005; Tokuda et al. 2006). There were no significant differences between the two procedures as regards the primary endpoints of mortality and surgery. Thus the benefits of fibrinolysis remain to some extent controversial and require further elaboration (Rahman et al. 2011).

11.3 Tuberculous Pleurisy

11.3.1 Clinical Background

Tuberculous pleural involvement may occur at any stage of the disease but is more likely to be associated with a primary pulmonary tuberculous infection. Most patients present with acute fever and the clinical picture mimics bacterial parapneumonic pleurisy, which is also the most important differential diagnosis. *Pleuritis exsudativa tuberculosa* is the classical term for this form of tuberculosis. The pleural fluid is serous and a high-grade exudate with a protein concentration usually greater than 5 g/dl. Pleural cellularity shows a prevalence of lymphocytes but may become transiently neutrophilic in the acute febrile and initial stages. Exudative pleuritis occurs unilaterally in the vast majority of cases and rarely, if ever, develops profuse or compressive features. Overt concomitant pulmonary involvement is often absent. Exudative pleuritis is unlike *tuberculous empyema*, which again may mimic nonspecific bacterial empyema. Tuberculous empyema is a sequel and complication of long-standing postprimary pulmonary tuberculosis that may be associated with the rupture of caseous pulmonary lesions, tuberculous fibrothorax, and calcareous pleural thickening.

11.3.2 Prethoracoscopic Investigations

Conventional microbiological investigation of pleural fluid for the diagnosis of pleural TB is associated with major limitations. The microbiological yield (culture) in the pleural fluid is as low as 25 % and may only reach 50 % in exceptional cases. In addition, biochemical changes in the pleural fluid are only suggestive and nonspecific, e.g., excessive LDH elevation and low glucose and pH values (Frank 2002). In the past decade, considerable progress has been made in the noninvasive diagnosis of tuberculous pleurisy from pleural fluid and tissue aspirates using novel-specific inflammatory markers and *nucleic acid amplification techniques* (*NAAT*). Today, the main methods used to support a diagnosis of TB include the determination of *adenosine deaminase (ADA)* and *IFN-γ*, both of which yield excellent results with roughly 95 % sensitivity and 90 % specificity (Valdes et al. 1995; Söderblom et al. 1996). Commercially available MTB gene probes such as the AMPLICOR MTB®, AMTDT®, or AccuProbe® sets, mostly of which use the IS 6110 DNA or 16S-rRNA target sequence, provide an optimum specificity of about 100 % (as might be expected) and overall sensitivities up to 80–90 %, in both fluid and tissue samples. However, major problems with a limited sensitivity (range 45–82 %) have also become apparent in the fairly common culture negative variety of paucibacillar pleurisy (Ruiz-Manzano et al. 2000).

11.3.3 The Role of Thoracoscopy

The future role of thoracoscopy in the management of tuberculous pleurisy needs to be redefined (1) in the setting of the new diagnostic techniques outlined above and (2) in light of its close historical association with TB. From the very beginnings of thoracoscopy, when it was introduced into medicine by Jacobaeus in 1910, tuberculosis has been a main focus of "pleuroscopy" – as it was renamed in the early 1920s in Western Europe (Jacobaeus 1910; Loddenkemper 2004). Anticipating a modern minimally invasive interventional technique, all of which are included under the term VATS, his pioneering approach to thoracoscopy was interventional with a view to optimizing pneumolysis and mechanical breaking of strands for artificial pneumothorax induction in TB ("Jacobaeus' operation") (Loddenkemper 2004). Medical thoracoscopy has been developed over the decades and is now a powerful and gold standard tool for the management of tuberculous pleurisy. A large body of data now testifies to the diagnostic efficacy of thoracoscopy. The ability to visualize major portions of the pleural surface, to intervene when membranes and septa are present, and the additional option of performing numerous dedicated biopsies ensure an optimum diagnostic

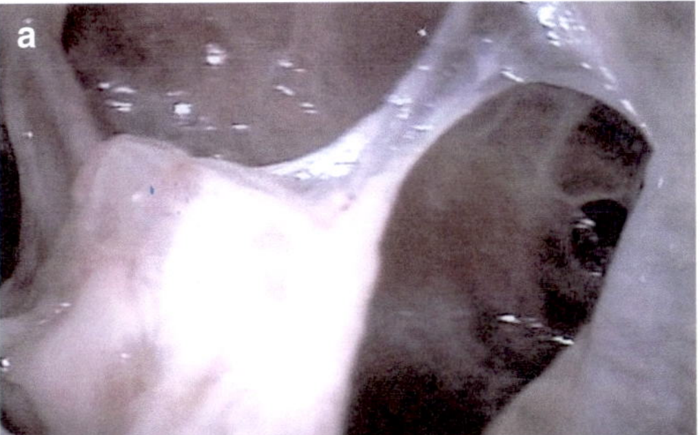
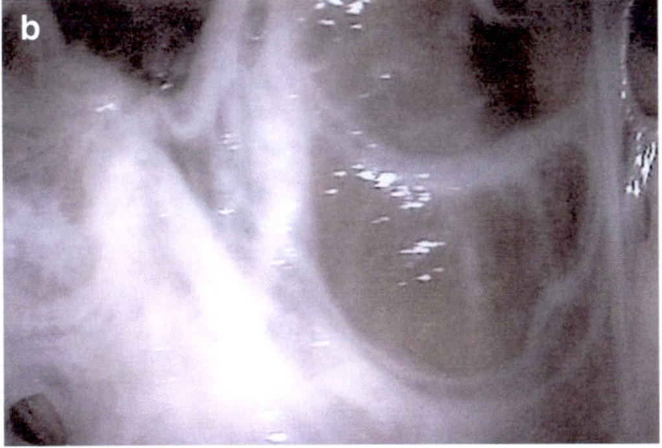

Fig. 11.6 Typical features of fibrin-type multiloculated effusion in tuberculous pleurisy. (**a**) Upper part of the pleural cavity. (**b**) Lower part of the pleural cavity

result. The combination of these features with the likely additional impact on outcome by thoracoscopy justifies the renewed interest and continued use of the traditional thoracoscopic approach in tuberculous pleurisy.

11.3.4 Procedure

The procedure employed is similar to that used in pleural effusion and parapneumonic effusion. At the time of visual exploration, as in bacterial empyema, three characteristic patterns may be found:

- First is the development of abundant fibrinous membranes, septa, and chambers with diffuse inflammation of the parietal pleura as the prevailing lesion. An example of this endoscopic aspect is shown in Fig. 11.6. Similar cautions should apply before introducing the thoracoscope as outlined previously in the section on multiloculated empyema, in order to prevent laceration of adhesive lung compartments.

Fig. 11.7 Typical features of disseminated, small sago-type nodules of the parietal pleura in tuberculous pleurisy (Courtesy C Boutin and Ph Astoul, Marseille, France)

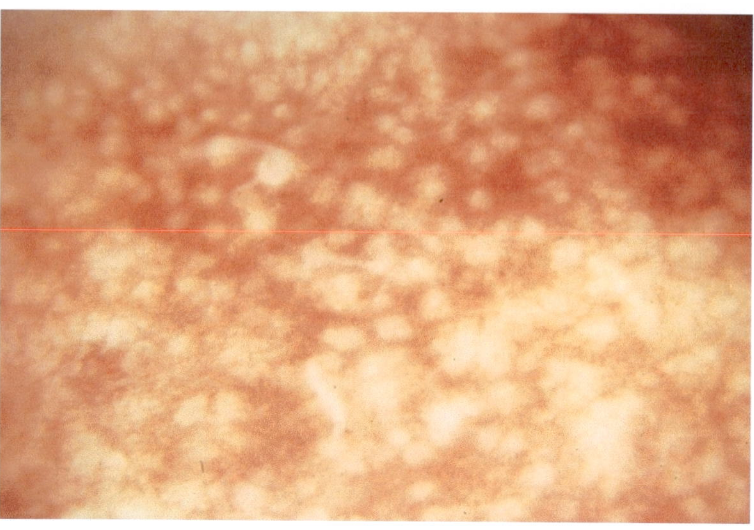

- A second characteristic feature is a varying degree of seeding of the pleural surface with solid or caseous, sago-like nodules and associated scanty fibrin deposits. A typical example is shown in Fig. 11.7. Although this is usually fairly small, when major or extensive lesions occur, they may easily be confused with disseminated malignant nodules (Fig. 11.8).

Tuberculous empyema may be indistinguishable from nonspecific empyema, unless visible calcifications, irreversible lung trapping, or suspect pulmonary changes suggest a tuberculous origin.

A sufficient number of biopsies should be obtained from the parietal pleura, i.e., at least six (Kirsch et al. 1997). This may often require debridement of membranes and opening of loculations to gain access to the inflamed parietal pleura. It is advisable to save recovered fibrinous material for additional microbiological investigations, since a positive culture yield has been described in a high proportion of these samples. Lung biopsies will usually not be required unless there is a suspect subvisceral lesion or evidence of spread of pulmonary disease to the pleura.

11.3.5 Diagnostic Yield

According to various authors, the overall diagnostic yield of thoracoscopy, including analysis of the pleural fluid, fibrinous membranes, and tissue specimens (combining microscopy, cultures, and histology together), is in the range of 94–99 % (Loddenkemper 1981, 2003; Loddenkemper and Boutin 1993; Colt 1999; Seijo and Sterman 2001). Thus, when thoracoscopic results are combined with the results of less invasive tests, the yield should be close to 100 % (Loddenkemper and Boutin 1993). The most important least invasive contribution is certainly provided by closed needle biopsy, which has a sensitivity of 50–60 %, as in the series reported by Loddenkemper (Loddenkemper and Boutin 1993). In one collective review, an average sensitivity of 69 % (28–88 %) is reported; however, these high sensitivities refer to areas of high prevalence of TB, which would suggest that the pretest probability was elevated (Seijo and Sterman 2001). In a recent study from South Africa, which combined conventional histological and microbiological investigations with novel methods (NAAT, ADA), a sensitivity of 93 % with 100 % specificity has been reported – this is approaching the diagnostic efficacy of thoracoscopy (Diacon et al. 2003). In future, it would therefore be wise to combine thoracoscopy and closed needle biopsy (which has the specific advantage of also exploring deeper chest wall structures) with novel biological methods. Needle biopsy is clearly advantageous if thoracoscopy is not available or in the presence of clinical obstacles such as an absolute contraindications to thoracoscopy or advanced obliteration

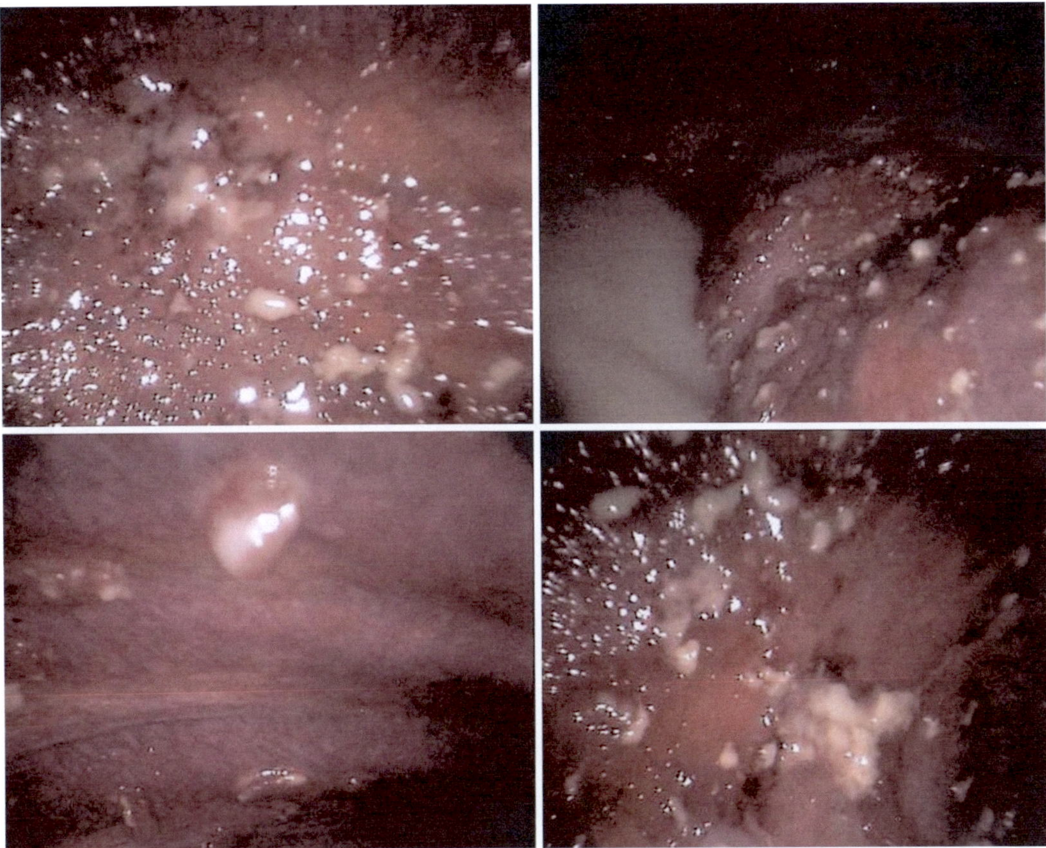

Fig. 11.8 Sago-type disseminated small and larger nodules on the parietal and visceral pleura concerning for malignancy

of the pleural space. In general, thoracoscopy and less invasive procedures should not be considered competitive alternatives but rather reciprocally supportive tools for obtaining optimum tissue specimens for mycobacterial cultures, susceptibility testing, and possibly also tissue-based NAAT. The importance of microbiological investigation of membranes and fibrinous material also needs to be emphasized, since with a maximum reported sensitivity of 87 % of this assessment, the yield may well exceed that of needle biopsy (Loddenkemper 1981).

11.3.6 Intervention Options and Outcome

Thoracoscopy not only allows but often even requires the opening of loculations and adhesions or even large-scale debridement and peeling of large membranes. While such efforts are not necessarily a regular part of the diagnostic exploration of the pleural cavity, they may be expected to modify and improve the clinical course in terms of more rapid resolution of effusion, shorter hospital stays, and improved outcomes and, in particular, avoid the development of long-term chest encasements and fibrothorax. However, no data exists from controlled clinical trials on this issue. In our view, the clinical benefit of complete evacuation of the pleura, including separation and removal of membranes, would seem evident. Similar beneficial effects certainly cannot be expected to result from the addition of an oral or parenteral steroid regimen to antituberculous drug therapy, since controlled studies did not demonstrate any impact on the endpoints – pleural sequelae and physiological abnormalities (Wyser et al. 1996).

11.4 Other Benign Inflammatory Effusions

11.4.1 Clinical Background

This group covers a number of heterogenous inflammatory conditions which may present with both specific and nonspecific biochemical and histological criteria. Their overall incidence is in the order of 10 % of all exudative effusions (although the incidences of some entities are purportedly higher). The clinical presentations of these conditions are highly variable, ranging from clinically silent cases to severe thoracic symptoms such as in acute thromboembolism. These effusions are rarely associated with a profuse collection and almost never displace the contralateral lung; however, they may occur bilaterally.

11.4.2 Prethoracoscopic Investigations

Once specific infectious etiologies can be consistently ruled out, the diagnostic investigation must focus on determining a series of immunologic and inflammatory parameters in both the pleural fluid and serum. Depending on the clinical background, these may include IgG and IgM rheumatoid factor, ADA, interleukin (IL)-2 receptors, complement components (3, 4, SC5b-9), antinuclear factors (ANA), c/p-ANCA, and double-stranded DNA and LE cells. The role of thoracoscopy in the management of this type of effusion may be considered to include attaining additional diagnostic certainty on the basis of dedicated tissue recovery and sometimes specific pathological macroscopic findings. Rarely there may be necessity for an intervention, such as draining a large compressive fluid collection. On the other hand, a small group of difficult-to-diagnose "idiopathic" effusions may even escape all combined diagnostic efforts.

11.4.3 Pulmonary Infarction

Epidemiological and clinical data on the frequency of thromboembolism-related pleural effusion is scarce and reports vary between different sources. According to Light and additional data originating from the Czech Republic, thromboembolism would appear to be the fourth leading cause of pleural effusion, i.e., it accounts for 18 % of all exudates, whereas in most series, it accounts for 5 % or less (Marel et al. 1993; Light 1995b). The issue is probably confounded by the fact that both hemodynamic and inflammatory mechanisms are involved, and hence the effusion may be both exudative and transudative. Nevertheless, these data imply that the clinical significance of thromboembolic effusion is probably largely underestimated, since many cases remain unidentified and are thus merged into a large subset of effusion of unclear ("idiopathic") origin. Key clues for the diagnosis include the sudden onset of chest symptoms, including hemoptysis, compatibility between laboratory and imaging findings such as a sharp rise in D-dimers, and high-probability lung scans. Pleural fluid analysis shows variable inflammatory patterns including eosinophilia, sometimes also hemorrhagic features, but in general, it is largely nonspecific. Thoracoscopy does not yield any specific findings. Even well-trained pulmonologists will rarely encounter an effusion that is unequivocally attributable to thromboembolism, and there is consequently a dearth of endoscopic pictorial documentation. Changes that give reason to suspect a thromboembolic origin of a nonmalignant effusion include a sanguineous or frankly hemorrhagic accumulation of fluid in the presence of sharply delineated hemorrhagic pulmonary changes or large-scale consolidation. Lung biopsies may finally confirm pulmonary infarction as the causative lesion.

11.4.4 Effusions Caused by Rheumatic and Collagen Vascular Disease

Effusions in *rheumatic and collagen vascular disease* share many features with those seen in thromboembolism, and their clinical significance is similarly likely to be underestimated. Pleural involvement is common in rheumatoid arthritis,

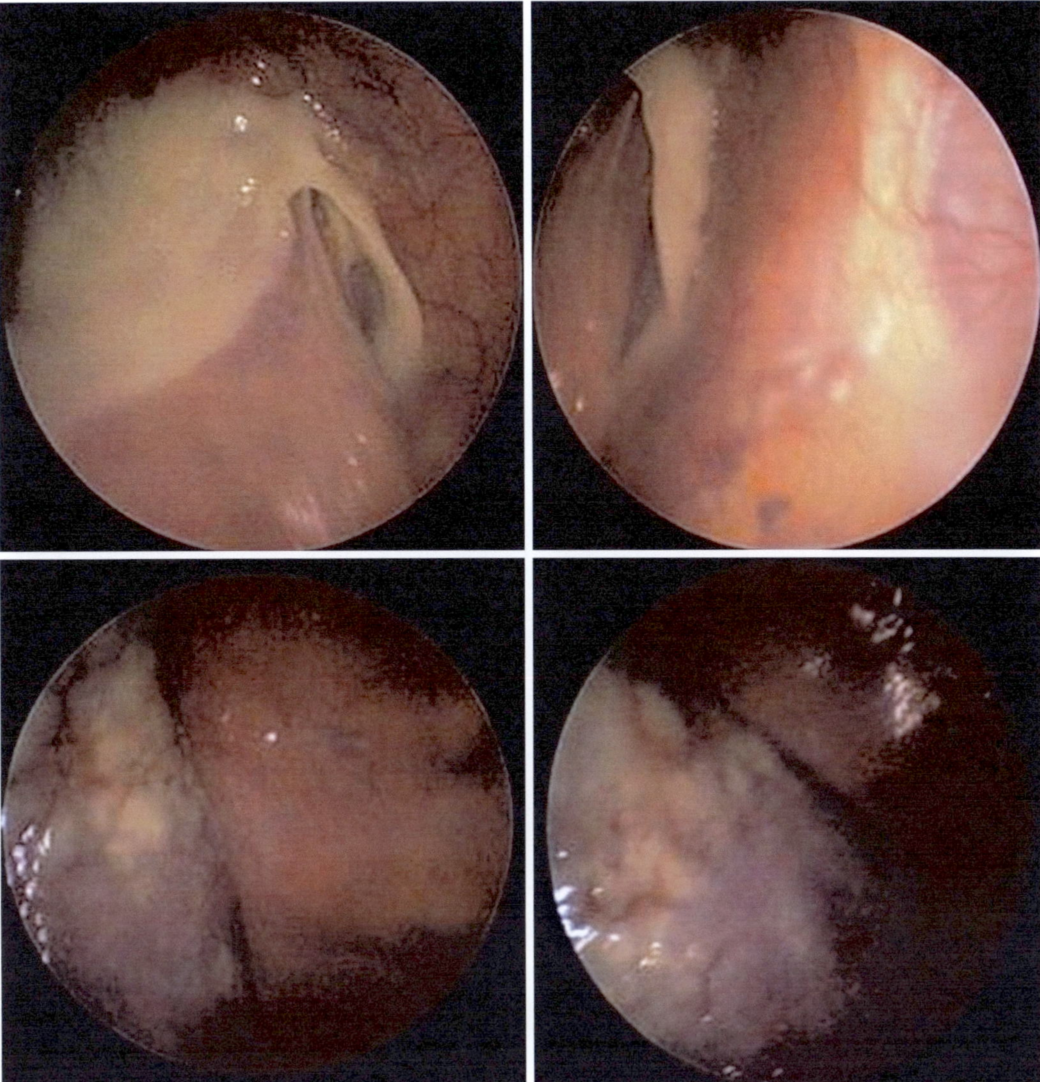

Fig. 11.9 A thoracoscopic image of an effusion in a patient with known rheumatoid arthritis showing both visceral and parietal fibrinous inflammation

occurring in about 5 % of patients, sometimes even as the primary manifestation (Joseph and Sahn 1993). However, in contrast to the situation with embolism, there are important inflammatory, immunologic, and histological markers and patterns which narrow or establish a diagnosis with sufficient certainty prior to thoracoscopy. One characteristic feature of rheumatoid effusions is a tendency for pleural fluids to have high cholesterol contents, hence the term "cholesterol pleurisy" a synonym for *pseudochylothorax*. The advantage of conducting thoracoscopy in rheumatic and connective tissue disease is that it provides visual guidance for obtaining more representative tissue specimens. Thoracoscopy frequently reveals diffuse or focal fibrinous lesions suggestive of rheumatoid arthritis with typical necrobiotic nodules on the visceral pleura (Fig. 11.9). The endoscopic equivalent of nongranulomatous collagen vascular disease is nonspecific diffuse pleural thickening and inflammation termed (*benign*) *pachypleuritis*; this often includes localized fibrin deposits. An

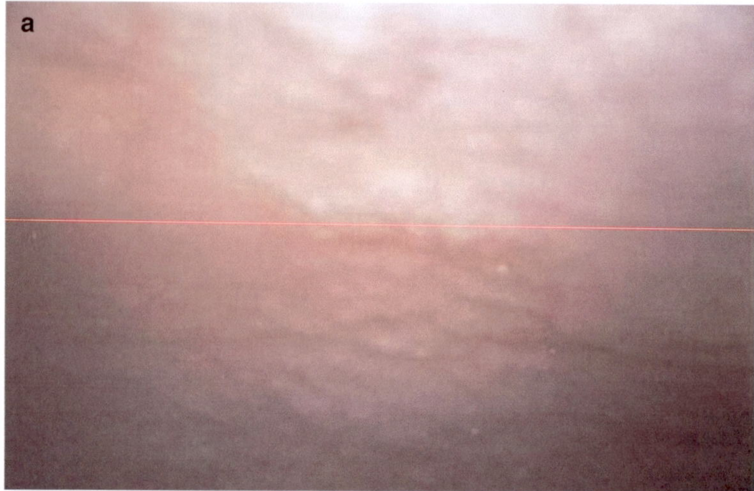

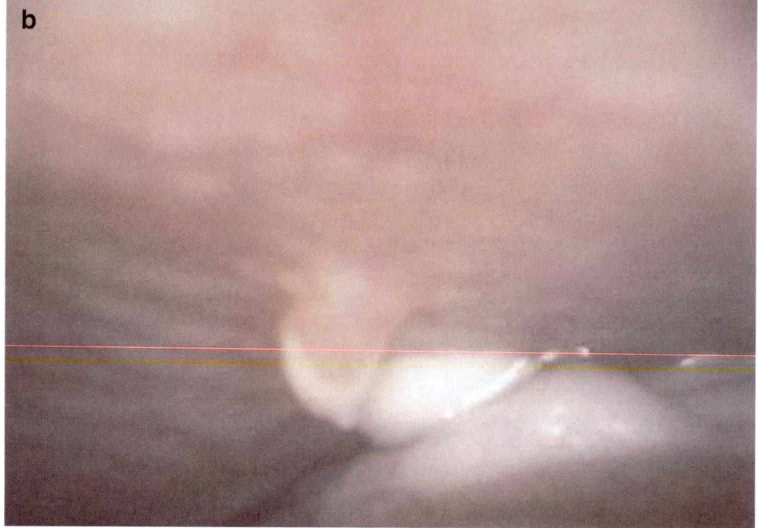

Fig. 11.10 A thoracoscopic image of an effusion in a patient with mixed connective tissue disease (MCTD) showing diffuse pleural thickening (pachypleuritis) and fibrin deposits. Female, 35 years, parietal pleura (**a**), chest wall, and diaphragm (**b**)

example of pleurisy in a case of mixed connective tissue disease (MCTD) is presented in Fig. 11.10). In systemic lupus erythematosus (SLE), the pleura is involved in approximately 40 % of patients. The presence of LE cells in the pleural fluid and tissue specimens is diagnostic for this disease, although the sensitivity is low (<50 %) (Orens et al. 1994).

11.4.5 Sarcoidosis

Sarcoidosis very rarely leads to pleural effusions (<1 %). The fluid is an exudate (and only in very rare cases a transudate) with a lymphocyte predominance. A small number of anecdotal cases with secondary *chylothorax* have also been described (Soskel and Sharma 2000). Nevertheless, occult sarcoidosis-related pleural involvement in the form of dry pleurisy is often clinically evident. When a thoracoscopy is performed to obtain a lung biopsy in undetermined interstitial lung disease, granulomas of the parietal and visceral pleura are not an uncommon incidental finding which strongly suggests sarcoidosis. The prevalence of nodules in sarcoidosis is reported between 11 and 71 %, depending on the source (Soskel and Sharma 2000). Figure 11.11 presents examples of typical parietal and visceral lesions which may be found in sarcoidosis.

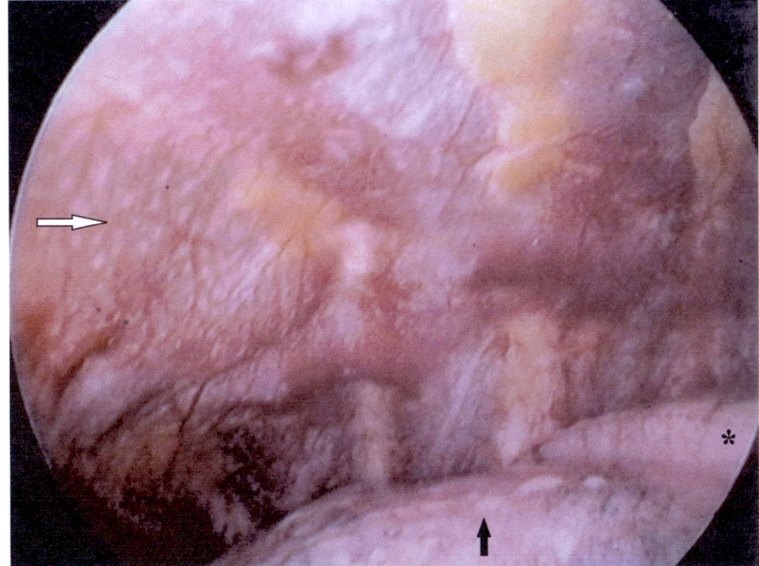

Fig. 11.11 Thoracoscopic image of pleural involvement in sarcoidosis showing disseminated nodules on the parietal pleural (*white arrow*) and on the surface of the lung (*black arrow*) – * fissure (Courtesy Ph Astoul, Marseille, France)

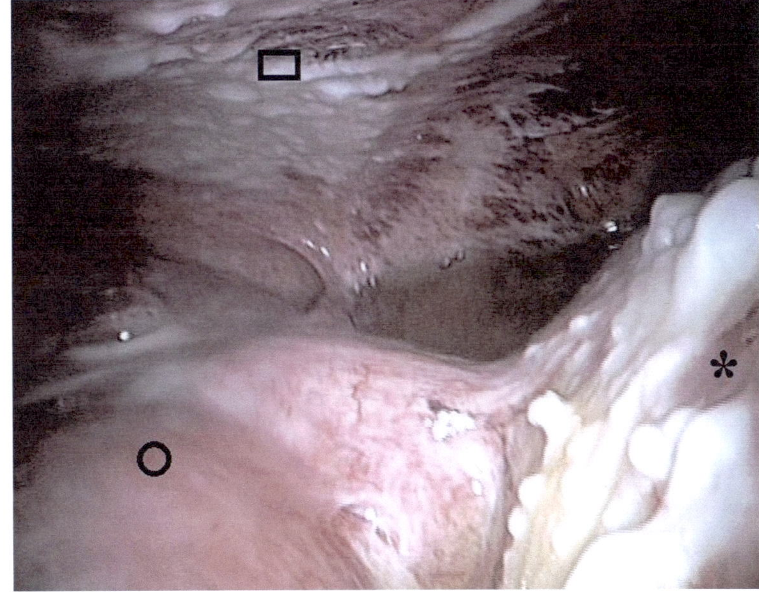

Fig. 11.12 A benign pleural effusion in asbestos-exposed patient. The left costodiaphragmatic gutter has residual fluid. Pleural plaques are located on the posterior parietal pleura (□). The left lower lobe is covered by a fibrotic layer (O). Pleural plaques are also visible on the diaphragm (*star*) (courtesy Ph Astoul, Marseille, France)

11.4.6 Benign Asbestos Pleurisy

Benign asbestos pleurisy is a component of the benign pleural asbestos complex. This also includes *pleural plaques, diffuse pleural thickening* (*pleural fibrosis*), and *rounded atelectasis*. Pleural effusions are believed to occur primarily in patients exposed to crocidolite and may coexist with pleural plaques. When exploring an otherwise undefined exudate during thoracoscopy or noninvasively with CT images, the finding of plaques strongly suggests an asbestos-related etiology. Since recurrent benign asbestos pleurisy, in particular, may be interpreted as a precursor of fibrosis and malignant transformation to mesothelioma, one objective of thoracoscopy is to scrutinize the pleural cavity carefully to exclude malignant lesions (Figs. 11.12 and 11.13). This may necessitate obtaining serial biopsies from all aspects of the parietal pleura (chest wall and

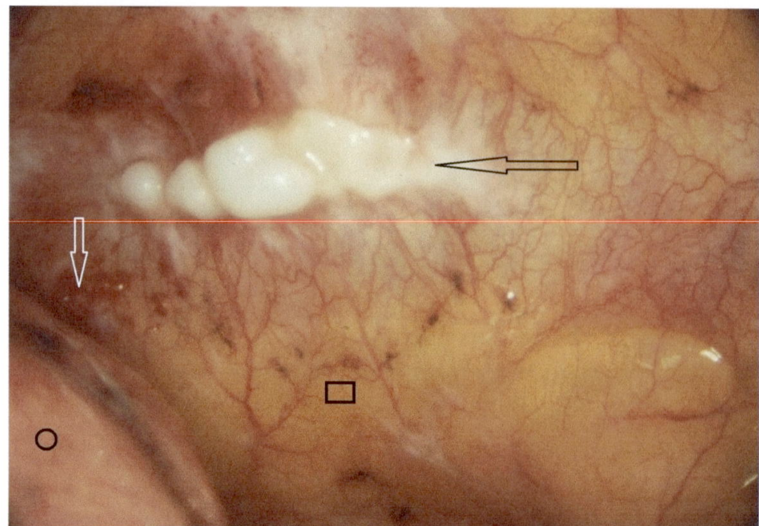

Fig. 11.13 A pleural effusion in an asbestos-exposed patient. Previous percutaneous pleural biopsies failed to obtain a diagnosis. A typical pleural plaque is visible on the posterior parietal pleura (*black arrow*). Careful examination of the pleural cavity identified anthracotic deposits (□) and small malignant nodules (*white arrow*). The diagnosis of epithelial malignant pleural mesothelioma was confirmed by pathological analysis. Lung (○) (Courtesy Ph Astoul, Marseille, France)

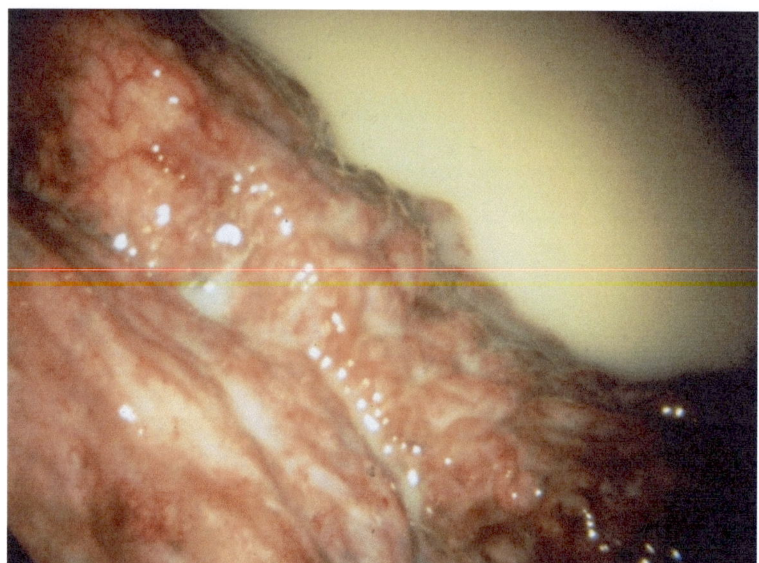

Fig. 11.14 A chylothorax is a rare cause of a pleural effusion. Thoracoscopy should rule out pleural lymphoma and multiple pleural biopsies are mandatory (Courtesy Ph Astoul, Marseille, France)

diaphragm). Apart from plaques, there are no characteristic findings in asbestos pleurisy except occasional eosinophilia, which may sometimes be marked. The establishment of the diagnosis depends largely on indirect evidence, i.e., confirmed evidence of asbestos exposure and exclusion of the differential diagnoses. Pleurodesis, performed either during thoracoscopy or surgically, has been suggested for recurrent effusion, but unless large-scale or total pleurectomy is carried out, this strategy forfeits the option of follow-up examinations for the early detection of mesothelioma.

11.4.7 Miscellaneous Rare Benign Effusions

The pleura may be affected by a large number of other extrapulmonary, systemic, and organ-related disease states such as gastrointestinal, renal, hepatic, heart, and even endocrine disease. The diagnosis of these conditions will usually concentrate on the primary organ, and pleural fluid studies and thoracoscopy have no specific contribution to make in cases with these underlying secondary disease states (Fig. 11.14). In some instances such effusions may be diagnosed incidentally when thoracoscopy is performed during the workup of an undiagnosed effusion.

11.5 Recurrent Idiopathic Pleural Effusion

Idiopathic pleural effusion, as pointed out earlier, is a collective term and merger of heterogenous benign, overwhelmingly exudative (i.e., inflammatory), occasionally transudative effusion which defies unequivocal allocation to defined disease states. The incidence varies in the literature from 5 to 17 %, obviously depending on the intensity of investigational efforts in excluding causative factors (Ryan et al. 1981; Menzies and Charbonneau 1991; Loddenkemper 2003). The "true" incidence of idiopathic effusion, or more importantly, whether it exists as an entity at all (!), remains basically contentious and unknown. Its quantitative significance may be analyzed in terms of follow-up and outcome studies after nondiagnostic thoracoscopy. The primary concern in this scenario is that of occult malignancy. When corrected for the false-negative rate of malignancy – which is in the range of 8 % – the remaining large fraction of true benign disease at thoracoscopy will contain a variable proportion of unexplained (idiopathic) effusions. In one series following 75 nonmalignant pleuritis cases at initial thoracoscopy for 34–48 months, the rate of unexplained pleuritis remained as high as 39 % (Venekamp et al. 2005). In another series which followed 66 patients with undiagnosed nonselected pleural effusion during the subsequent 12 months, 19 cases (29 %) were identified as truly benign. However in only 8 of these, the causative etiology could be convincingly established, 11 cases, i.e., a fraction as high as 17 % of nonselected exudates remained unexplained. For some undiagnosed effusions which were previously considered to be "idiopathic," the causative condition has been identified over time, for example, the *postcardiotomy syndrome*. Others cases may become apparent after an intensified search for remote causes of effusion such as familial *Mediterranean fever*, *yellow nail syndrome*, or a manifestation of various *drug adverse reactions*. In general, such "difficult-to-diagnose" cryptogenic effusions are rarely profuse, often bilateral and prone to spontaneous remissions but also recurrences. In clinical practice, the diagnosis should be made employing a pragmatic approach using a defined exclusion sequence where the level of diagnostic invasiveness will largely depend on the clinical presentation in terms of the extent and dynamics of the fluid collection. Spontaneous resolution of undetermined small effusions will usually obviate such efforts. On the other hand in profuse, persistent, or recurrent effusion of unexplained origin, an active strategy such as second-look ("redo") thoracoscopy or invasive escalation to surgery (VATS or even formal thoracotomy) may be an essential part of the diagnostic workup (Breen et al. 2008). The prognostic focus and diagnostic aim in these instances will be to definitively exclude occult malignancy. A final diagnosis of idiopathic benign effusion in cases presenting with either recurrent or chronic effusion should only be made reasonable after a thorough thoracoscopic exclusion process.

Endoscopic findings in nonmalignant effusion of unexplained origin may show highly variable but nonspecific features. One should keep in mind that chronic effusion from a number of completely different etiologies may induce similar secondary changes of the pleura. These include diffuse pleural thickening such as *pachypleuritis* or *diffuse fibrinous pleuritis*, which produces a characteristic "sugar powder" appearance of both pleural surfaces, and this is even true for long-standing transudates. Alternatively, the generation of membranous pleural thickening and loculations may eventually give rise to metabolic changes of the pleural fluid with the formation of "cholesterol pleurisy" (*pseudochylothorax*) as (and more typically) described in rheumatoid-associated pleural disease.

As for all exudative effusion, extensive sampling of the pleura is a mandatory part of the thoracoscopic exploration to exclude previously unsuspected specific tissue lesions and thus a distinct etiologic diagnosis.

References

Alfageme I, Munoz F, Pena N et al (1993) Empyema of the thorax in adults. Etiology, microbiologic findings, and management. Chest 103:839–843

Antunes G, Neville E, Duffy J et al (2003) BTS guidelines for the management of malignant pleural effusions. Thorax 58:ii29

Bouros JG, Schiza S, Patrurakis G et al (1997) Intrapleural streptokinase versus urokinase in the treatment of complicated parapneumonic effusions: a prospective double blind study. Am J Respir Crit Care Med 155:291–295

Boutin C, Viallat JR, Aelony Y (1991) Diagnostic thoracoscopy for pleural effusions. In: Boutin C, Viallat JR, Aelony Y (eds) Practical thoracoscopy. Springer, Berlin, pp 51–64

Breen D, Fraticelli A, Greillier L et al (2008) Redo medical thoracoscopy is feasible in patients with pleural disease: a series. Interact Cardiovasc Thorac Surg 8:330–338

Brutsche MH, Tassi GF, Gjörik S et al (2005) Treatment of sonographically stratified multiloculated thoracic empyema by medical thoracoscopy. Chest 128: 3303–3309

Colice GL, Curtis A, Deslauriers J et al (2000) Medical and surgical treatment of parapneumonic effusions: an evidence-based guideline. Chest 118:1158–1171

Colt HG (1999) Thoracoscopy: window to the pleural space. Chest 116:1409–1415

Davies CWH, Lok S, Davies RJ (1998) The systemic fibrinolytic activity of intrapleural streptokinase. Am J Respir Crit Care Med 157:328–330

Davies CWH, Gleeson FV, Davies RJO (2003) BTS guidelines for the management of pleural infection. Thorax 58(Suppl I):ii18–ii28

Diacon AH, van de Wal BW, Wyser C et al (2003) Diagnostic tools in tuberculous pleurisy: a direct comparative study. Eur Respir J 22:589–591

Diacon AH, Theron J, Schuurmans MM et al (2004) Intrapleural Streptokinase for Empyema and complicated parapneumonic effusions. Am J Respir Crit Care Med 170:49–53

Frank W (2002) Tuberculous pleural effusion. In: Loddenkemper R, Anthony VB (eds) Pleural diseases, European respiratory monograph, 22. European Respiratory Society Journals, Sheffield, pp 219–233

Heffner JE, Brown LK, Barbieri C et al (1995) Pleural fluid chemical analysis in parapneumonic effusions. A meta-analysis. Am J Respir Crit Care Med 151:1700–1708

Heffner JE, Brown LK, Barbieri C (1997) Diagnostic value of tests that discriminate exudative and transudative pleural effusions. Chest 111:970–979

Hersh CP, Feller-Kopman D, Wahidi M et al (2003) Ultrasound guidance for medical thoracoscopy: a novel approach. Respiration 70:299–301

Jacobaeus HC (1910) Über die Möglichkeit, die Zystoskopie bei Untersuchung seröser Höhlungen anzuwenden. Münch Med Wochenschr 40:2090–2092

Jacobaeus HC (1925) Die Thorakoskopie und ihre praktische Bedeutung. Ergeb Ges Med 7:112–166

Joseph J, Sahn SA (1993) Connective tissue disease and the pleura. Chest 104:262–270

Kirsch CM, Kroe DM, Azzi RL et al (1997) The optimal number of pleural biopsy specimens for a diagnosis of tuberculous pleurisy. Chest 112:334–343

Kolditz M, Halank M, Schiemanck CS et al (2006) High diagnostic accuracy of NT-pro BNP for cardiac origin of pleural effusions. Eur Respir J 28:144–150

Landreneau RJ, Keenan RJ, Hazelrigg SR et al (1995) Thoracoscopy for empyema. Chest 109:18–24

Light RW, Macgregor MI, Luchsinger PC et al (1972) Pleural effusions: the diagnostic separation of transudates and exudates. Ann Intern Med 77:507–513

Light RW (1995a) Pleural disease, 3rd edn. Williams & Wilkins, Baltimore, pp 36–74

Light RW (1995b) Approach to the patient. In: Light RW (ed) Pleural disease, 3rd edn. Williams & Wilkinson, Baltimore, pp 75–82

Loddenkemper R (1981) Thoracoscopy: results in noncancerous and idiopathic pleural effusions. Poumon Coeur 37:261–264

Loddenkemper R (2003) Medical thoracoscopy. In: Light RW, Lee GYC (eds) Textbook of pleural Diseases. Arnold, London, pp 505–509

Loddenkemper R (2004) Zur Geschichte und Zukunft der Thorakoskopie. Pneumologie 58:42–49

Loddenkemper R, Boutin C (1993) Thoracoscopy: present diagnostic and therapeutic indications. Eur Respir J 6:1544–1555

Loddenkemper R, Frank W (2006) Chest tubes and thoracoscopy. In: Fein AM, Kamholz S, Ost D (eds) Respiratory emergencies. Hodder Arnold, London, pp 123–143

Marel M, Arustova M, Stasny B et al (1993) Incidence of pleural effusion in a well-defined region: epidemiologic study in central Bohemia. Chest 104:1486–1489

Maskell NA, Davies RJO (2003) Effusions from parapneumonic infection and empyema. In: Light RW, Lee GYC (eds) Textbook of pleural diseases. Hodder Arnold, London, pp 310–328

Maskell NA, Davies CW, Nunn AJ et al (2005) First Multicenter Intrapleural Sepsis Trial (MIST1) Group. UK controlled trial of intrapleural streptokinase for pleural infection. N Engl J Med 352:865–874

Menzies R, Charbonneau M (1991) Thoracoscopy for the diagnosis of pleural disease. Ann Intern Med 114:271–276

Orens JB, Martinez FJ, Lynch JP (1994) Pleuropulmonary manifestations of systemic lupus erythematosus. Rheum Dis Clin North Am 20:159–193

Rahman NM, Maskell NA, West A et al (2011) Intrapleural use of tissue plasminogen activator and DNase in pleural infection. N Engl J Med 365:518–526

Ruiz-Manzano J, Monterola JM, Gamboa F et al (2000) Detection of mycobacterium tuberculosis in paraffin-embedded pleural biopsy specimens by commercial ribosomal RNA and DNA amplification kits. Chest 118:648–655

Ryan CJ, Rodgers RF, Unni KK et al (1981) The outcome of patients with pleural effusion of indeterminate cause at thoracotomy. Mayo Clin Proc 56:145–149

Seijo LM, Sterman DH (2001) Interventional pulmonology. N Engl J Med 344:740–749

Simpson G, Roomes D, Heron M (2000) Effects of streptokinase and desoxyribonuclease on the viscosity of human surgical and empyema pus. Chest 117:1728–1732

Söderblom T, Nyberg P, Am T et al (1996) Pleural fluid interferon gamma and tumor necrosis factor in tuberculous and rheumatoid pleurisy. Eur Respir J 9:1652–1655

Solèr M, Wyser C, Bolliger CT et al (1997) Treatment of early parapneumonic empyema by "medical" thoracoscopy. Schweiz Med Wochenschr 127:1748–1753

Soskel NT, Sharma OP (2000) Pleural involvement in sarcoidosis. Curr Opin Pulm Med 6:455–468

Tokuda Y, Matsushima D, Stein GH et al (2006) Intrapleural fibrinolytic agents for empyema and complicated parapneumonic effusions: a meta-analysis. Chest 129:783–790

Valdes L, Alvares D, San Jose E (1995) Value of adenosin deaminase in the diagnosis of tuberculous pleural effusions in young patients in a region of high prevalence of tuberculosis. Thorax 50:600–603

Venekamp LN, Velkeniers B, Noppen M (2005) Does 'Idiopathic Pleuritis' exist? Natural history of nonspecific pleuritis diagnosed after thoracoscopy. Respiration 72:74–78

Weiss JM, Spodick DH (1984) Laterality of pleural effusion in congestive heart failure. Am J Cardiol 53:951–953

Weissberg D (1980) Diagnostic and therapeutic pleuroscopy. Chest 78:732–735

Wyser C, Walzl G, Smedema JP (1996) Corticosteroids in the treatment of tuberculous pleurisy: a double-blind, placebo-controlled randomised study. Chest 110:333–338

Management of Spontaneous Pneumothorax: Common Sense Should Prevail

Jean-Marie Tschopp and Philippe Astoul

The management of spontaneous pneumothorax (SP) has been debated over the last two decades and lacks from good scientific evidence (Schramel et al. 1997; Miller 2008). However most will agree that the choice of treatment offered to patients with SP should be cost-effective and based on robust scientific evidence. The primary principle should be primum non nocere, first do no harm, i.e., the basis of medicine over the centuries. In other words, our responsibility should be to offer a beneficial treatment with minimal side effects. In addition, most experts agree that there are two aims when treating SP: to evacuate air, if necessary, and to prevent recurrences.

There is a general consensus that the first episode of primary SP, if occurring without symptoms, can be treated with either observation or simple aspiration, and this is supported by good evidence from many randomized controlled trials (Harvey and Prescott 1994; Andrivet et al. 1995; Noppen et al. 2002a). However this is not reflected in daily hospital practice as documented by Grundy and Bentley (see chapter 13). We also know that many patients who present with a first episode of primary SP still receive, as routine treatment, a chest tube insertion, although it has been clearly shown that a chest tube does not bring more benefit to the patient and indeed is more painful than simple aspiration (Ayed et al. 2006; Marquette et al. 2006). Recently, Miller advised a more evolved view on the treatment of pneumothorax than immediately using a large-bore intercostal tube (Miller 2008). This initial method of drainage of primary spontaneous pneumothorax should now be considered as unacceptable medical practice (Astoul 2010).

Irrespective of the type of drainage used, it is of critical important to manage the pain associated with the chosen treatment. When the first randomized controlled trial comparing chest tube drainage with simple thoracoscopic talc poudrage was performed, we learned an important lesson (Tschopp et al. 2002). Seven European institutions participated in this study; two out of the seven centers did not give any opioids at all – even to patients undergoing talc poudrage. Pain score as measured by VAS was significantly greater after talc poudrage than chest tube insertion. This finding disappeared when patients from the two centers were excluded from the analysis. These were European reference centers for the treatment of pleural diseases. This demonstrates that as clinicians, we sometimes forget to ask patients about pain, although it is accepted that opioids are safe and efficient to treat this unpleasant symptom.

The second aim in the management of SP is therefore to prevent recurrence; this occurs in about

J.-M. Tschopp (✉)
Département de Médecine Interne
Centre valaisan de pneumologie,
CHCVs, Montana 3963, Switzerland
e-mail: jean-marie.tschopp@hopitalvs.ch

P. Astoul
Division of Thoracic Oncology,
Pleural Diseases, and Interventional Pulmonology,
Hôpital NORD, Marseille, France
e-mail: pastoul@ap-hm.fr

P. Astoul et al. (eds.), *Thoracoscopy for Pulmonologists*,
DOI 10.1007/978-3-642-38351-9_12, © Springer-Verlag Berlin Heidelberg 2014

30 % of patients after a first episode of primary SP. As discussed in the next article, there are many approaches to prevent recurrences ranging from surgery such as thoracotomy, minithoracotomy, or video-assisted thoracic surgery (VATS) to noninvasive techniques such as medical thoracoscopy with talc poudrage. It has been clearly shown for many decades (Almind et al. 1989; Boutin et al. 1991; Bresticker et al. 1993; Tschopp et al. 1997) that the recurrence rate after performing simple talc poudrage under thoracoscopy is similar to the recurrence rate associated with the surgical treatment of SP. Therefore medical thoracoscopy is truly mininvasive, cost-effective, and safe as no serious side effects have ever been recorded with the graded talc we commonly use in Europe (Janssen et al. 2007; Bridevaux et al. 2011). This is contrary to the safety profile associated with the talc used in USA or Brazil (Werebe et al. 1999; Campos et al. 1997). Moreover the cost of this simple procedure performed under local anesthesia is about one fifth that of any surgical treatment including VATS as suggested in a noncontrolled study (Schramel et al. 1996) and later confirmed in our multicenter European randomized study (Tschopp et al. 2002). There was no difference in total calculated costs between the arm with chest tube drainage and the arm with talc poudrage. Moreover, in this cost calculation, costs of hospital readmission were not taken into account, although it was certainly higher in the group who only had chest tube drainage as compared with the group who had pleurodesis via talc poudrage (the observed relapse rate of SP after 5 years of follow-up was 27 % (chest tube drainage) versus 5 % (talc poudrage)). Cardillo et al. confirmed these results by presenting a prospective study which enrolled more than 800 cases and confirmed the previous reported findings already shown by an Israeli group (Cardillo et al. 2006; Weissberg and Refaely 2000). One explanation to the paucity of scientific evidence might be that talc is considered as dangerous, based on many studies performed in English-speaking countries, which contrasts with the results obtained in Europe over the last 50 years. Short-term safety was questionable; even serious complications are extremely rare and have only been observed in studies from the USA, Brazil, and New Zealand (Sahn 2002). The

occurrence of these serious complications seemed to be independent of the underlying disorder (malignant effusion or pneumothorax), the volume of talc used (2–10 g), or the method of administration (slurry or poudrage). Talc dissemination has been observed in virtually all organs when North American or Brazilian talc was used (Kennedy et al. 1995; Werebe et al. 1999) but not when extremely high doses were used (Montes et al. 2003), whereas no talc dissemination occurred when European, size-calibrated talc was used (Fraticelli et al. 2002). These differences can be attributed to the variations in talc preparations due to the number or proportion of small-sized talc particles (Ferrer et al. 2001). Small particle-sized talc causes lung damages, more inflammation, and impaired gas exchange than large particle-sized talc (Maskell et al. 2004). There has been now many animal and clinical studies demonstrating that the talc used in Europe is safe and does not provoke ARDS when used in the management of cases with recurrent SP (Noppen 2007; Bridevaux 2011) and as already published in the higher risk patient population with poor performance status, i.e., in patients with malignant pleural effusion (Janssen et al. 2007), and more recently the safety profile was also confirmed in more than 350 patients treated by simple talc poudrage after recurrence of SP, i.e., young patients in good health (Bridevaux et al. 2011). Nowadays regarding to the long-term safety of talc poudrage, we can briefly summarize this procedure does not cause pulmonary fibrosis, significant impairment of pulmonary function, and pleural cancer (Tschopp 1997; Lange et al. 1988; Viskum et al. 1989) and does not preclude VATS re-intervention (Doddoli et al. 2004).

References

Almind M, Lange P, Viskum K (1989) Spontaneous pneumothorax: comparison of simple drainage, talc pleurodesis, and tetracycline pleurodesis. Thorax 44:627–630

Andrivet P, Djedaini K, Teboul JL et al (1995) Spontaneous pneumothorax. Comparison of thoracic drainage vs immediate or delayed needle aspiration. Chest 108: 335–339

Astoul P (2010) Editorial comment: management of primary spontaneous pneumothorax: a plea for a mini-invasive approach. Eur J Cardiothorac Surg 37:1135–1136

Ayed AK, Chandrasekaran C, Sukumar M (2006) Video-assisted thoracoscopic surgery for primary spontaneous pneumothorax: clinicopathological correlation. Eur J Cardiotorac Surg 29:221–225

Boutin C, Viallat JR, Aelony Y (1991) Diagnostic thoracoscopy for pleural effusions. In: Boutin C, Viallat JR, Aelony Y (eds) Practical thoracoscopy. Springer, Berlin, pp 51–64

Bresticker MA, Oba J, LoCicero J 3rd (1993) Optimal pleurodesis: a comparison study. Ann Thorac Surg 55:364–366

Bridevaux PO, Tschopp JM, Cardillo G et al (2011) Short-term safety of thoracoscopic talc pleurodesis for recurrent primary spontaneous pneumothorax: a prospective European multicentre study. Eur Respir J 38:770–773

Campos JR, Werebe EC, Vargas FS et al (1997) Respiratory failure due to insufflated talc. Lancet 349:251–252

Cardillo G, Carleo F, Giunti R et al (2006) Videothoracoscopic talc poudrage in primary spontaneous pneumothorax: a single-institution experience in 861 cases. J Thorac Cardiovasc Surg 131:322–328

Doddoli C, Barlési F, Fraticelli A, Thomas P, Astoul P, Giudicelli R, Fuentes P (2004) Video-assisted thoracoscopic management of recurrent primary spontaneous pneumothorax after prior talc pleurodesis: a feasible, safe and efficient treatment option. Eur J Cardiothorac Surg 26:889–892

Ferrer J, Villarino MA, Tura JM (2001) Talc preparations used for pleurodesis vary markedly from one preparation to another. Chest 119:1901–1905

Fraticelli A, Robaglia-Schlupp A, Riera A et al (2002) Distribution of calibrated talc after intrapleural administration: an experimental study in rats. Chest 122:1737–1741

Harvey J, Prescott RJ (1994) Simple aspiration versus intercostal tube drainage for spontaneous pneumothorax in patients with normal lungs. British Thoracic Society Research Committee. BMJ 309:1338–1339

Janssen JP, Collier G, Astoul P et al (2007) Safety of pleurodesis with talc poudrage in malignant pleural effusion: a prospective cohort study. Lancet 369:1535–1539

Kennedy L, Harley RA, Sahn SA et al (1995) Talc slurry pleurodesis: pleural fluid and histologic analysis. Chest 107:1707–1712

Lange P, Mortensen J, Groth S (1988) Lung function 22–35 years after treatment of idiopathic spontaneous pneumothorax with talc poudrage or simple drainage. Thorax 43:559–561

Marquette CH, Marx A, Leroy S et al (2006) Simplified stepwise management of primary spontaneous pneumothorax: a pilot study. Eur Respir J 27:470–476

Maskell NA, Lee YC, Gleeson FV et al (2004) Randomized trials describing lung inflammation after pleurodesis with talc of varying particle size. Am J Respir Crit Care Med 170:377–382

Miller AC (2008) Spontaneous pneumothorax. In: Light RW, Garry Lee Lee YC (eds) Textbook of pleural diseases, 2nd edn. Hodder Arnold, London, pp 515–532

Montes JF, Ferrer J, Villarino MA et al (2003) Influence of talc dose on extrapleural talc dissemination after talc pleurodesis. Am J Respir Crit Care Med 168:1648–1654

Noppen M (2007) Who's (still) afraid of talc? Eur Respir J 29:619–621

Noppen M, Alexander P, Driesen P et al (2002a) Manual aspiration versus chest tube drainage in first episodes of primary spontaneous pneumothorax: a multicenter, prospective, randomized pilot study. Am J Respir Crit Care Med 165:1240–1244

Noppen M et al (2002b) Pleural diseases: pneumothorax. Eur Respir Mon 22:279–296

Sahn SA (2002) Is talc indicated for pleurodesis? Pro: talc should be used for pleurodesis. J Bronchol 61:35–38

Schramel FM, Sutedja TG, Braber JC et al (1996) Cost-effectiveness of video-assisted thoracoscopic surgery versus conservative treatment for first time or recurrent spontaneous pneumothorax. Eur Respir J 9:1821–1825

Schramel FM et al (1997) Current aspects of spontaneous pneumothorax. Eur Respir J 10:1372–1379

Tschopp JM, Brutsche M, Frey JG (1997) Treatment of complicated spontaneous pneumothorax by simple talc pleurodesis under thoracoscopy and local anaesthesia. Thorax 52:329–332

Tschopp JM, Boutin C, Astoul P et al (2002) Talcage by medical thoracoscopy for primary spontaneous pneumothorax is more cost-effective than drainage: a randomised study. Eur Respir J 20:1003–1009

Viskum K, Lange P, Mortensen J (1989) Long-term sequelae after talc pleurodesis for spontaneous pneumothorax. Pneumologie 43:105–106

Weissberg D, Refaely Y (2000) Pneumothorax: experience with 1,199 patients. Chest 117:1279–1285

Werebe EC, Pazetti R, Milanez de Campos JR et al (1999) Systemic distribution of talc after intrapleural administration in rats. Chest 115:190–193

Thoracoscopy for Spontaneous Pneumothorax

13

Seamus Grundy and Andrew Bentley

13.1 Introduction

Spontaneous pneumothorax is a relatively common disease with an incidence for primary spontaneous pneumothorax (PSP) of 18–28/100,000 per year in males and 1.8–6/100,000 per year in females (Henry et al. 2003) and rates for secondary spontaneous pneumothorax (SSP) of 6.3/100,000 in males and 2.0/100,000 in females (Melton et al. 1979). Despite the publication of numerous national and international guidelines, there remains debate over the best way to manage both primary and secondary pneumothorax. After a first episode of primary pneumothorax, the 5-year recurrence rate without pleurodesis/pleural abrasion is 30–50 % (Sadicot et al. 1997). Debate remains over the best time for a definitive procedure to prevent recurrence and indeed what the best form of intervention is either apical pleurectomy/pleural abrasion +/- bullectomy via VATS or thoracotomy or medical thoracoscopy with talc poudrage. Medical thoracoscopy can be a safe and effective method for offering recurrence prevention (Boutin et al. 1991), but is not widely accepted. Current UK guidelines do not include medical thoracoscopy for definitive recurrence prevention of PSP (Henry et al. 2003).

In this chapter we will review the classification and pathology of spontaneous pneumothorax and summarise the management strategies for the initial management of pneumothorax. Recurrence prevention strategies for spontaneous pneumothoraces will be discussed, in particular the role of medical thoracoscopy compared with surgical techniques. An outline of the practicalities of medical thoracoscopy will also be described.

13.2 Classification

Pneumothorax can be classified as spontaneous or traumatic (Table 13.1). Spontaneous pneumothorax is then further subclassified into primary and secondary spontaneous pneumothorax (Miller 2008). Primary spontaneous pneumothorax occurs

S. Grundy (✉)
NIHR Translational Research Facility,
University Hospital of South Manchester,
Manchester M23 9LT, UK
e-mail: seamus.grandy@manchester.ac.uk

A. Bentley
Department of Respiratory & Intensive Care
Medicine, North West Lung Center, Manchester
Academic Health Science Centre, University Hospital
of South Manchester, Manchester, UK
e-mail: andrew.bentley@manchester.ac.uk

Table 13.1 Classification of pneumothorax

Type	Aetiology
Primary spontaneous	No underlying lung disease (but blebs/bullae commonly present)
Secondary spontaneous	Associated with underlying lung disease, e.g. COPD, Cystic Fibrosis, AIDS
Traumatic	Related to trauma to the thorax
Iatrogenic	Secondary to transthoracic or transbronchial lung biopsy (10 %), central venous catheterisation, supraclavicular nerve block

P. Astoul et al. (eds.), *Thoracoscopy for Pulmonologists*,
DOI 10.1007/978-3-642-38351-9_13, © Springer-Verlag Berlin Heidelberg 2014

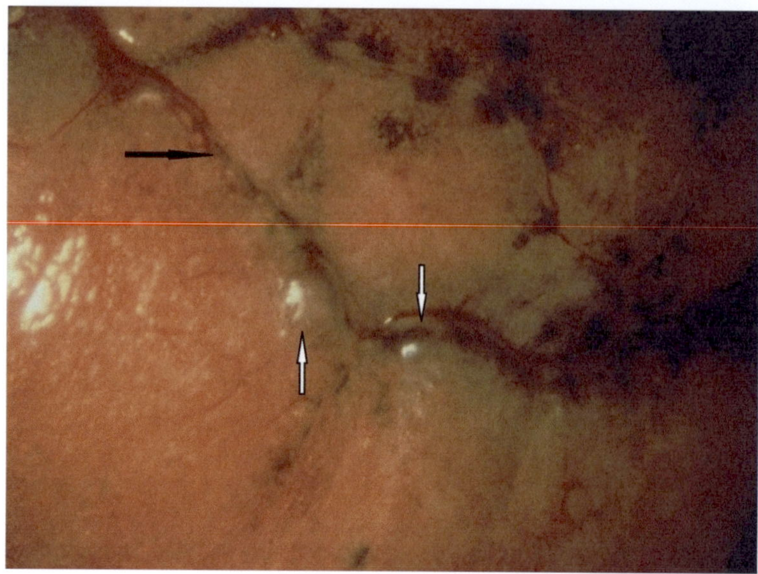

Fig. 13.1 Small blebs in spontaneous pneumothorax. The blebs (*white arrows*), close to the fissure (*black arrow*) and are visible at thoracoscopy with high-quality optical magnification. Anthracotic deposits are located on the surface of the lung (Courtesy C Boutin and Ph Astoul, Marseille, France)

in the presence of no underlying lung disease, whereas secondary pneumothorax occurs in association with underlying lung disease. The most common associated pathologies are COPD, emphysema and in association with AIDS and asthma. However secondary pneumothorax can occur in association with any pulmonary pathology.

13.3 Pathology

Spontaneous pneumothorax, both primary and secondary, has been shown to be associated with the presence of pleural blebs/bullae – also termed 'emphysema like changes' (Figs. 13.1, 13.2, and 13.3). Blebs/bullae are visible on CT scanning in 89 % of patients with PSP (Mitlehner et al. 1992), in 90 % of cases at visual inspection using video-assisted thoracoscopy (Mouroux et al. 1996) and up to 100 % of cases at thoracotomy (Donohue et al. 1993). It has long been assumed that the cause of spontaneous pneumothorax is rupture of these blebs/bullae (Light 2001). Despite this widely held opinion, there is no direct evidence which confirms rupture of blebs/bullae as the cause of SP. An Electron microscopy study of resected tissue has failed to confirm the presence of rupture in any blebs/bullae (Ohata et al. 1980). More recently, an elegant study using

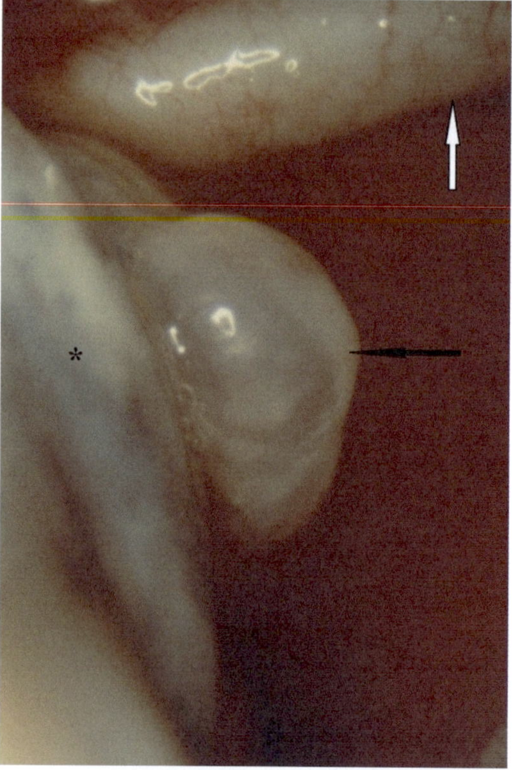

Fig. 13.2 Blebs (*black arrow*) on the apical surface of the lung (*). This translucent and fragile blister has a very thin, nonvascularised wall and is very frequently found in patient with primary spontaneous pneumothorax. In this case it is very close to the subclavian artery (*white arrow*) (Courtesy C Boutin and Ph Astoul, Marseille, France)

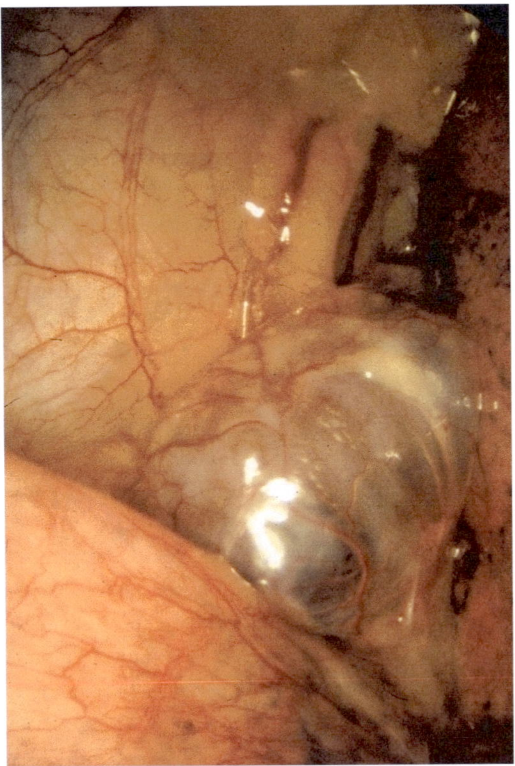

Fig. 13.3 Emphysematous bullae with a vascularised surface and a size usually superior than 2 cm in diameter. In this case, the bullae are inflated and therefore it is not the cause of the spontaneous pneumothorax (Courtesy Ph Astoul, Marseille, France)

fluorescein-enhanced autofluorescence at thoracoscopy to study the visceral pleura of patients with spontaneous pneumothorax has shown that patients who have spontaneous pneumothorax have evidence of diffuse pleural abnormalities at sites not associated with pleural blebs/bullae. Interestingly this study noted areas of air leak in a small proportion of patients. None of the observed air leaks were directly associated with pleural bullae (Noppen et al. 2006).

PSP has been shown to be associated with an inflammatory process within the lung, with increased numbers of inflammatory cells, particularly macrophages present in bronchoalveolar lavage (Schramel et al. 1995), and the histology of resected lung reveals the presence of an obstructive bronchiolitis (Lichter et al. 1971). Furthermore, the risk of recurrence cannot be predicted by the presence of blebs/bullae either at thoracoscopy (Janssen et al. 1995) or on CT imaging (Martinez-Ramos et al. 2007). It has been hypothesised that the site of air leak is actually distant to the blebs/bullae and related to increased distal airways pressures consequent to obstructive bronchiolitis (Noppen et al. 2002b). It is important to bear in mind that the site of air leak is unlikely to be solely from the blebs/bullae when we later consider recurrence prevention techniques (Fig. 13.4).

Fig. 13.4 Spontaneous pneumothorax due to the rupture (*black arrow*) of a large emphysematous bullae on the lung apex (*white arrow*). However the site of air leak is unlikely to be solely from the blebs/bullae when we consider recurrence prevention techniques (* parietal pleura) (Courtesy C Boutin and Ph Astoul, Marseille, France)

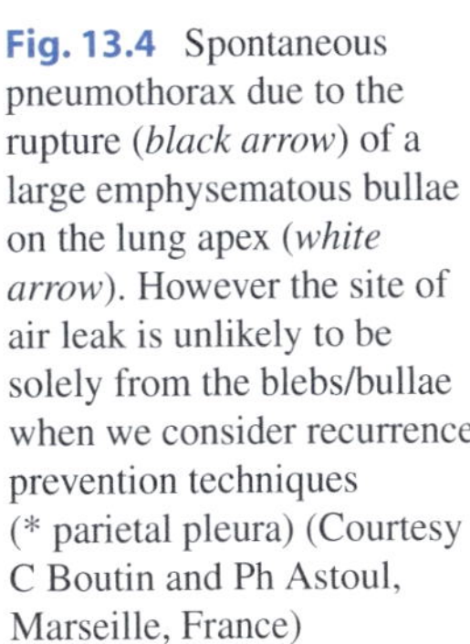

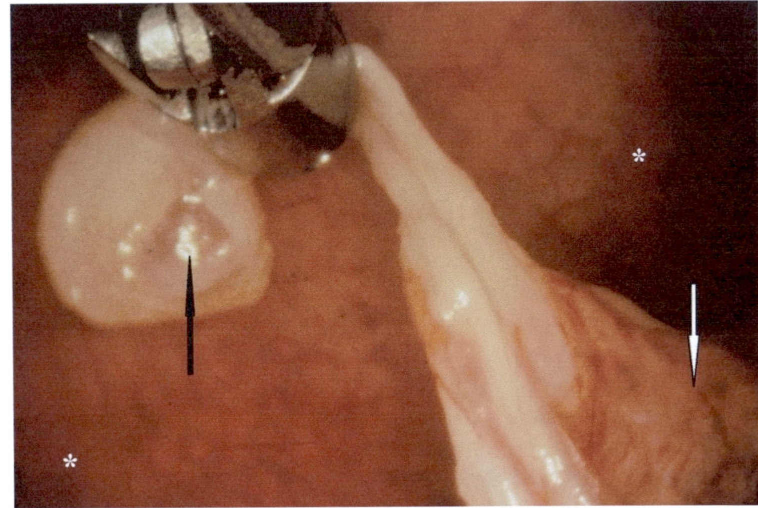

13.4 Management of Spontaneous Pneumothorax

13.4.1 Initial Treatment

There are a number of published guidelines which make recommendations regarding the management of both primary and secondary spontaneous pneumothorax (Henry et al. 2003; Baumann et al. 2001). There are differences between the guidelines which highlight the fact that the optimal management strategy for spontaneous pneumothorax is yet to be defined. Detailed discussion of the initial management of spontaneous pneumothorax is beyond the scope of this chapter but includes observation, pleural aspiration and intercostal drainage. The choice of initial treatment option depends upon the size of the pneumothorax, the physiological impact on the patient and whether there is underlying pulmonary disease (Marquette et al. 2006). Small pneumothoraces which have minimal physiological impact on the patient can safely be observed without invasive intervention. If removal of air is warranted, then the initial approach should be simple aspiration (Astoul 2010). This has been conclusively shown in randomised controlled trials to be equally effective as intercostal drain insertion with a success rate of approximately 80 % (Noppen et al. 2003; Andrivet et al. 1995; Ayed et al. 2006; Harvey and Prescott 1994). If aspiration is unsuccessful or the patient is severely compromised, then an intercostal drain should be inserted. The presence of underlying pulmonary disease lowers the threshold for consideration of insertion of an intercostal drain rather than simple aspiration. Accurate estimation of the size of a pneumothorax on a plain chest radiograph can be difficult but for clinical purposes is guided by the distance of the lung edge from the cupola/chest wall. A distance of >2 cm should be regarded as significant.

13.4.2 Recurrence Prevention

Spontaneous pneumothorax is associated with a significant recurrence rate. After a first primary spontaneous pneumothorax treated without any form of pleurodesis, the recurrence rate is approximately 30 % with most recurrences occurring in the first 2 years (Schramel et al. 1997). The recurrence rate increases significantly after a second and third episode to 62 and 83 % respectively (Gobbel et al. 1963). Independent risk factors for recurrence of a primary spontaneous pneumothorax include ongoing cigarette smoking, increasing age and height (Lippert et al. 1991). The risk of recurrence after a secondary spontaneous pneumothorax is higher than that for a primary spontaneous pneumothorax (Lippert et al. 1991) approaching 40–50 % with similar independent risk factors to PSP. Importantly, the presence of blebs/bullae either ipsilaterally or contralaterally is not predictive of recurrence (Martinez-Ramos et al. 2007) and hence should not be used to guide management decisions. Given the risk of recurrence, particularly after a second PSP, recurrence prevention is an important aspect of the management of spontaneous pneumothorax.

Procedures available for recurrence prevention include pleurodesis through an intercostal drain with talc (Almind et al. 1989), medical thoracoscopy with talc poudrage and surgical intervention with a combination of treatment of blebs/bullae (bullectomy/wedge resection/stapling of bullae) and a form of pleurodesis either chemical or with abrasion or subtotal pleurectomy. The surgical interventions can be carried out through video-assisted thoracic surgery (VATS) or via thoracotomy. Table 13.2 summarises the reported efficacy of these different approaches.

Pleurodesis through an intercostal drain is less effective than other treatment options with a recurrence rate of 8–13 % depending on the pleurodesing agent used – with talc shown to be the most effective agent (Almind et al. 1989). However this technique should be considered for those either unwilling or unfit to undergo more invasive procedures (Kennedy et al. 1995). The reason for the lower efficacy of pleurodesis without visualisation of the pleura (slurry) may be related to the inability to confirm diffuse spread of the pleurodesing agent.

For all other patients, a more invasive approach should be taken. There are proponents for both

Table 13.2 Different approaches for the management of recurrent spontaneous pneumothorax

Reference	Technique	Procedure	PSP/SSP/mixed	Success rate (%)
Athanassiadi et al. (1998)	Thoracotomy	Stapling of bullae + pleural abrasion	Mixed	99
Korner et al. (1996)	Thoracotomy	Wedge resection	Mixed	95
Ayed and Raghunathan (2000)	VATS	Stapling of bullae + pleural abrasion	Mixed	95
Lang-Lazdunski (2003)	VATS	Bleb excision/pleural abrasion	PSP	97
Maskell et al. (2004)	MT	TP	SSP	95
Tschopp et al. (1997)	MT	TP	Mixed	95
Tschopp et al. (2002)	MT	TP	PSP	95

Abbreviations: *MT* medical thoracoscopy, *PSP* primary spontaneous pneumothorax, *SSP* secondary spontaneous pneumothorax, *TP* talc poudrage

surgical intervention and medical thoracoscopy. A dearth of randomised controlled trials comparing the different approaches makes it difficult to say with certainty what the best approach is. The 'gold standard' in terms of recurrence prevention remains intervention via thoracotomy (Henry et al. 2003) as this has been shown to have a very high success rate approaching 100 % in some series (Nkere et al. 1994; Athanassiadi et al. 1998), but most surgeons prefer VATS (Baumann et al. 2001) which is associated with less cost and has lower rates of morbidity and mortality (Crisci et al. 1996). VATS procedures are much more commonly performed in the current era compared to thoracotomy. VATS procedures are acknowledged to have a slightly lower success rate with a long-term recurrence rate of approximately 5 % (Ayed and Raghunathan 2000) and a relative risk of recurrence of 4.7 when compared to thoracotomy (Barker et al. 2007), but this is balanced by the lower morbidity/mortality.

There are two key differences between a surgical approach (VATS or thoracotomy) and medical thoracoscopy. The first is that surgical therapies require a general anaesthetic with its inherent risks and secondly most surgeons will carry out both pleurodesis of some form and a treatment directed at removing/repairing any blebs/bullae. As discussed earlier, there is no evidence to support the view that blebs/bullae are the sole site of air leak and indeed there is a body of evidence to support the fact that they are not the source of air leak. Although there has been no randomised controlled trial comparing pleurodesis + surgical

repair of blebs/bullae with pleurodesis alone, a number of surgical studies have clearly shown that the risk of recurrence of pneumothorax is significantly higher if some form of pleurodesis is not carried out irrespective of the other surgical interventions performed (Hatz et al. 2000; Liu et al. 1995; Korner et al. 1996).

The timing of intervention is a further area of debate. There is a broad consensus that any patient presenting with a recurrent or contralateral pneumothorax, be it primary or secondary, should be offered some form of recurrence prevention as the risk of a further pneumothorax after a first recurrence is significantly higher than after a first event (Gobbel et al. 1963). Some guidelines recommend recurrence prevention for all secondary spontaneous pneumothoraces on the grounds that the clinical impact of a pneumothorax on a patient with underlying lung disease is much greater (Baumann et al. 2001). The area of greatest debate is whether or not to offer recurrence prevention to patients after a first PSP. In this situation we have to balance the risk of recurrence (approximately 30 %) against the risk of carrying out invasive pleural procedures. It has been shown that carrying out VATS on first time PSP is a cost-effective strategy as compared with conservative treatment, as the costs of treating recurrent pneumothoraces are significant (Schramel et al. 1996). These authors recognised that the cost of medical thoracoscopy and talc poudrage is 62 % less than VATS and would be even more cost-effective. This is supported by similar evidence from other groups (Tschopp et al. 2002).

13.5 The Role of Medical Thoracoscopy in the Management of Spontaneous Pneumothorax

Medical thoracoscopy and talc poudrage has been employed, with good effect, as a method of recurrence prevention for both primary and secondary spontaneous pneumothorax for over three decades (Guerin and Boutin 1999). More invasive procedures such as pleurectomy or bullectomy cannot be performed without either general anaesthesia with single-lung ventilation or epidural anaesthesia. We discuss in detail here the supporting evidence for and the role of medical thoracoscopy–talc poudrage (MT–TP) in the management of both primary and secondary pneumothorax and follow on from this with a discussion of the technical aspects of talc poudrage via medical thoracoscopy for pneumothorax (Campos et al. 1997; Ferrer et al. 2001).

13.5.1 Primary Spontaneous Pneumothorax

Given that the aetiology of primary spontaneous pneumothorax has never been shown to be directly related to rupture of bullae and that the pleura of patients with spontaneous pneumothorax has been shown to be diffusely abnormal at areas distant to any bullae or blebs, the requirement for anything more than effective pleurodesis can be debated. It has been shown that a diffuse form of pleurodesis, i.e. talc poudrage, is more effective than a local form of pleurodesis, i.e. subtotal pleurectomy (Bresticker et al. 1993; Cardillo et al. 2006). Talc poudrage was first described in 1935 and has been used successfully as a sole method of recurrence prevention by cardiothoracic surgeons carrying out thoracoscopy under general anaesthetic (Nandi 1980; van de Brekel 1993). The early case series reported in the medical literature for MT–TP reported on its use for either complicated pneumothorax (i.e. prolonged air leak) or recurrent pneumothorax. These series treated both primary and secondary pneumothora-

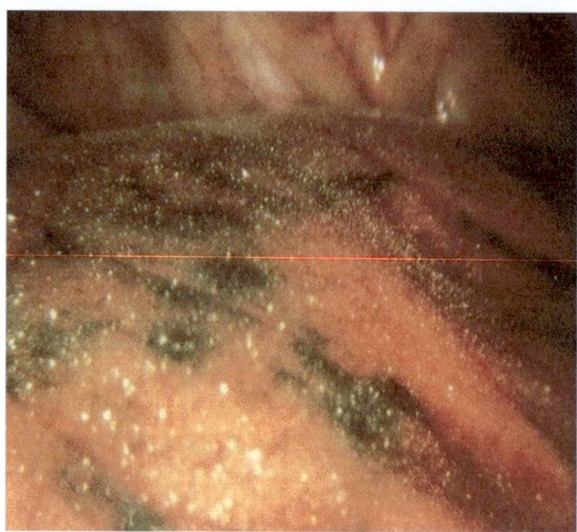

Fig. 13.5 View of the apex after talc poudrage procedure. The particles of talc have been gently spread on the surface of the lung with a talc atomiser. This technique uses asbestos-free calibrated talc and is the gold standard to induce pleurodesis (Courtesy Ph Astoul, Marseille, France)

ces. They reported good long-term efficacy with recurrence rates of 7 % (Guerin and Boutin 1999; El Khawand 1995). More recently a prospective study evaluating the safety and efficacy of MT–TP for both complicated pneumothorax and recurrent pneumothorax showed MT–TP to be a safe and effective method of recurrence prevention (Tschopp et al. 1997). This study recruited 89 patients, and after a mean follow-up of 5.1 years, there was a recurrence rate of 5 %, which are on a par with the efficacy rates quoted for VATS procedures for pneumothorax recurrence prevention (Ayed and Raghunathan 2000). This study did note that recurrence of pneumothorax was significantly more likely in the presence of bullae greater than 2 cm in diameter.

The first, and to date only, multicentre randomised controlled study evaluating MT–TP has compared the efficacy, complications and cost-effectiveness of MT–TP with simple pleural drainage for the management of primary spontaneous pneumothorax (Tschopp et al. 2002). This study recruited 108 patients with either first episode or recurrent PSP who had failed aspiration and randomised them to either intercostal drain or MT–TP (Fig. 13.5). This study showed that the early success rate of MT–TP was significantly higher than intercostal drain alone (1.6 % vs 21.7 %), and late recurrence with a mean follow-up of 5 years was significantly lower for those patients who underwent MT–TP (5 % vs 34 %). The length of hospital stay and total costs were similar between the two groups, and if a calculation is included for the cost of recurrent episodes, then early intervention with MT–TP is more cost-effective than intercostal drain alone. Those who underwent MT–TP did suffer slightly more pain than those who underwent intercostal drain alone, but in the centres which provided opiate analgesia routinely to all patients, this difference was negated. In support of this data, another study which evaluated the efficacy and cost-effectiveness of VATS surgery with conservative treatment in a similar patient group found VATS to be both more cost-effective than conservative treatment with a 2-year recurrence rate of 4 %. The authors of this study recognised that MT–TP would be 62 % less costly than VATS and thus expected to be even more cost-effective (Schramel et al. 1996). This data would support a more aggressive policy of intervention than is currently standard, and perhaps the risk of recurrence against the side effects of MT–TP should be discussed with all patients with PSP to allow them to make an informed decision about how they wish to be managed (Sahn 2002).

13.5.2 Secondary Spontaneous Pneumothorax

Secondary spontaneous pneumothorax has a higher recurrence rate after the first episode due to the presence of underlying lung disease and therefore carries significantly greater risk to the patient than a primary spontaneous pneumothorax. As recognition of this, some major guidelines for pneumothorax recommend recurrence prevention after a first episode (Baumann et al. 2001). VATS surgery with bullectomy/pleurectomy is the standard recommendation. However, this requires a general anaesthetic with single-lung ventilation which carries significant risk of morbidity and mortality, particularly for patients with underlying severe lung disease. For patients deemed unfit for a general anaesthetic or for those who would prefer not to undergo

general anaesthetic, then medical thoracoscopy–talc poudrage is a safe and effective treatment alternative. This has been shown in a study evaluating the safety and efficacy of MT–TP for patients with moderate to severe COPD (mean FEV_1 0.88 l). The long-term success rate in this group was 95 % at 35 months (Maskell et al. 2004; Lee et al 2004). However, this study did reveal a significant 30-day mortality rate of 10 %. The early mortality was directly related to severe underlying lung disease, low BMI and associated ischaemic heart disease. These risks should be discussed with individual patients and weighed up against the significant risk of pneumothorax recurrence after a first episode. As the risk of recurrence of pneumothorax seems to be higher in the presence of large bullae (>2 cm) and this may be particularly important for patients with bullous emphysema.

13.5.2.1 Summary

The available data supports MT–TP to be both a safe method and an effective method for offering recurrence prevention to patients with both primary and secondary pneumothorax. Many patients (Bridevaux et al. 2011; Doddoli et al. 2004; Fraticelli et al. 2002; Lange et al. 1988), with secondary pneumothorax are deemed unsuitable for surgical intervention, and as such, MT–TP would be the most effective method for this, with better results than simple talc pleurodesis via intercostal drain.

There is an argument in favour of being more invasive in the treatment of first episode PSP, and MT–TP can have a significant role in this situation as it is safe and effective and carries significantly lower healthcare costs when compared to either VATS or thoracotomy (Viskum et al. 1989; Weissberg and Refaely 2000).

13.5.3 Technical Aspects

The technique for MT–TP for the treatment of spontaneous pneumothorax is similar to thoracoscopy for the diagnosis and treatment of pleural effusions. It should be carried out at the time of the pneumothorax whilst an intercostal drain is in situ to allow insufflation of air to collapse the underlying lung prior to port insertion. Premedication with atropine and morphine/pethidine with titrated midazolam is often employed as analgesia and conscious sedation. Continuous monitoring of blood pressure, electrocardiogram and pulse oximetry is required. With the patient in the lateral decubitus position, a single port is inserted into the third or fourth intercostal space after checking the lung is properly collapsed. After inspection of both the parietal and visceral pleura, 1–2 g of graded talc is gently insufflated into the pleural space paying attention to achieving spread of talc diffusely over the pleura and diaphragm. Talc poudrage in the setting of pneumothorax management can be intensely painful, and patients should be administered additional analgesia prior to insufflation. Post-procedure the intercostal drain should be attached to an underwater seal with 10–20 cm H_2O suction. The drain can be removed when the air leak has ceased and the lung expanded. If there is persistent air leak after 1 week of suction, a repeat procedure should be considered.

Conclusions

Although there is evidence supporting medical thoracoscopy–talc poudrage to be a safe and effective treatment modality for pneumothorax recurrence prevention, currently VATS surgery with pleurectomy/bullectomy remains the procedure of choice in many centres. However, there remains a dearth of evidence to support the use of resection of blebs/bullae over and above a pleurodesis. A randomised controlled study of the efficacy of VATS bullectomy talc poudrage compared with medical thoracoscopy–talc poudrage would be undertaken in an ideal world. Medical thoracoscopy–talc poudrage has been shown to be a cost-effective method of treating primary spontaneous pneumothorax. It has low morbidity/mortality rates when compared with VATS surgery and avoids the need for general anaesthesia. In these circumstances there is no reason why MT–TP could not be more formally regarded as a definitive treatment option for prevention of recurrence of pneumothoraces including PSP.

References

Almind M, Lange P, Viskum K (1989) Spontaneous pneumothorax: comparison of simple drainage, talc pleurodesis, and tetracycline pleurodesis. Thorax 44: 627–630

Andrivet P, Djedaini K, Teboul JL et al (1995) Spontaneous pneumothorax. Comparison of thoracic drainage vs immediate or delayed needle aspiration. Chest 108: 335–339

Astoul P (2010) Editorial comment: management of primary spontaneous pneumothorax: a plea for a mini-invasive approach. Eur J Cardiothorac Surg 37: 1135–1136

Athanassiadi K et al (1998) Surgical treatment of spontaneous pneumothorax: ten-year experience. World J Surg 22:803–806

Ayed A, Raghunathan R (2000) Thoracoscopy versus open lung biopsy in the diagnosis of interstitial lung disease: a randomized controlled trial. J R Coll Surg Edinb 45:159–163

Ayed AK, Chandrasekaran C, Sukumar M (2006) Aspiration versus tube drainage in primary spontaneous pneumothorax: a randomised study. Eur Respir J 27:477–482

Barker A et al (2007) Recurrence rates of video-assisted thoracoscopic versus open surgery in the prevention of recurrent pneumothoraces: a systematic review of randomised and non-randomised trials. Lancet 370: 329–335

Baumann M et al (2001) Management of spontaneous pneumothorax: an American College of Chest Physicians Delphi consensus statement. Chest 119:590–602

Boutin C, Viallat JR, Aelony Y (1991) Diagnostic thoracoscopy for pleural effusions. In: Boutin C, Viallat JR, Aelony Y (eds) Practical thoracoscopy. Springer, Berlin, p 51

Bresticker MA, Oba J, LoCicero J 3rd (1993) Optimal pleurodesis: a comparison study. Ann Thorac Surg 55:364–366

Bridevaux PO, Tschopp JM, Cardillo G et al (2011) Short-term safety of thoracoscopic talc pleurodesis for recurrent primary spontaneous pneumothorax: a prospective European multicentre study. Eur Respir J 38: 770–773

Campos JR, Werebe EC, Vargas FS et al (1997) Respiratory failure due to insufflated talc. Lancet 349: 251–252

Cardillo G, Carleo F, Giunti R et al (2006) Videothoracoscopic talc poudrage in primary spontaneous pneumothorax: a single-institution experience in 861 cases. J Thorac Cardiovasc Surg 131: 322–328

Crisci R et al (1996) Video-assisted thoracoscopic surgery versus thoracotomy for recurrent spontaneous pneumothorax. A comparison of results and costs. Eur J Cardiothorac Surg 10:556–560

Doddoli C, Barlési F, Fraticelli A, Thomas P, Astoul P, Giudicelli R, Fuentes P (2004) Video-assisted thoracoscopic management of recurrent primary spontaneous pneumothorax after prior talc pleurodesis: a feasible, safe and efficient treatment option. Eur J Cardiothorac Surg 26:889–892

Donohue DM et al (1993) Resection of pulmonary blebs and pleurodesis for spontaneous pneumothorax. Chest 104:1767–1769

El Khawand C (1995) Spontaneous pneumothorax. Results of pleural talc therapy using thoracoscopy. Rev Mal Respir 12:275–281

Ferrer J, Villarino MA, Tura JM (2001) Talc preparations used for pleurodesis vary markedly from one preparation to another. Chest 119:1901–1905

Fraticelli A, Robaglia-Schlupp A, Riera A et al (2002) Distribution of calibrated talc after intrapleural administration: an experimental study in rats. Chest 122: 1737–1741

Gobbel WG et al (1963) Spontaneous pneumothorax. J Thorac Cardiovasc Surg 46:331–345

Guerin JC, Boutin C (1999) Interventional medical thoracoscopy. Rev Mal Respir 16:703–708

Harvey J, Prescott RJ (1994) Simple aspiration versus intercostal tube drainage for spontaneous pneumothorax in patients with normal lungs. British Thoracic Society Research Committee. BMJ 309:1338–1339

Hatz RA et al (2000) Long-term results after video-assisted thoracoscopic surgery for first-time and recurrent spontaneous pneumothorax. Ann Thorac Surg 70:253–257

Henry M et al (2003) BTS guidelines for the management of spontaneous pneumothorax. Thorax 58(Suppl II):ii39–ii52

Janssen JP et al (1995) Videothoracoscopic appearance of first and recurrent pneumothorax. Chest 108: 330–334

Kennedy L, Harley RA, Sahn SA et al (1995) Talc slurry pleurodesis: pleural fluid and histologic analysis. Chest 107:1707–1712

Korner H et al (1996) Surgical treatment of spontaneous pneumothorax by wedge resection without pleurodesis or pleurectomy. Eur J Cardiothorac Surg 10:656–659

Lange P, Mortensen J, Groth S (1988) Lung function 22–35 years after treatment of idiopathic spontaneous pneumothorax with talc poudrage or simple drainage. Thorax 43:559–561

Lang-Lazdunski L, Chapuis O et al (2003) Videothoracoscopic bleb excision and pleural abrasion for the treatment of primary spontaneous pneumothorax: long-term results. Ann Thorac Surg 75:960–965

Lee P, Yap WS, Pek WY et al (2004) An Audit of medical thoracoscopy and talc poudrage for pneumothorax prevention in advanced COPD. Chest 125:1315–1320

Lichter I et al (1971) Spontaneous pneumothorax in young subjects. A clinical and pathological study. Thorax 26:409–417

Light RW (2001) Pneumothorax. Pleural diseases. Lippincott/ Williams & Wilkins, Philadelphia, pp 284–319

Lippert HL et al (1991) Independent risk factors for cumulative recurrence rate after first spontaneous pneumothorax. Eur Respir J 4:324–331

Liu HP et al (1995) Thoracoscopic surgery as a routine procedure for spontaneous pneumothorax. Results from 82 patients. Chest 107:559–562

Marquette CH, Marx A, Leroy S et al (2006) Simplified stepwise management of primary spontaneous pneumothorax: a pilot study. Eur Respir J 27:470–476

Martinez-Ramos D et al (2007) Usefulness of computed tomography in determining risk of recurrence after a first episode of primary spontaneous pneumothorax: therapeutic implications. Arch Bronconeumol 43: 304–308

Maskell NA, Lee YC, Gleeson FV et al (2004) Randomized trials describing lung inflammation after pleurodesis with talc of varying particle size. Am J Respir Crit Care Med 170:377–382

Melton L et al (1979) Incidence of spontaneous pneumothorax in Olmsted County, Minnesota: 1950 to 1974. Am Rev Respir Dis 20:1379–1382

Miller AC (2008) Spontaneous pneumothorax. In: Garry Lee YC, Light RW (eds) Textbook of pleural diseases, 2nd edn. Hodder Arnold, London, pp 515–532

Mitlehner W et al (1992) Value of computer tomography in the detection of bullae and blebs in patients with primary spontaneous pneumothorax. Respiration 59:221–227

Mouroux J et al (1996) Video-assisted thoracoscopic treatment of spontaneous pneumothorax: technique and results of one hundred cases. J Thorac Cardiovasc Surg 112:385–391

Nandi P (1980) Recurrent spontaneous pneumothorax; an effective method of talc poudrage. Chest 77:493–495

Nkere UU et al (1994) Surgical management of spontaneous pneumothorax. Thorac Cardiovasc Surg 42: 45–50

Noppen M, Alexander P, Driesen P et al (2002a) Manual aspiration versus chest tube drainage in first episodes of primary spontaneous pneumothorax: a multicenter, prospective, randomized pilot study. Am J Respir Crit Care Med 165:1240–1244

Noppen M et al (2002b) Pleural diseases: pneumothorax. Eur Respir Mon 22:279–296

Noppen M et al (2003) Pathogenesis and treatment of primary spontaneous pneumothorax: an overview. Respiration 70:431–438

Noppen M, Dekeukeleire T, Hanon S et al (2006) Fluorescein-enhanced autofluorescence thoracoscopy in patients with primary spontaneous pneumothorax and normal subjects. Am J Respir Crit Care Med 174:26–30

Ohata M et al (1980) Pathogenesis of spontaneous pneumothorax. With special reference to the ultrastructure of emphysematous bullae. Chest 77:771–776

Sadicot R et al (1997) Recurrence of primary spontaneous pneumothorax. Thorax 52:805–809

Sahn SA (2002) Is talc indicated for pleurodesis? Pro: talc should be used for pleurodesis. J Bronchol 61:35–38

Schramel FM et al (1995) Inflammation as cause of spontaneous pneumothorax and emphysematous like changes: results of bronchoalveolar lavage. Eur Respir J 19:397s

Schramel FM, Sutedja TG, Braber JC et al (1996) Cost-effectiveness of video-assisted thoracoscopic surgery versus conservative treatment for first time or recurrent spontaneous pneumothorax. Eur Respir J 9:1821–1825

Schramel FM, Postmus PE, Vanderschueren RG (1997) Current aspects of spontaneous pneumothorax. Eur Respir J 10:1372–1379

Tschopp JM, Brutsche M, Frey JG (1997) Treatment of complicated spontaneous pneumothorax by simple talc pleurodesis under thoracoscopy and local anaesthesia. Thorax 52:329–332

Tschopp JM, Boutin C, Astoul P et al (2002) Talcage by medical thoracoscopy for primary spontaneous pneumothorax is more cost-effective than drainage: a randomised study. Eur Respir J 20:1003–1009

Van de Brekel JA (1993) Pneumothorax. Results of thoracoscopy and pleurodesis with talc poudrage and thoracotomy. Chest 103:345–347

Viskum K, Lange P, Mortensen J (1989) Long-term sequelae after talc pleurodesis for spontaneous pneumothorax. Pneumologie 43:105–106

Weissberg D, Refaely Y (2000) Pneumothorax: experience with 1,199 patients. Chest 117:1279–1285

Management of Recurrent Pleurisies by Thoracoscopy

14

Felix Herth

14.1 Introduction

Recurrent pleural effusion is commonly seen in clinical practice and results from the anatomical and/or functional impairment of the pleural surfaces by benign or malignant processes. There is a wide range of clinical entities responsible for the production of these effusions and can be subgrouped according to the biochemistry of the fluid into transudates (resulting, in particular, from heart, liver, or kidney failure) and exudates (principally generated by nonspecific infections, tuberculosis, or neoplasms).

In this context, the significant predominance of cancer, which accounts for approximately 50 % of the total number of these cases, must be highlighted (DiBonito et al. 1992). It is estimated that there are approximately 200,000 new cases of malignant pleural effusion per year in the USA (Light 1995).

The treatment for recurrent pleural effusion is complex and is aimed at preventing fluid collection and maintaining the pleural cavity free from new fluid accumulation. The first step is to address the pathological process responsible for the formation of the effusion. In the case of transudates, the treatment is aimed at treating the heart, kidney, or liver failure, whereas it is aimed at treating the infection or cancer in the case of exudates. However, when the systemic treatment of the condition responsible for the formation of the effusion does not control the fluid accumulation and does not prevent its recurrence, local treatment should be recommended, allowing the free expansion of the lung with subsequent functional improvement. Methods include initial thoracentesis, pleural drainage, pleuroperitoneal shunt, pleurectomy, and pleurodesis.

The objective of the initial thoracentesis is the removal of fluid from the pleural cavity in order to achieve lung expansion and subsequent functional improvement. However, due to the potential risks of this procedure, caution is needed regarding the volume to be removed from the pleural cavity. Therefore, it is recommended that, even in large effusions, fluid removal should not exceed 1,500 ml since the removal of larger volumes of fluid increases the risk of developing pulmonary edema, in addition to respiratory or hemodynamic alterations that can ultimately result in respiratory distress syndrome or hemodynamic shock.

Pleural fluid removal, performed with all the necessary precautions, is well tolerated and significantly improves the dyspnea caused by the effusion. Nevertheless, since the fluid can rapidly reaccumulate, performing multiple thoracenteses becomes a temporary alternative in the control of a recurrent pleural effusion. The need for multiple punctures is physically and emotionally invasive, resulting in protein and electrolyte depletion.

F. Herth
Department of Pneumology
and Critical Care Medicine,
Thoraxklinik/University of Heidelberg,
Heidelberg, Germany
e-mail: felix.herth@thoraxklinik-heidelberg.de

P. Astoul et al. (eds.), *Thoracoscopy for Pulmonologists*,
DOI 10.1007/978-3-642-38351-9_14, © Springer-Verlag Berlin Heidelberg 2014

The second option to be considered is prolonged drainage to maintain the pleural cavity free of fluid. It should be noted that leaving a drain in place for long periods (a month or more) can, in itself, result in symphysis of the pleural surfaces, which is positive outcome. Nonetheless, prolonged drainage results in great nutritional deprivation, increases the risk of pleural infections, and can decrease survival (Vargas et al. 2004). Until recently, such drainage was performed with large-bore thoracic drains (34–40 F), which have now been replaced by small-caliber catheters in most institutions (maximum, 16 F).

The third option is using a pleuroperitoneal shunt, which is nothing more than a thin catheter with a receptacle (a unidirectional valve) at its midpoint. The extremities of the shunt are placed in the pleural and peritoneal cavities, and the catheter, including the receptacle, follows a subcutaneous path. When the patient presents worsening of symptoms (basically dyspnea), the receptacle is repeatedly compressed, removing fluid from the pleural cavity and, by virtue of its unidirectionality, sending it to the peritoneal cavity. The inconvenience of this system lies in the small volume of the valve chamber (+2 ml), which can require an exhaustive number of compressions of this compartment. For the removal of 400 ml pleural fluid, for example, more than 200 compressions are necessary. Other negative aspects of the system are the high valve obstruction rate, the risk of neoplastic implantation in the abdominal cavity, and the high costs (Genc et al. 2000).

The fourth option is pleurectomy. It is undoubtedly the most effective procedure.

However, it is often contraindicated due to the accompanying high rates of morbidity and mortality (Vargas and Teixeira 1996).

In fact, the high risk of complications is justifiable since it is major surgery and the candidates are patients with impaired general health status. It represents a highly aggressive treatment option in a group of patients with limited survival.

Finally, there is pleurodesis, that is, the intentional collapse of the pleural surfaces (visceral and parietal) resulting in the symphysis of the pleural space, which hinders the accumulation of fluid. This has been the procedure most often used when there is complete pulmonary re-expansion and the general condition of the patient is good. It is currently the best option for the control of recurrent malignant pleural effusion (Dikensoy and Light 2005).

Pleurodesis reduces the dyspnea caused by fluid accumulation in the pleural space and consequently results in greater functional capacity and a better quality of life.

The aim of this chapter is to discuss the strategies for inducing pleurodesis in patients with recurrent pleural effusion, especially those of neoplastic origin.

In this review, due to the current tendency toward simplification of the pleurodesis procedure, the integration of the skills of clinical pulmonologists, thoracic surgeons, and oncologists will be discussed in a joint section, in order to promote effective and minimally invasive pleurodesis.

14.2 Indications

14.2.1 Recurrent Benign Pleural Effusions

The performance of pleurodesis in recurrent benign (transudative) pleural effusion is controversial and should be regarded as a procedure reserved for use in exceptional cases (de Campos et al. 2001).

There exist no controlled, randomized, or comparative studies evaluating the efficacy and safety of pleurodesis in benign processes. The findings of observational studies suggest that, in these situations, pleurodesis is efficacious and safe.

However, there is the theoretical fear that, after pleurodesis of the transudates, the pleural fluid will begin to accumulate in other tissues, such as those of the pulmonary parenchyma (Webb et al. 1992). Therefore, pleurodesis is performed in recurrent benign pleural effusion in those rare situations in which there is an absolute failure of the clinical treatment of the underlying disease.

Liver, kidney, and heart failure account for the majority of recurrent benign pleural effusion; however, hypoproteinemia and previous myocardial revascularization should also be included in the differential.

14.2.2 Recurrent Malignant Pleural Effusions

The main indication for pleurodesis resides with this group of patients. However, not all the patients with malignant pleural effusion benefit from the procedure. In some situations, there is a consensus regarding the induction of pleurodesis; in others, it is absolutely controversial.

Once an indication for pleurodesis has been satisfied, the ideal moment at which to perform the procedure should be analyzed. Some authors argue that pleurodesis should be performed as soon as possible after the diagnosis has been confirmed (Marrazzo et al. 2005). Others recommend performing pleurodesis only if chemotherapy fails to control the pleural effusion. However, there is no evidence to support the use of the latter strategy. In this situation, the assessment for control of the pleural effusion (radiological regression of the effusion and decreased number of thoracenteses to maintain relief of dyspnea) can be undertaken after one or two cycles of chemotherapy.

Although there are factors in favor of and against these approaches, both indications are currently accepted.

Once the timing of pleurodesis has been decided, other factors, despite not enjoying a consensus, can modify the indications for pleurodesis and therefore should be considered, since they can interfere with the expected result. Low pH (<7.3) (Crnjac et al. 2004), low glucose level (<60 mg/dl), and the presence of a chylothorax have been related to a poorer prognosis and decreased efficacy of pleurodesis (Fig. 14.1), independent of the technique and of the agent used (Vargas and Teixeira 1996).

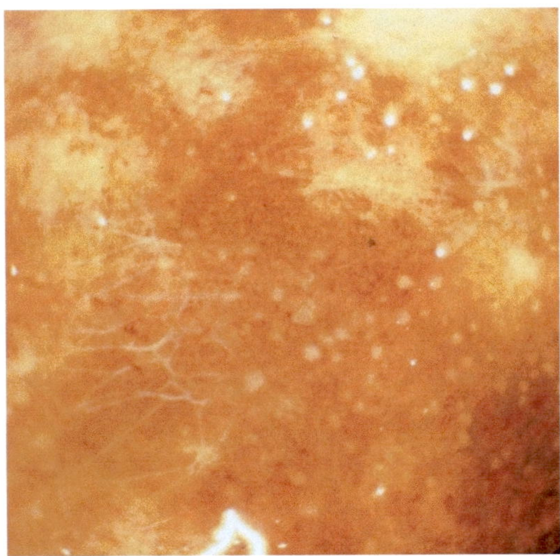

Fig. 14.1 Pleural lymphangitis in a chylothorax. The parietal pleura is covered with a network of ectatic lymphatic vessels (Courtesy C Boutin, Marseille, France)

The presence of lymphangitis (Figs. 14.2, 14.3, and 14.4), a disseminated pleural carcinomatosis (Fig. 14.5), and a performance status index lower than 70 have been associated with a poorer clinical course after the induction of pleurodesis (Vargas and Teixeira 1996). Finally, lung entrapment (Figs. 14.6, 14.7 ,and 14.8), either due to pleural loculations or to failure of pulmonary expansion, reduces the efficacy of pleurodesis, as well as increasing the risk of infections in the pleural space. Therefore, pleurodesis is not recommended under these conditions (Vargas et al. 2004).

14.3 Types of Procedures

Pleurodesis can be achieved using a variety of stimuli: direct physical abrasion, instillation of caustic or irritating chemical substances (talc, doxycycline, silver nitrate, or bleomycin) into the pleural space, or immunological induction with Corynebacterium parvum, transforming growth factor beta (TGF-ß) or interferon-alpha 2 (IFN-a 2).

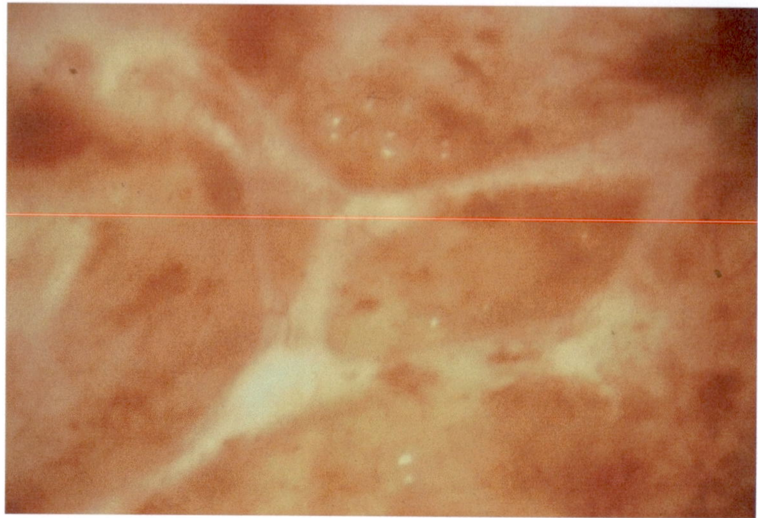

Fig. 14.2 Lymphangitis is frequently seen in cases of malignant pleural effusion. In some situations the lymphangitis can become thicker, resembling candle wax droppings (Courtesy C Boutin, Marseille, France)

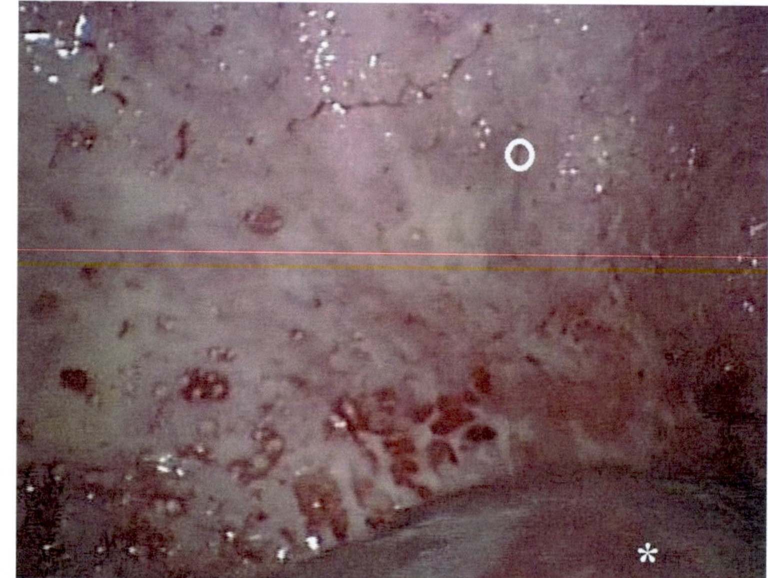

Fig. 14.3 In this case of malignant pleural effusion due to a primary lung adenocarcinoma, an irregular white network can be seen over the posterior parietal pleura (O). Fibrin deposits are visible on the lung (*star*) (Courtesy Ph Astoul, Marseille, France)

14.3.1 Mechanical Stimuli

Among the mechanical techniques employed, abrasion is the principal method. Abrasion is carried out during a surgical intervention, whether conventional or video-assisted, where the surgeon exfoliates the pleural mesothelium, creating friction with a rough-surfaced material (e.g., gauze). This irritation results in the desquamation of the mesothelium and activation of the inflammatory and coagulation pathways, with subsequent proliferation of fibroblasts and collagen deposition. This will result in pleural symphysis.

Pleural abrasion is not currently used in the control of recurrent neoplastic pleural effusions due to its lower efficacy, as well as to the high risk of bleeding in the regions involved by tumor and in addition, due to the theoretical possibility of malignant dissemination. Another inconvenience of pleural abrasion is that it requires surgical intervention.

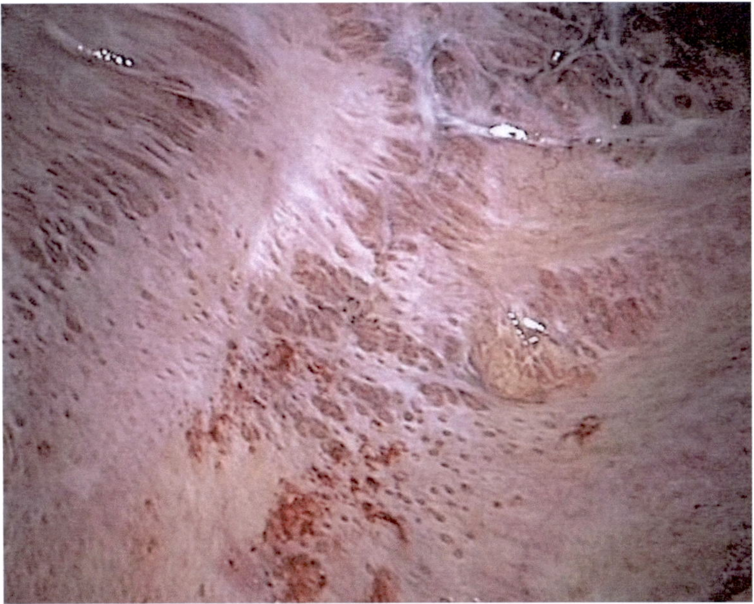

Fig. 14.4 Malignant lymphangitis on the parietal pleura and costodiaphragmatic gutter (Courtesy Ph Astoul, Marseille, France)

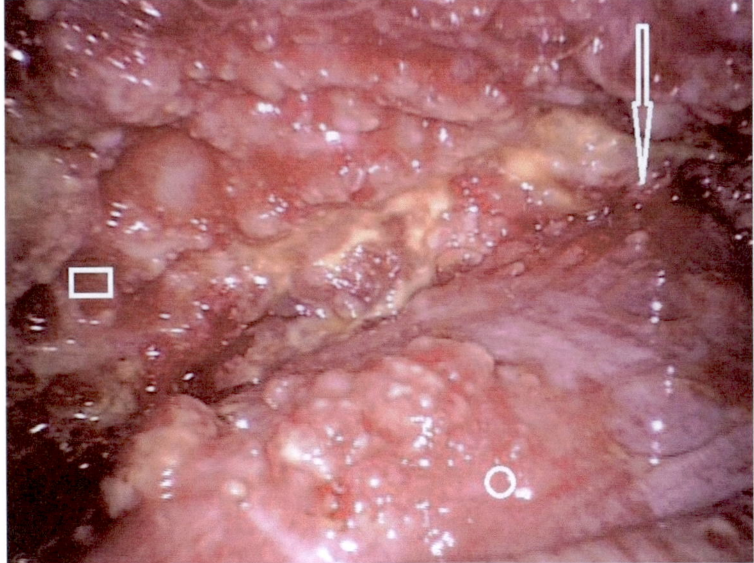

Fig. 14.5 A view of the costophrenic angle (*arrow*). The lung ($\bigcirc$) and the posterior parietal pleura ($\square$) are covered by multiple nodules (Courtesy Ph Astoul, Marseille, France)

14.3.2 Chemical Stimuli

Pleurodesis induced by chemical stimuli was first carried out at the beginning of the last century. There are references that, in 1901, Spengler injected silver nitrate into the pleural cavity for the control of recurrent pneumothorax (Vargas and Teixeira 1996).

Apparently, talc was first introduced into the pleural cavity, with the objective of collapsing the existing residual space after pulmonary TB by Bethune in 1935 (Vargas and Teixeira 1996).

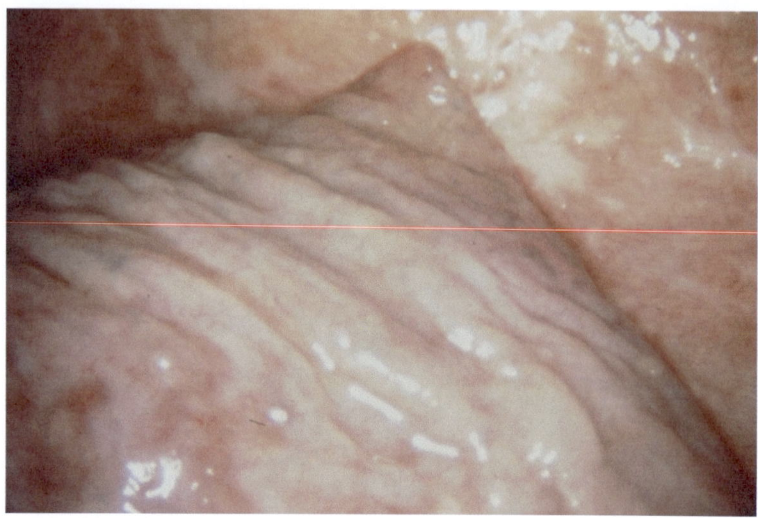

Fig. 14.6 Trapped lung (lower lobe) in a patient with a malignant pleural effusion (Courtesy C Boutin and Ph Astoul, Marseille, France)

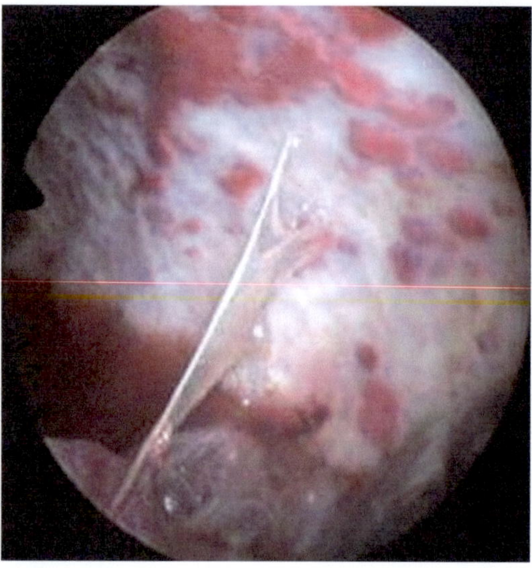

Fig. 14.7 This picture shows pleural lymphangitis, nodules, and fibrin deposits. There is an adhesion between the posterior parietal pleural (lower part of the pleural cavity) and the lower lobe of the left lung (Courtesy C Boutin, Marseille, France)

Since then, various substances have been used to induce pleurodesis. Chemical stimulation can be performed through various routes of access – pleurodesis can be achieved thoracosopically or through simple drainage.

Talc is classically considered the most efficacious sclerosant. When compared with other agents, it presents a relative risk of 1.34 for therapeutic success (95 % confidence interval: 1.16–1.55) with a success rate of over 90 % in most studies (Shaw and Agarwal 2004; Dresler et al. 2005). Talc has been considered the agent of choice, since it presents many of the characteristics cited in the definition of an ideal agent (low cost, wide distribution, easy administration, high efficacy, and low rate of side effects). Despite its low rate of complications, its use has been associated with acute respiratory distress syndrome. It is believed that this complication is related to the size of the talc particles. The smaller ones would be more easily absorbed from the pleural cavity and distributed throughout the circulation, resulting in a greater risk of remote complications and induction of cytokine-based systemic inflammatory reactions (Rehse et al. 1999; Maskell et al. 2004).

Doxycycline has proven efficacious and safe for the induction of pleurodesis. However, it is not available in many countries. Silver nitrate was the first substance utilized in the induction of pleurodesis; however, it was abandoned, for reasons that remain unclear, in the 1980s (Paschoalini et al. 2005). In studies with laboratory animals (rabbits), 0.5 % silver nitrate proved highly efficacious with a low rate of complications (Vargas et al. 2002). The pathophysiological mechanism involved in the induction of pleurodesis by silver nitrate appears to be, to a certain extent, different from that observed with talc, since, in this rabbit

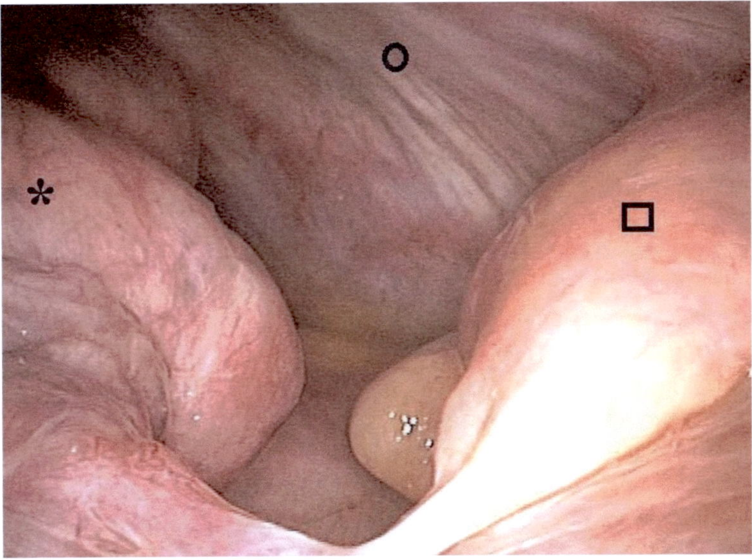

Fig. 14.8 Even without a fibrotic inflammatory reaction of the visceral pleura, the lung can be trapped. This patient was diagnosed with a lung tumor of the lower lobe (*star*). This view shows the costodiaphragmatic angle with the lower part of the posterior parietal pleura (○) and the diaphragm (□) (Courtesy Ph Astoul, Marseille, France)

model, corticosteroids did not reduce the efficacy of the pleurodesis obtained with silver nitrate, in contrast to what occurs with talc. A recently published study involving human subjects with neoplastic pleural effusion, and utilizing 0.5 % silver nitrate, demonstrated efficacy indices similar to those found for talc, with low rates of side effects (Paschoalini et al. 2005).

Bleomycin is an antineoplastic agent that was used to induce pleurodesis in the past decades. However, its low efficacy and high cost have significantly limited its use.

14.3.3 Immunological Stimuli

Chief among the immunostimulants is C. parvum. Its principal advantage is that it does not require thoracoscopic intervention or pleural drainage and can be introduced into the pleural space through a simple puncture. However, there are currently difficulties in its production, and there is no defined distribution network.

Other immunostimulant agents include interleukin-2 alpha, staphylococcal superantigen, and TGF-β. In a comparative, randomized, prospective, parallel study carried out in 2004, IFN-a 2b was found to be less efficacious than bleomycin (Sartori et al. 2004), and its use was not indicated for induction of pleurodesis. Staphylococcal superantigen seems to be a promising agent, despite limited investigations. In a study carried out in 2004 (Ren et al. 2004), staphylococcal superantigen was instilled in 14 patients with a low performance status. It was successful in 11 patients (71 %), without any side effects. Its principal advantage is ease of administration, not requiring hospitalization or thoracic drainage. Since these results are still preliminary, further studies of efficacy and safety are required. Finally, TGF-β is a cytokine that stimulates tissue proliferation and collagen formation, without inducing an inflammatory reaction or tissue lesion. The major concern regarding its use is related to its systemic absorption, with development of fibrosis in other organs, including the lung. It was successfully tested in experimental animals with low short-term complication rates (Gary Lee et al. 2001). However, studies analyzing its efficacy and safety in humans have yet to be carried out.

14.3.4 Route of Access

The route of access is defined as the route of administration of the sclerosing agent into the pleural space, either through classical thoracotomy, video-assisted surgery, thoracic drainage with local anesthesia, or thoracic drainage with thoracic puncture and a small-caliber catheter.

All of these techniques present advantages and disadvantages that can affect the final result of the procedure. Among the advantages, colleagues cite the importance of complete drainage of the pleural cavity and the more homogeneous distribution of the sclerosing agent in the pleural space. It is also important to have a minimally aggressive procedure and short periods of hospitalization. These factors influence the choice of the technique performed for a given patient.

Over the last few years, the route of access for pleurodesis has been thoroughly studied. There is a tendency to reduce the aggressiveness of the treatment, migrating from talc insufflation during thoracotomy to video-assisted insufflation and eventually to the instillation of sclerosant through a thoracic drain. Even when the thoracic drain is used as a route of access to the pleural cavity, there is a tendency toward reducing its complexity and morbidity (pain).

However, in parallel with a reduction in procedure aggressiveness, the efficacy of the treatment must be maintained. The ideal route of access for the sclerosant which strikes a balance between efficacy and safety has yet to be defined. Unfortunately, many studies comparing routes of access have not employed the same sclerosing agent for each route, thereby making interpretation difficult. A meta-analysis carried out in 2004 by the Pain, Palliative Care and Supportive Care Group of the Cochrane Database of Systematic Reviews (112 patients) evaluated the efficacy of talc pleurodesis using video-assisted surgery or via drainage/talc slurry (talc in suspension) (Clemensten et al. 1998). The authors showed that the instillation through video-assisted surgery was more efficacious, with a favorable relative risk of 1.19 (95 % confidence interval, 1.04–1.36), with a similar mortality rate in the two groups. Unfortunately, medical thoracoscopy was not examined, and in this meta-analysis, it was not possible to compare the adverse effects of the two treatments due to the lack of pertinent data in the studies involved. Despite the fact that video-assisted surgery was found to be more efficacious than slurry pleurodesis, the level of success for both procedures was over 90 %, which is quite acceptable in clinical terms.

14.4 Conclusions and Recommendations

The principal indication for pleurodesis is recurrent malignant pleural effusions, after full pulmonary re-expansion, in patients with good performance status indices.

Pleurodesis using a chemical sclerosant, especially talc, remains the first option for the treatment of recurrent malignant pleural effusion.

Silver nitrate seems to be a reasonable alternative, although more studies looking at the safety profile are needed.

The most efficacious route of access is the thoracoscope. However, the use of small-caliber thoracic drains (catheters) provides a good cost-effectiveness/comfort ratio, especially for patients in advanced stages of neoplastic disease.

The goal is that pleurodesis becomes a procedure carried out in outpatient clinics by physicians. This would considerably simplify its execution while maintaining efficacy. Therefore, there is no need for hospitalization, which would deprive patients, during this difficult phase of their life, of contact with their families and in turn adversely affect quality of life.

References

Clemensten P, Evald T, Grode G et al (1998) Treatment of malignant pleural effusion: pleurodesis using a small percutaneous catheter. A prospective randomised study. Respir Med 92:593–596

Crnjac A, Sok M, Kamenik M (2004) Impact of pleural effusion pH on the efficacy of thoracoscopic mechanical pleurodesis in patients with breast carcinoma. Eur J Cardiothorac Surg 26:432–436

De Campos JR, Vargas FS, de Campos Werebe E, Cardoso P, Teixeira LR, Jatene FB, Light RW (2001) Thoracoscopy talc poudrage: a 15-year experience. Chest 119:801–806

DiBonito L, Falconieri G, Colautti I et al (1992) The positive pleural effusion. A retrospective study of cytopathologic diagnoses with autopsy confirmation. Acta Cytol 36:329–332

Dikensoy O, Light RW (2005) Alternative widely available, inexpensive agents for pleurodesis. Curr Opin Pulm Med 11:340–344

Dresler CM, Olak J, Herndon JE 2nd et al, Cooperative Groups Cancer and Leukemia Group B; Eastern Cooperative Oncology Group; North Central

Cooperative Oncology Group; Radiation Therapy Oncology Group (2005) Phase III intergroup study of talc poudrage vs talc slurry sclerosis for malignant pleural effusion. Chest 127: 909–915

Gary Lee YC, Teixeira LR, Devin CJ et al (2001) Transforming growth factor-beta2 induces pleurodesis significantly faster than talc. Am J Respir Crit Care Med 163:640–644

Genc O, Petrou M, Ladas G et al (2000) The long-term morbidity of pleuroperitoneal shunts in the management of recurrent malignant effusions. Eur J Cardiothorac Surg 18:143–146

Light RW (1995) Pleural disease, 3rd edn. Williams & Wilkins, Baltimore, pp 36–74

Marrazzo A, Noto A, Casa L et al (2005) Video-thoracoscopic surgical pleurodesis in the management of malignant pleural effusion: the importance of an early intervention. J Pain Symptom Manage 30:75–79

Maskell NA, Lee YC, Gleeson FV et al (2004) Randomized trials describing lung inflammation after pleurodesis with talc of varying particle size. Am J Respir Crit Care Med 170:377–382

Paschoalini MS, Vargas FS, Marchi E et al (2005) Prospective randomized trial of silver nitrate vs talc slurry in pleurodesis for symptomatic malignant pleural effusions. Chest 128:684–689

Rehse DH, Aye RW, Florence MG (1999) Respiratory failure following talc pleurodesis. Am J Surg 177:437–440

Ren S, Terman DS, Bohach G et al (2004) Intrapleural staphylococcal superantigen induces resolution of malignant pleural effusions and a survival benefit in non-small cell lung cancer. Chest 126:1529–1539

Sartori S, Tassinari D, Ceccotti P et al (2004) Prospective randomized trial of intrapleural bleomycin versus interferon alfa-2b via ultrasound-guided small-bore chest tube in the palliative treatment of malignant pleural effusions. J Clin Oncol 22:1228–1233

Shaw P, Agarwal R (2004) Pleurodesis for malignant pleural effusions. Cochrane Database Syst Rev 1, CD002916

Vargas FS, Teixeira LR (1996) Pleural malignancies. Curr Opin Pulm Med 2:335–340

Vargas FS, Antonangelo L, Capelozzi V et al (2002) Lung damage in experimental pleurodesis induced by silver nitrate or talc: 1-year follow-up. Chest 122:2122–2126

Vargas FS, Teixeira LR, Marchi E (2004) Derrame pleural, 4a edn. Roca, São Paulo

Webb WR, Ozmen V, Moulder PV et al (1992) Iodized talc pleurodesis for the treatment of pleural effusions. J Thorac Cardiovasc Surg 103:881–885

Part III

Interventional Thoracoscopy ('The Grey Zone')

Advanced Application of Medical Thoracoscopy

15

Philippe Astoul, GianFranco Tassi, and Jean-Marie Tschopp

This section, identified as a "grey zone," marks the transition from the common indications of thoracoscopy in the management of pleural effusion and pneumothorax, which are accepted into practice, and as discussed in the preceding chapters, to more complex applications. They should be limited to centers with extensive thoracoscopic experience.

The treatment of infections of the pleural space still represents a field in which medical thoracoscopy, if correctly and expeditiously carried out, can allow for a complete recovery in highly selected cases and in turn avoid chronic evolution, more invasive interventions, and long-term functional limitations.

Forceps lung biopsy during thoracoscopy has been used for many years by pulmonologists, but with the advent of video-assisted thoracoscopic surgery (VATS), its employment in the diagnostic work-up of diffuse interstitial lung disease has been considerably reduced. Depending on the institutional habits and local expertise, it can be an alternative to a surgical procedure, as long as the physician is aware of the limitations of the technique. These diagnostic limitations are mainly due to the suboptimal specimen quality—often with a small proportion of small vessels.

P. Astoul (✉)
Division of Thoracic Oncology,
Pleural Diseases, and Interventional Pulmonology,
Hôpital NORD, Marseille, France
e-mail: pastoul@ap-hm.fr

G. Tassi
Division of Pneumology,
Spedali Civili di Brescia, Brescia, Italy
e-mail: gf.tassi@tin.it

J.-M. Tschopp
Département de Médecine Interne
Centre valaisan de pneumologie,
CHCVs, Montana 3963, Switzerland
e-mail: jean-marie.tschopp@hopitalvs.ch

P. Astoul et al. (eds.), *Thoracoscopy for Pulmonologists*,
DOI 10.1007/978-3-642-38351-9_15, © Springer-Verlag Berlin Heidelberg 2014

GianFranco Tassi, Martin H. Brutsche,
and Robert J.O. Davies

16.1 Introduction

Parapneumonic effusion and empyema are still an important medical problem since they remain a significant cause of morbidity and mortality (Davies et al. 1999; Farjah et al. 2007). Risk factors for the development of empyema include alcohol abuse, aspiration and poor dental hygiene, chronic lung disease, diabetes mellitus, gastroesophageal reflux, rheumatoid arthritis, and intravenous drug abuse (Ferguson et al. 1996). About one third of cases occur without any identified risk factors (Ferguson et al. 1996; Davies et al. 2003), suggesting that the host immune defense system or modification in bacterial virulence may also play important roles.

Empyema can arise as a complication of pneumonia or may follow iatrogenic procedures, surgery, trauma, or, rarely, bronchial obstruction from a tumor or foreign body. Pleural infection can also develop as a "primary" infection,

G. Tassi (✉)
Division of Pneumology,
Spedali Civili di Brescia, Brescia, Italy
e-mail: gf.tassi@tin.it

M.H. Brutsche
Division of Pneumology,
Kantonsspital St. Gallen, St. Gallen, Switzerland
e-mail: martin.brutsche@kssg.ch

R.J.O. Davies
Department of Respiratory Medicine, Oxford Pleural Unit, Oxford Centre for Respiratory Medicine,
Oxford Radcliffe Hospital,
Churchill Hospital Site, Oxford, UK

without evidence of lung parenchymal infection (Alfageme et al. 1993).

The first to describe pleuritis and empyema was Hippocrates in his aphorisms – short sentences which were for many years the only source of information for practising doctors. He stated: "pleuritis that does not clear up in 14 days results in empyema." and "pains and fevers occur rather at the formation of pus than when it is already formed." Other aphorisms refer to the therapy: "When empyema is treated either by the cautery or incision, if pure and white pus flow from the wound, the patients recover; but if mixed with blood, slimy and fetid, they die" (Tassi and Marchetti 2008).

16.2 Guidelines

Evidence-based guidelines for the management of complicated parapneumonic effusion and empyema, discussing the approach to diagnosis and treatment, are available in the literature (Colice et al. 2000; Davies et al. 2003).

In 2000 a panel convened by the American College of Chest Physicians drew up guidelines (Colice et al. 2000) on the medical and surgical management of parapneumonic effusions, developing an annotated table for evaluating the risk for poor outcome. Estimates of the risk were based on the clinical judgment that, without adequate drainage of the pleural space, the patient with a parapneumonic effusion would be likely to develop any or all of the following: prolonged hospitalization,

P. Astoul et al. (eds.), *Thoracoscopy for Pulmonologists*,
DOI 10.1007/978-3-642-38351-9_16, © Springer-Verlag Berlin Heidelberg 2014

prolonged evidence of systemic toxicity, increased morbidity from any drainage procedure, increased risk for residual ventilatory impairment, increased risk for local spread of the inflammatory reaction, and increased mortality. Three variables – pleural space anatomy, pleural fluid bacteriology, and pleural fluid chemistry – were used in this annotated table to categorize patients into four separate risk levels for poor outcome: categories 1 (very low risk), 2 (low risk), 3 (moderate risk), and 4 (high risk). A category three patient was characterized by the presence of pus in the pleural cavity, therefore including "true" empyemas. The guideline examined the results of randomized, controlled trials and historically controlled series. Based on these papers and consensus opinion, the panel suggested different approaches to managing parapneumonic effusions, including empyemas.

The British Thoracic Society guidelines for the management of pleural diseases (Davies et al. 2003, 2010a) attempted to integrate the available objective evidence with clinical experience relating to the investigation and treatment of these complex patients. They were researched and drafted by a subgroup of the Pleural Diseases Group (itself a subcommittee of the BTS Standards of Care Committee). An algorithm for clinical management based on a typical patient's diagnostic and therapeutic path was then drafted by the subgroup. This draft was based, where possible, on the published evidence, but this was then combined with clinical expertise as required.

Neither of these guidelines mention medical thoracoscopy, even though the comments regarding VATS could be indirectly extended to it.

16.3 Pathogenesis

The natural history of the disease includes three distinct phases or stages as described in the 1962 classification of empyema proposal of the American Thoracic Society (Andrews et al. 1962). This classification is still employed because it remains clinically useful. Empyema was subdivided into three stages: exudative, fibropurulent, and organized. The acute or exudative phase lasts for several days and is characterized by an effusion that is free-flowing in the pleural cavity.

Progression to the fibropurulent phase is characterized by reduced endocavitary fibrinolysis which causes fibrin deposition on the pleural surfaces and by alteration of fluid which becomes cloudy and viscous.

The chronic or organized phase follows on from the fibrin and collagen deposition and creates a fibrous thickening of the pleura, a sort of "peel" which entraps the lung. This differentiation into stages is of course a simplification of a biological process which evolves progressively, but it is useful in practice because the therapeutic approach is very different at each stage.

16.4 Diagnostic Approach

16.4.1 Pleural Fluid Analysis

Thoracocentesis in the setting of a pleural space infection is always useful when there is sufficient quantity of fluid to allow safe sampling (i.e., a free effusion when it is more than 1 cm on the lateral chest radiograph (Colice et al. 2000). This allows visual examination (the discovery of purulent fluid signifies empyema), biochemical analysis, in particular the measurement of pH, glucose, and pleural lactate dehydrogenase (LDH) (Heffner et al. 1995), and microbiologic analysis. Pleural fluid pH is considered clinically significant and the ACCP guidelines suggest the placement of a chest tube in the presence of a pH <7.20 (Colice et al. 2000). However there is the possibility of varying pH values in different loculations of a parapneumonic effusion. A low pH can be also present in neoplastic pleurisies, in tuberculosis, and in collagen vascular disease.

16.4.2 Bacteriology

The percentage of cases where the pleural fluid cultures are positive is significantly variable through different series (it was, e.g., 54 % in a case study of 430 patients (Maskell et al. 2005)). This depends on the characteristics of the infection, community-acquired or nosocomial, and the antibiotic treatment administered prior to thoracocentesis.

In recent years bacteria more frequently isolated (Davies et al. 2003; Maskell et al. 2005) include Gram-positive aerobes, Streptococcus group (in particular Streptococcus pneumoniae), and Staphylococcus group (mainly Staphylococcus aureus); less frequently Gram-negative aerobes and anaerobic bacteria are isolated. Also, the finding of multiple organisms is not rare. It is rare to isolate mycobacteria and fungi in immunocompetent.

16.4.3 Diagnostic Imaging

The diagnostic imaging of infectious pleurisies (Levin and Klein 1999) principally uses chest radiography, ultrasonography, and CT scan. It is employed mainly to confirm a suspected diagnosis but also as a guide for interventional procedures and to aid with the diagnosis of complex cases, such as the infectious effusions associated with other thoracic or extrathoracic pathologies.

16.4.3.1 Chest Radiography
Chest radiography is the most important examination for the patient with a suspected pleural infection. It is economical, rapidly available in all hospitals, can be carried out at the patient's bed, and is easily repeatable.

16.4.3.2 Ultrasonography
Ultrasonography is an inexpensive and easy method which can be carried out at the patient's bed. It can accurately differentiate between a free effusion and a loculated effusion and guide thoracocentesis or, if necessary, the introduction of a chest drain. Its main advantages are the absence of radiation and the possibility to explore both the pleural cavity and the abdominal cavity. The limits are the dependency on the experience of the operator and the presence of blind areas like the normal lung and bone structures.

16.4.3.3 Computed Tomography (CT)
This examination is characterized by high cost not only financial but also the health risks involved for the patient due to X-ray exposure and potential adverse reaction to contrast medium. Therefore its use should be preceded by ultrasonographic evaluation. The advantage of CT scan is that it allows for simultaneous exploration of the pleural space, chest wall, lungs and mediastinum, as well as the subdiaphragmatic region. Therefore this method is indicated in difficult cases, especially to identify possible lesions which may be associated with the pleural effusion.

16.5 Treatment

The treatment, as a rule, is based on antibiotic therapy and complete drainage of the liquid to allow total lung re-expansion. But the treatment choice in individual cases is more often guided by available resources and philosophy of individual physicians, rather than scientific data, and varies considerably between different hospitals, regions, and countries.

16.5.1 Antibiotics

The selection of antibiotics should be based on the results of blood and pleural fluid culture and sensitivity testing, however, since there is a low rate of positive results from bacteriology (~30 %) in the setting of empyema; therefore the initial antibiotic therapy is empirical and frequently continues to be empirical and only in a minority of cases should be adapted to the positive laboratory results. However it is important to remember when selecting appropriate antibiotics (Davies et al. 2003) that community-acquired infection normally exhibits a different microbiological spectrum from hospital-acquired infections. Therefore it requires different antibiotics at presentation: antibiotics for community-acquired empyema include beta-lactams and quinolones; while in hospital-acquired empyema, the therapy needs to cover both Gram-positive and Gram-negative aerobic organisms as well as anaerobes and therefore should include tazobactam, carbapenems, or third-generation cephalosporins with metronidazole. Aminoglycosides should be avoided due to poor penetration in the pleural space and reduced efficacy in acidic surroundings.

16.5.2 Chest Tube Drainage and Serial Thoracocentesis

A lack of response to antibiotics, as suggested by a failure to obtain clinical and radiological improvements, is a strong indication for chest tube drainage. The optimal size of chest tube and duration of drainage remain controversial. In parapneumonic effusions, small-bore (12–14 F) drains are easier to insert, more comfortable and adequate for the drainage of infected pleural collections, but this is not the case in the presence of frank pus, where larger tubes (20–24 F) are needed. The role of therapeutic thoracocentesis as an alternative to formal chest tube placement in pleural infection remains unclear. Treatment with serial thoracocentesis is attractive, as it may avoid the complications of chest drainage and perhaps allow outpatient management of selected cases. Successful treatment of empyema with therapeutic thoracocentesis and antibiotics has been reported (Storm et al. 1992), but has not been compared with formal drainage in randomized controlled trials.

16.5.3 Intrapleural Fibrinolytics

The role of intrapleural fibrinolytics remains uncertain. A meta-analysis (Tokuda et al. 2006) provides no evidence of benefit of intrapleural fibrinolytic therapy for reduction of mortality and need for surgery in adult patients with empyema and complicated parapneumonic effusions. Less definite are the conclusions of the recent review performed by the Cochrane Collaboration (Cameron and Davies 2008) which affirms that intrapleural fibrinolytic therapy confers significant benefit in reducing the requirement for surgical intervention for patients. However this was not supported by the large 2005 MIST1 study (Maskell et al. 2005).

16.6 Thoracoscopy

16.6.1 Indications

The correct use of thoracoscopy in pleural infectious disease has yet to be established unanimously (Waller 2002). Its exact position in the treatment algorithm remains unclear. Its utilization has been recommended prior to the placement of a chest drain (Loddenkemper 1998), while another application might be when the chest drain has failed to reduce the fever or the complete evacuation of pleural fluid within a few days (Kohman 1994; Yim 1999). Yet another approach makes reference to multiloculated effusions and considers thoracoscopy to be indicated to divide loculations both for parapneumonic effusion (Huang et al. 1999; Solèr et al. 1997) and for empyema (Silen and Naunheim 1996; Solèr et al. 1997; Wait et al. 1997; Cassina et al. 1999). More recently, in the surgical field the treatment has been extended to chronic organizing empyema, to clean the cavity both prior to formal thoracotomy and decortication (Lawrence et al. 1997) and for the actual decortication (Waller and Rengarajan 2001).

The guidelines of the American College of Chest Physicians (ACCP) (Colice et al. 2000) only consider the role of surgical thoracoscopy and video-assisted thoracoscopic surgery (VATS). VATS is advised for patients defined as at high risk of poor outcome (categories 3 and 4). Category 3 includes effusion larger than half of the hemithorax, which may be loculated or characterized pleural thickening. In category 4 there is the presence of pus in the pleural cavity. These recommendations are, however, based on a single randomized study of only 20 patients (Wait et al. 1997) and on a retrospective case study of 64 patients (Angelillo Mackinlay et al. 1996). A similar approach is described in the 2003 British Thoracic Society guidelines for the management of pleural infection (Davies et al. 2003, 2010b) and again only considers the role of surgical thoracoscopy. Moreover these papers do not discuss medical thoracoscopy, even if the discussion on VATS could be inferred to thoracoscopy.

16.6.2 Instruments and Techniques

Medical thoracoscopy and surgical thoracoscopy (VATS), both used to treat infections of the pleural space, are different in the kind of anesthesia, equipment, and technique as previously described elsewhere (Loddenkemper 1998).

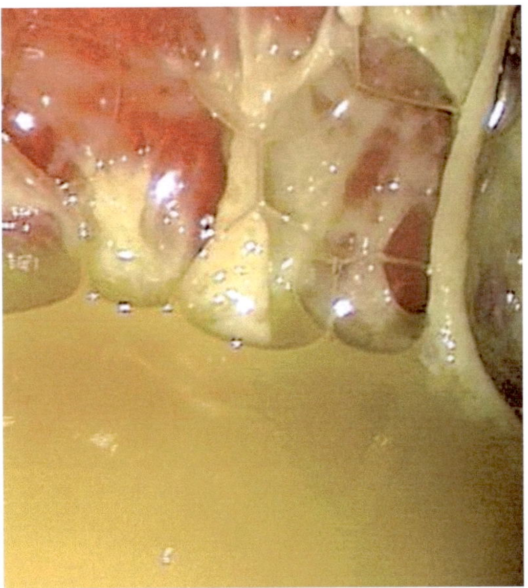

Fig. 16.1 A typical empyematous collection

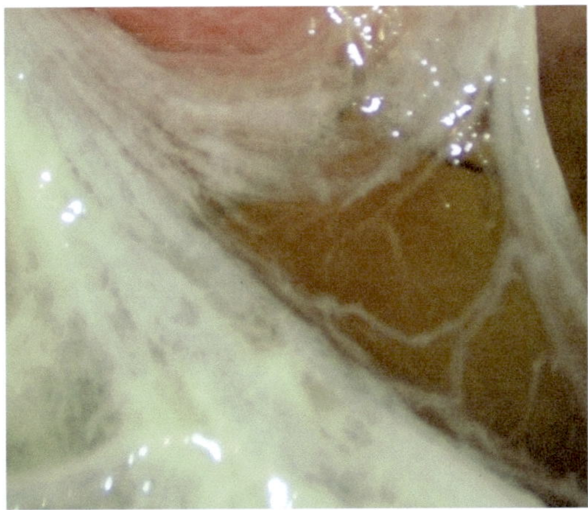

Fig. 16.2 Fibrin membranes in the pleural cavity

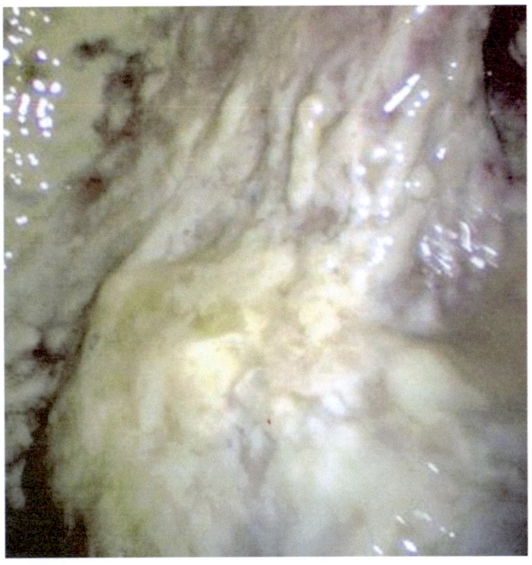

Fig. 16.3 An empyematous loculation in the left pleural cavity

In our experience with medical thoracoscopy, it is advisable to determine the trocar entry point by ultrasonography by detecting where the effusion is more abundant and to establish the location of the diaphragm, which is often elevated.

Thoracoscopy should be performed step by step and includes:

- Removal of pus (Fig. 16.1).
- Exploration of the pleural cavity to identify fibrin membranes (Fig. 16.2) and to detect loculations (Fig. 16.3), as well as possible neoplastic nodules, or intrapleural bubbling which may be an indirect sign of fistula (Fig. 16.4).
- Opening of loculations (Fig. 16.5).
- Removal of fibrinous membranes (Fig. 16.6) and purulent material from the cavity (Fig. 16.7) and, in addition, from the parietal and visceral pleural surfaces.
- Pleural biopsy.
- Pleural space lavage with saline solution.
- Introduction of a chest tube, with a caliber large enough (>24 F) to remove dense and viscous pus and fibrin detritus. This can be performed, if necessary, under visual control (Fig. 16.8).

16.6.3 Results

The published case studies on thoracoscopy in the infection of the pleural space (Table 16.1) deal principally with empyema and include both medical and surgical techniques, of which the latter is undoubtedly more numerous.

In general these studies report positive results, with rates of primary success (meaning recovery without subsequent thoracotomy or conversion from thoracoscopy to thoracotomy) between 60

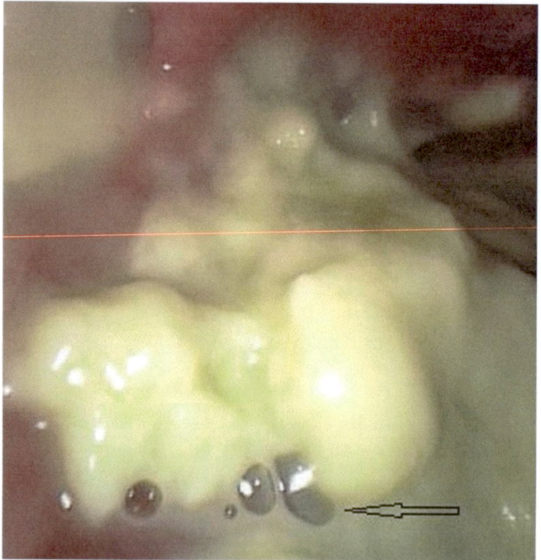

Fig. 16.4 Bubbles (*arrow*) indicating an associated lung parenchymal fistula

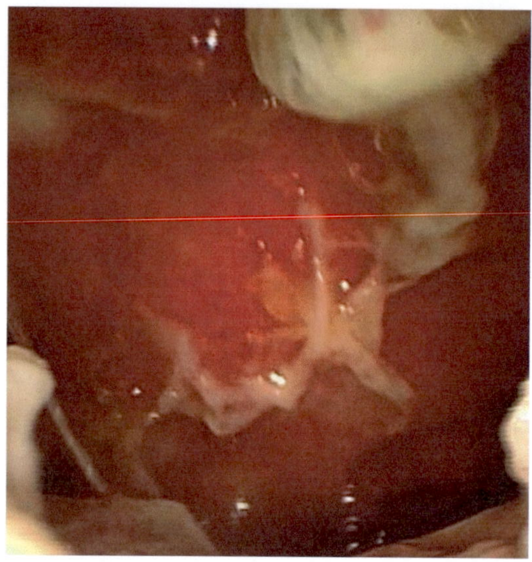

Fig. 16.6 The pleural cavity after the removal of the fibrinous membranes

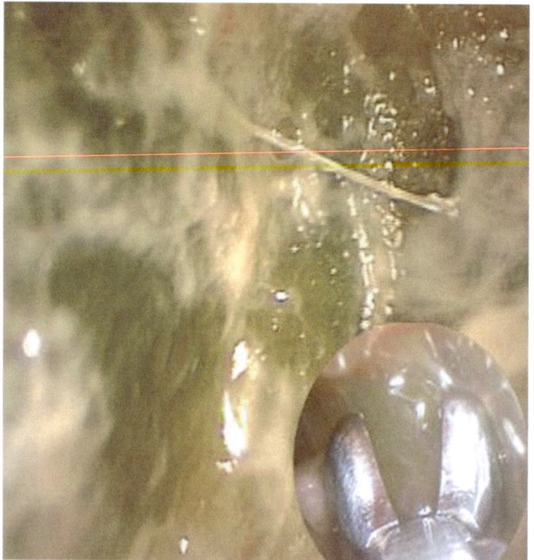

Fig. 16.5 Loculations dissected by forceps

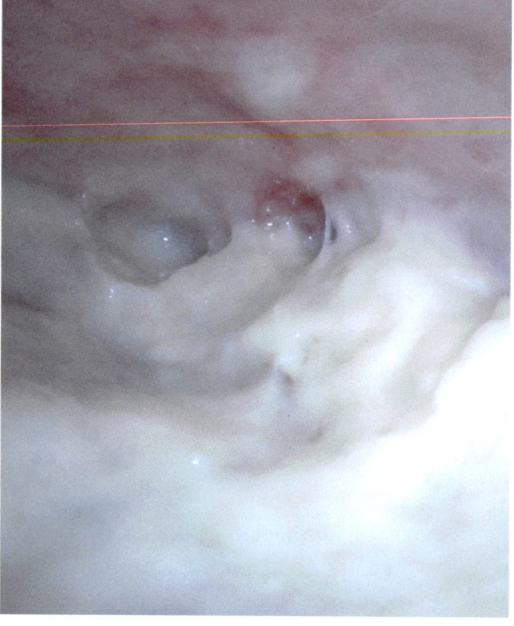

Fig. 16.7 Purulent material in the pleural cavity

and 100 % and higher if the procedure was performed earlier in the clinical course. However the number of patients treated was generally small, and only a few authors present case series with more than 100 patients.

In general there is total agreement about the advantages of VATS over thoracotomy, with shorter hospitalization, lower cost, and better cosmetic results.

The medical thoracoscopy experience outline the minimal invasive nature of the method,

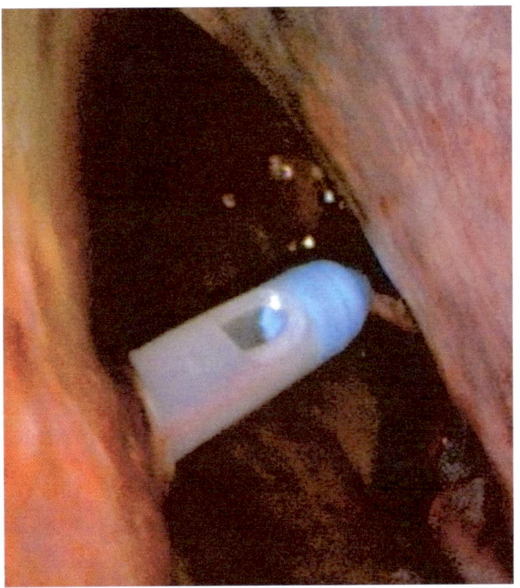

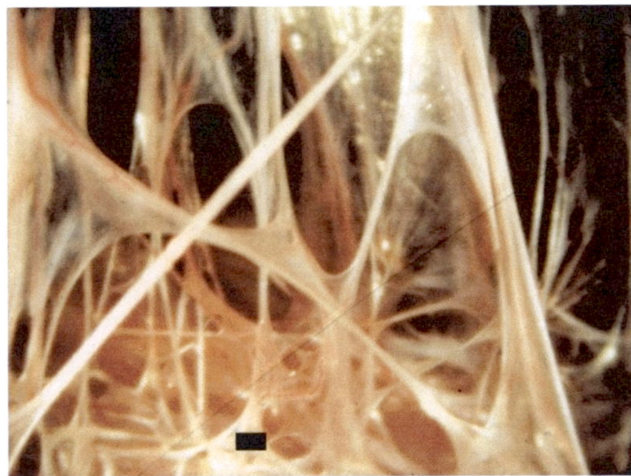

Fig. 16.9 An empyema at an early stage. There are multiple nonvascularized fibrotic adhesions, between the lung (■) and the chest wall. It is easy to severe such adhesions with the tip of optical biopsy forceps (Courtesy Ph Astoul – Marseille – France)

Table 16.1 Medical (M) and surgical thoracoscopy (S) in parapneumonic effusion and empyema

Author	Year	Patients	% of success	% of complications
Colt (M)	1995	7	86	14
Solèr (M)	1997	16	73	0
Striffeler (S)	1998	67	72	4
Reynard (M)	2004	5	100	0
Brutsche (M)	2005	127	91	9
Luh (S)	2005	234	86.3	8.3
Wurnig (S)	2006	130	91	9
Solaini (S)	2007	120	91.8	11

together with lower cost compared to VATS. In addition it has advantages in high-risk anesthetic groups such as frail patients.

Complications were strictly related to the complexity of the cases treated and were represented mainly by bleeding and extensive air leaks, with reported incidence between 0 % (Sendt et al. 1995; Cassina et al. 1999) and 16 % (Angelillo Mackinlay et al. 1996). In some surgical series which included subjects with serious comorbidity, deaths did occur (Angelillo Mackinlay et al. 1996; Landreneau et al. 1996; Weissberg and Refaely 1996; Lawrence et al. 1997; Wait et al. 1997).

Conclusions

Thoracoscopy is certainly effective in the treatment of pleural infections, especially in multiloculated empyema, preventing progression to thoracotomy (Silen and Naunheim 1996), even if large randomized studies have yet to be performed to confirm this finding (Waller 2002).

Medical thoracoscopy can play an important role in patients in poor health and high surgical risk. It is an intermediate drain procedure between chest tube placement and surgical thoracoscopy (VATS) performed under general anesthesia. Moreover, it is an efficacious procedure with associated low cost. It should be performed early in the disease to try to avoid chronic evolution of the disease.

16.7 Pleural Infections – Mini-Atlas

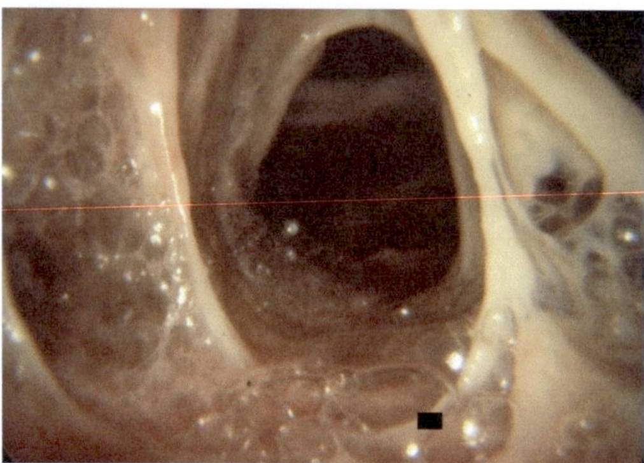

Fig. 16.10 Multilocular empyema at the fibrinopurulent stage. The thick adhesions can create pockets of pus with different fluid pH, degree of infection, and microbial culture which makes management difficult, in particular puncture and drainage, even when image-guided. These adhesions can be broken down during thoracoscopy in order to obtain a single cavity which may allow for better drainage and pleural lavage, (■■) parietal pleura (Courtesy C Boutin, Ph Astoul – Marseille – France)

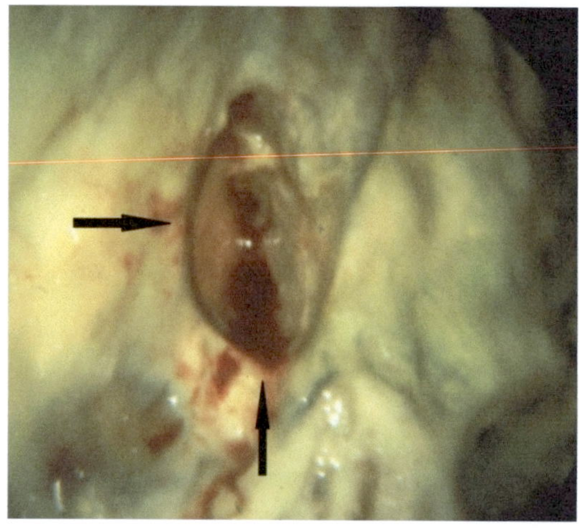

Fig. 16.12 An empyema at an advanced stage. A bronchopleural fistula (*arrows*) is a dreaded complication of infectious pleurisy (Courtesy C Boutin, Ph Astoul – Marseille – France)

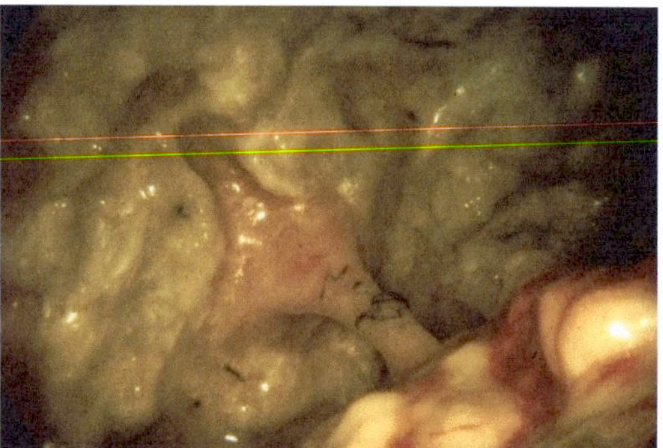

Fig. 16.11 An empyema after resection of adhesions. The parietal pleura and the lung are covered by a purulent layer as seen on the bottom right of the figure (Courtesy C Boutin, Ph Astoul – Marseille – France)

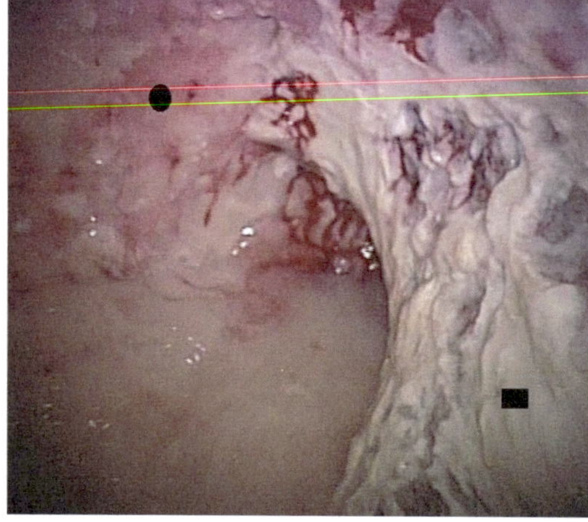

Fig. 16.13 An empyema caused by *Streptococcus intermedius* in a former drug user, HIV- negative young man. After resection of adhesions, the posterior parietal pleura (●) and the diaphragm (■) at the level of the left costodiaphragmatic gutter are covered with a fibrinopurulent layer (Courtesy Ph Astoul – Marseille – France)

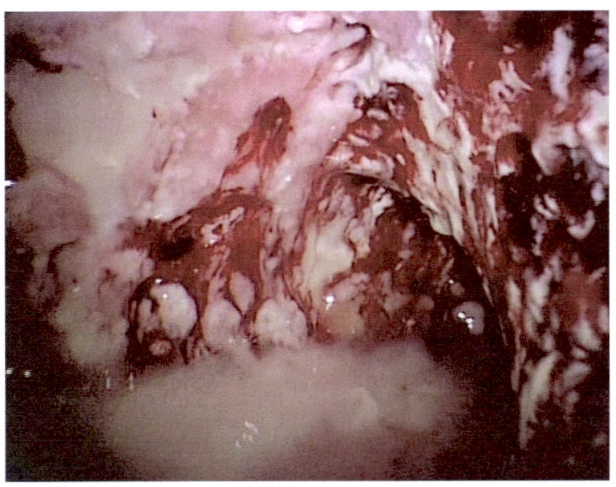

Fig. 16.14 Same patient. In this case, multiple biopsies were done using optical biopsy forceps through a single point of entry. No underlying disease was found (Courtesy Ph Astoul – Marseille – France)

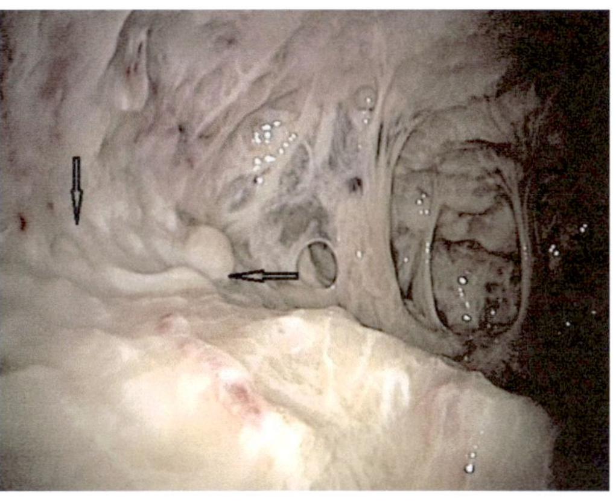

Fig. 16.16 Empyema (*left side* – upper part of the pleural cavity). Pus deposits on the lung (*bottom*) and the posterior parietal pleura (*top*). Purulent adhesions are visible between the lung and the chest wall. There is a complete symphysis (*arrow*) between the upper part of the lung and the chest wall (Courtesy Ph Astoul – Marseille – France)

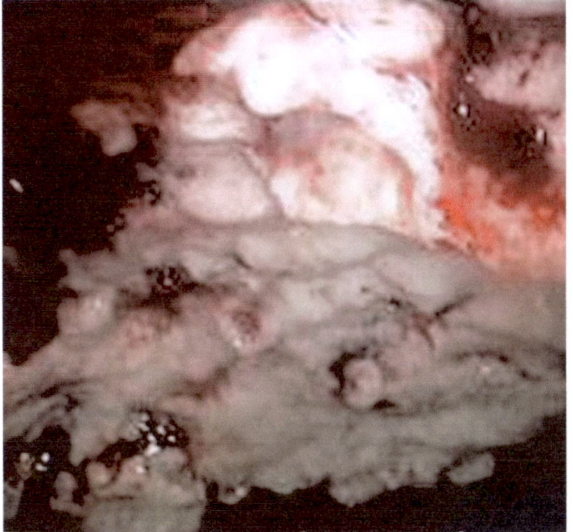

Fig. 16.15 Hemorrhagic empyema (Courtesy Ph Astoul – Marseille – France)

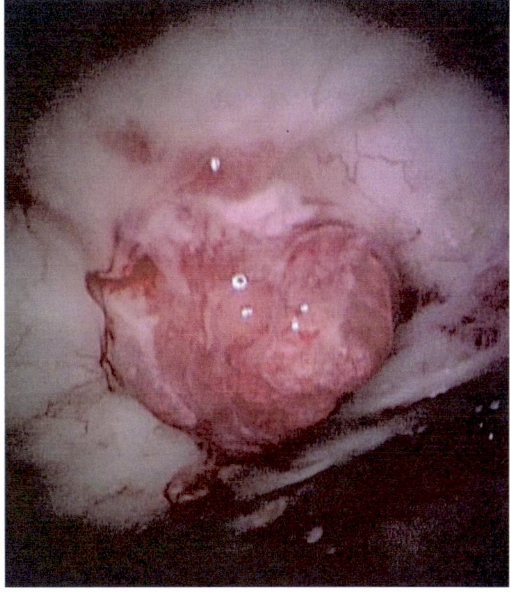

Fig. 16.17 A malignant nodule in patient managed for an empyema. In addition to resection of the multiple pleural adhesions, the thoracoscopist should perform a careful examination of the pleural cavity in order to rule out an underlying disease (Courtesy Ph Astoul – Marseille – France)

References

Alfageme I, Munoz F, Pena N et al (1993) Empyema of the thorax in adults. Etiology, microbiologic findings, and management. Chest 103:839–843

Andrews NC, Parker EF, Shaw RP et al (1962) Management of nontuberculous empyema. A statement of the subcommittee on surgery. Am Rev Respir Dis 85:935–936

Angelillo Mackinlay TA, Lyons GA, Chimondeguy DJ et al (1996) VATS debridement versus thoracotomy in the treatment of loculated postpneumonia empyema. Ann Thorac Surg 61:1626–1630

Cameron R, Davies HR (2008) Intra-pleural fibrinolytic therapy versus conservative management in the treatment of adult parapneumonic effusions and empyema. Cochrane Database Syst Rev 2, CD002312

Cassina PC, Hauser M, Hillejan L et al (1999) Video-assisted thoracoscopy in the treatment of pleural empyema: stage-based management and outcome. J Thorac Cardiovasc Surg 117:234–238

Colice GL, Curtis A, Deslauriers J et al (2000) Medical and surgical treatment of parapneumonic effusions: an evidence-based guideline. Chest 118:1158–1171

Davies CWH, Kearney SE, Gleeson FV et al (1999) Predictors of outcome and long-term survival in patients with pleural infection. Am J Respir Crit Care Med 160:1682–1687

Davies CWH, Gleeson FV, Davies RJO (2003) BTS guidelines for the management of pleural infection. Thorax 58(Suppl II):ii18–ii28

Davies HE, Davies ROJ, Davies CWH et al (2010a) Management of pleural infection in adults: British Thoracic Society pleural disease guideline 2010. Thorax 65(Suppl II):ii41–ii53

Davies HE, Davies RJ, Davies CW, BTS Pleural Disease Guideline Group (2010b) Management of pleural infection in adults. British Thoracic Society Pleural Disease Guideline 2010. Thorax 65(Suppl 2): ii41–ii53, Review

Farjah F, Symons RG, Krishnadasan B et al (2007) Management of pleural space infections: a population-based analysis. J Thorac Cardiovasc Surg 133: 346–351

Ferguson AD, Prescott RJ, Selkon JB et al (1996) The clinical course and management of thoracic empyema. QJM 89:285–289

Heffner JE, Brown LK, Barbieri C et al (1995) Pleural fluid chemical analysis in parapneumonic effusions. A meta-analysis. Am J Respir Crit Care Med 151: 1700–1708

Huang HC, Chang HY, Chen CW et al (1999) Predicting factors for outcome of tube thoracostomy in complicated parapneumonic effusion or empyema. Chest 115:751–756

Kohman LJ (1994) Thoracoscopy for the evaluation and treatment of pleural space disease. Chest Surg Clin N Am 4:467–479

Landreneau RJ, Keenan RJ, Hazelrigg SR et al (1996) Thoracoscopy for empyema and hemothorax. Chest 109:18–24

Lawrence DR, Ohri SK, Moxon RE et al (1997) Thoracoscopic debridement of empyema thoracis. Ann Thorac Surg 64:1448–1450

Levin DL, Klein JS (1999) Imaging techniques for pleural space infections. Semin Respir Infect 14:31–38

Loddenkemper R (1998) Thoracoscopy: state of the art. Eur Respir J 11:213–221

Maskell NA, Davies CW, Nunn AJ, First Multicenter Intrapleural Sepsis Trial (MIST1) Group et al (2005) UK controlled trial of intrapleural streptokinase for pleural infection. N Engl J Med 352:865–874

Sendt W, Forster E, Hau T (1995) Early thoracoscopic debridement and drainage as definite treatment for pleural empyema. Eur J Surg 161:73–76

Silen ML, Naunheim KS (1996) Thoracoscopic approach to the management of empyema thoracis. Indications and results. Chest Surg Clin N Am 6:491–499

Solèr M, Wyser C, Bolliger CT et al (1997) Treatment of early parapneumonic empyema by "medical" thoracoscopy. Schweiz Med Wochenschr 127: 1748–1753

Storm HK, Krasnik M, Bang K et al (1992) Treatment of pleural empyema secondary to pneumonia: thoracocentesis regimen versus tube drainage. Thorax 47:821–824

Tassi GF, Marchetti GP (2008) Pleural disease: historic perspective. In: Light RW, Gary Lee YC (eds) Textbook of pleural diseases, 2nd edn. Hodder Arnold, London

Tokuda Y, Matsushima D, Stein GH et al (2006) Intrapleural fibrinolytic agents for empyema and complicated parapneumonic effusions: a meta-analysis. Chest 129:783–790

Wait MA, Sharma S, Hohn J et al (1997) A randomized trial of empyema therapy. Chest 111:1548–1551

Waller DA (2002) Thoracoscopy in management of postpneumonic pleural infections. Curr Opin Pulm Med 8:323–326

Waller DA, Rengarajan A (2001) Thoracoscopic decortication: a role for video-assisted surgery in chronic postpneumonic pleural empyema. Ann Thorac Surg 71:1813–1816

Weissberg D, Refaely Y (1996) Pleural empyema: 24-year experience. Ann Thorac Surg 62:1026–1029

Yim AP (1999) Paradigm shift in empyema management. Chest 115:611–612

Christophe Dooms and Johan Vansteenkiste

17.1 Introduction

Diffuse or focal interstitial lung disease, peripheral nodular lesions of unknown etiology, and pulmonary infection do sometimes require invasive tissue sampling after an inconclusive bronchoscopy with bronchoalveolar lavage (BAL) and/or transbronchial lung biopsies (TBLB). The decision to perform a lung biopsy has to be based on the probability that the examination will yield a specific diagnosis leading to a specific and/or change in treatment.

17.2 Equipment and Techniques

A surgical open lung biopsy requires general anesthesia, a single-lumen endotracheal tube, and a conventional thoracotomy usually with a limited (50 mm cutaneous) incision. A surgical lung biopsy specimen should be at least 4 cm in maximum diameter when aerated and a depth (distance from pleural surface) of 3–5 cm. An open lung biopsy is taken using bistouries and sutures. This

is certainly the method of choice if there is obliteration of the pleural space or if the patient is too unwell to tolerate single-lung ventilation.

A video-assisted thoracoscopic surgery (VATS) requires general anesthesia, a double-lumen endotracheal tube for one-lung ventilation, and two small (approximately 15 mm) and one larger incision to obtain three ports of entry. The lung edge of the lobe of interest is mobilized with a nontraumatic grasping forceps, and a disposable linear stapler/cutter is used to take one or two lung specimens of about 10×20 mm. Two randomized trials did not show clinical or pathological differences in outcomes for open surgical compared to thoracoscopic surgical approaches (Miller et al. 2000; Ayed and Raghunathan 2000).

A video-assisted medical thoracoscopy (VAMT) was originally described by Boutin (Boutin et al. 1982). It can be performed under light sedation and spontaneous breathing without needing an endotracheal tube or general anesthesia. After the induction of an artificial pneumothorax, two small (<10 mm) incisions are made for the insertion of two trocars. One to seven biopsies from different lobes are performed using a double-spoon forceps (5 mm in diameter) connected to a diathermy apparatus while applying thermocoagulation at 40–60 W (Fig. 17.1). It is important to keep the coagulation time as short as possible (<2 s) to avoid tissue artifacts. There is an ongoing controversy over the most suitable site for biopsy in diffuse interstitial lung disease. Lung biopsies should be performed in places distant from the interlobar fissures and bullae to reduce

C. Dooms (✉)
Pulmonology Department,
University Hospital Gasthuisberg, Leuven, Belgium
e-mail: christophe.dooms@uzleuven.be

J. Vansteenkiste
Respiratory Oncology Unit (Pulmonology)
and Leuven Lung Cancer Group,
University Hospital Gasthuisberg, Leuven, Belgium
e-mail: johan.vansteenkiste@uzleuven.be

P. Astoul et al. (eds.), *Thoracoscopy for Pulmonologists*,
DOI 10.1007/978-3-642-38351-9_17, © Springer-Verlag Berlin Heidelberg 2014

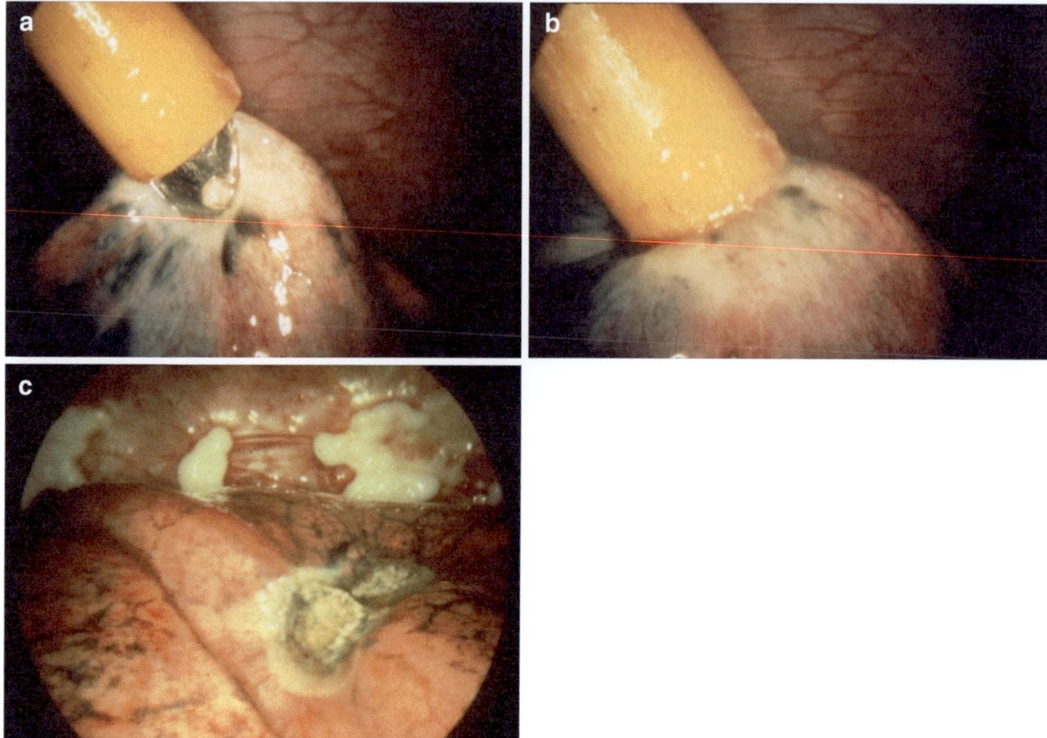

Fig. 17.1 The pulmonary biopsy technique. The biopsy area is grasped with the forceps perpendicular to the pulmonary surface (**a**). The forceps are closed for 1–2 s and pulled towards the 5-mm insulated trocar. Simultaneously the operator applies a brief current (approximately 1 s) using a foot pedal while pulling the forceps through the distal end of the trocar. The sharp distal tip of the trocar cuts the specimen (**b**). After this maneuver, the biopsy site blanches and retracts without bleeding or evidence of an air leak (**c**). A recent experimental study in animal subjects showed that subpleural biopsies obtained during pleuroscopy and deep lung biopsy specimens obtained by electrocautery provided satisfactory material for histologic examination (Emam et al. 2012) (Courtesy C Boutin and Ph Astoul – Marseille – France)

complications. In addition, biopsies should not be performed if there is obvious honeycombing or entirely normal-appearing parenchyma. In this regard, the HRCT provides valuable information that should be used to guide biopsy sites. Areas of intermediate abnormality or comparatively the normal lung adjacent to the honeycomb lung should be targeted. At the end of the procedure, a chest drain should be left in the pleural space to re-expand the lung and to check for air leaks or possible bleeding. In most cases the patients can be discharged from hospital within 3 days. Despite encouraging results from parenchymal lung biopsies in the diagnosis of interstitial lung disease by forceps biopsy during VAMT (Boutin et al. 1982; Dijkman et al. 1982), the technique gained little popularity among pulmonologists as thermocoagulatory closure of the air leaks may necessitate prolonged chest tube drainage, and in addition, the diagnostic yield may be inadequate in certain circumstances.

17.3 Indications and Contraindications

17.3.1 Diffuse Lung Disease

In patients with diffuse interstitial lung disease in whom the multidisciplinary integration of clinical and high-resolution computed tomography (HRCT) data, with the addition of BAL and TBLB data, is insufficient to yield a confident diagnosis, current guidelines recommend a surgical lung biopsy in the absence of medical contraindications (Wells and Hirani 2008). A dedicated chest radiologist and chest physician should discuss the HRCT images in advance and decide upon the most appropriate target area to biopsy. There are no randomized controlled trials comparing the three different biopsy techniques (wedge biopsy during VATS, forceps biopsy during VAMT, surgical open lung biopsy). Forceps lung biopsy during VAMT has been used for many years by pulmonologists (Boutin et al. 1982; Loddenkemper and Boutin 1993; Mathur and Loddenkemper 1995). Nevertheless the range of indications for forceps lung biopsies at VAMT in diffuse lung disease has steadily decreased over the last three decades; this has been demonstrated by the change in clinical practice at the Lungenklinik of Berlin where forceps lung biopsy accounted for 22 % of all thoracoscopies in 1971–1979, decreasing to 8 % in 1980–1988, and only 1 % in 1989–1996 (Loddenkemper 1998).

Most studies on VAMT discuss the technical characteristics, diagnostic yield, and potential complications (Boutin et al. 1982; Dijkman et al. 1982), but the diagnostic accuracy of the technique depends on the distribution pattern of the interstitial lung disease, and thus the lobular compartment involved (Fig. 17.2), and the histological specificity of the disease (Vansteenkiste et al. 1999). Only a few papers addressed the issue of biopsy size and histopathological quality (Vansteenkiste et al. 1999; Colt 1995).

A direct comparison of stapled wedge biopsy by VATS to thermocoagulation-assisted forceps biopsy by VAMT has been performed in adult swine with healthy lungs (Colt 1995). Transbronchial biopsy specimens by bronchoscopy are usually <2 mm² in size, forceps biopsies by VAMT are round-ovoid and range from 2.1 to 6.6 mm in longest diameter or 5–30 mm² in cross-sectional area, and wedge biopsies by VATS range from 27 to 146 mm in longest diameter (Ayed and Raghunathan 2000). The forceps biopsies contain 300–3,000 readily identifiable alveoli in the specimen, while a wedge biopsy

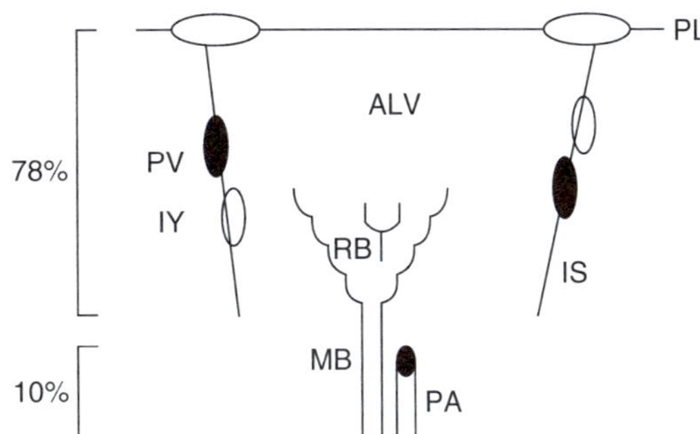

Fig. 17.2 Schematic drawing of the anatomy of the secondary lobule supplied by the bronchovascular bundle with a membranous bronchiole (*MB*) and a pulmonary artery (*PA*). The MB branches into the respiratory bronchioles (*RB*) in the centrilobular region. At the distal end there is the alveolated parenchyma (*ALV*) with the precapillary arterioles. The lobule is surrounded by the pleura (*PL*) and the interlobular septum (*IS*) containing the pulmonary veins (*PV*) and lymphatics (*LY*), the latter are also being present in the bronchovascular bundle. During medical thoracoscopy with lung biopsy procedure, the bronchovascular bundle is sampled in 10 % of the specimens and the periphery of the lobule, the IS, and the PL in 78 % of cases (From Vansteenkiste et al. 1999)

section contains at least 8,000 alveoli. No difference in the number of respiratory bronchioles per mm² was noted between forceps and wedge biopsy. A greater number of vessels per mm² were found in wedge biopsies compared to forceps biopsies.

Only one paper addressed the issue of histopathological quality of the forceps biopsies by VAMT in human interstitial lung disease. This demonstrated that the alveolar compartment (including the respiratory bronchiole, interlobular septa, and alveolar parenchyma; Fig. 17.2) was present in 2/3 of the biopsies, while the membranous bronchiole and central pulmonary arteries are present in only 10 % of the biopsies (Vansteenkiste et al. 1999). Consequently central pulmonary lesions (such as BOOP) and pulmonary vascular disorders (such as vasculitis, pulmonary microemboli) remain a difficult challenge and are thus poor indications for forceps biopsies during VAMT. The histological specificity of a forceps biopsy at VAMT is high in cases of involvement of the alveolar compartment such as in UIP, NSIP, DIP, granulomatous diseases such as sarcoidosis, and carcinomatous lymphangitis.

A thoracoscopic procedure should be avoided in cases with suspected major pleural adhesions or bullous degeneration of the lung based on the radiological features, in severe pulmonary hypertension, in patients on mechanical ventilation, and/or severe respiratory insufficiency with dependence on oxygen therapy (pO_2 <55 mmHg and/or pCO_2 >60 mmHg) (Vansteenkiste et al. 1999; Kreider et al. 2007).

17.3.2 Localized Lung Disease

The use of a thoracoscopic forceps lung biopsy in localized peripheral lung lesions has disappeared as surgical VATS with wedge resection has become the procedure of choice in these situations.

17.4 Complications

No major complications such as procedure-related death, lung bleeding, or persistent fistula are described in forceps biopsies by VAMT for ILD. The most important minor complication is a prolonged air leak which correlated to the total lung capacity and thus can be anticipated in patients with very stiff or honeycomb lungs (Vansteenkiste et al. 1999).

Conclusion

A medical thoracoscopy with forceps biopsy is a safe procedure in the hands of a well-trained interventional pulmonologist. Depending on the institutional habits and local expertise, it can be an alternative to a surgical procedure in the diagnostic work-up of diffuse interstitial lung disease, but one has to be aware of the limitations of the technique. The major reason why VAMT has not become a routine clinical practice for lung biopsy in diffuse interstitial lung disease is, in our opinion, the suboptimal specimen quality in terms of the small precapillary arterioles, central pulmonary arteries, and membranous arterioles.

References

Ayed A, Raghunathan R (2000) Thoracoscopy versus open lung biopsy in the diagnosis of interstitial lung disease: a randomized controlled trial. J R Coll Surg Edinb 45:159–163

Boutin C, Viallat J, Cargnino P et al (1982) Thoracoscopic lung biopsy. Experimental and clinical preliminary study. Chest 82:44–48

Colt HG (1995) Thoracoscopy. A prospective study of safety and outcome. Chest 108:324–329

Dijkman J, van der Meer J, Bakker W et al (1982) Transpleural lung biopsy by the thoracoscopic route in patients with diffuse interstitial pulmonary disease. Chest 82:76–83

Emam RH, Froudarakis ME, Refaat AI, et al (2012) Subpleural versus deep lung biopsies obtained during pleuroscopy for histological examination: an experimental animal study. Respiration 84:423–428

Kreider M, Hansen-Flaschen J, Ahmad N et al (2007) Complications of video-assisted thoracoscopic lung biopsy in patients with interstitial lung disease. Ann Thorac Surg 83:1140–1144

Loddenkemper R (1998) Thoracoscopy: state of the art. Eur Respir J 11:213–221

Loddenkemper R, Boutin C (1993) Thoracoscopy: present diagnostic and therapeutic indications. Eur Respir J 6:1544–1555

Mathur PN, Loddenkemper R (1995) Medical thoracoscopy. Role in pleural and lung diseases. Clin Chest Med 16:487–496

Miller J, Urschel J, Cox G et al (2000) A randomized, controlled trial comparing thoracoscopy and limited thoracotomy for lung biopsy in interstitial lung disease. Ann Thorac Surg 70:1647–1650

Vansteenkiste J, Verbeken E, Thomeer M et al (1999) Medical thoracoscopic lung biopsy in interstitial lung disease: a prospective study of biopsy quality. Eur Respir J 14:585–590

Wells A, Hirani N (2008) Interstitial lung disease guideline: the British Thoracic Society in collaboration with the Thoracic Society of Australia and New Zealand and the Irish Thoracic Society. Thorax 63 Suppl 5:v1–v58

The Frontier of Medical Thoracoscopy

18

Philippe Astoul, GianFranco Tassi, and Jean-Marie Tschopp

Advanced procedures in medical thoracoscopy are best described as nonroutine. They are interventions associated with greater complexity and lie somewhere between the medical procedure of thoracoscopy and the surgical procedure of VATS. The current advanced indications as described in the literature include sympathectomy and pericardial window. At the present time, thoracoscopic sympathectomy is minimally invasive and is an accepted intervention for patients with a variety of autonomous nervous system disturbances. Patients with essential hyperhidrosis as well as highly selected subjects with other defined disorders can be symptomatically improved with this procedure.

They can be performed by interventional pulmonologists, but it must be noted that when performed as a "medical thoracoscopy" they should be categorized as an advanced technique—a "red zone" procedure. A pericardial window can be performed at thoracoscopy, as previously described in the literature. However, VATS should be considered as the gold standard, and the dedicated chapter in this book is to remind the reader of the historical aspects and limits of medical thoracoscopy. For these advanced procedures expert skills are mandatory from performing the basic procedures, simulated training, and hands-on training under the supervision of an experienced trainer.

P. Astoul (✉)
Division of Thoracic Oncology,
Pleural Diseases, and Interventional Pulmonology,
Hôpital NORD, Marseille, France
e-mail: pastoul@ap-hm.fr

G. Tassi
Division of Pneumology,
Spedali Civili di Brescia, Brescia, Italy
e-mail: gf.tassi@tin.it

J.-M. Tschopp
Département de Médecine Interne
Centre valaisan de pneumologie,
CHCVs, Montana 3963, Switzerland
e-mail: jean-marie.tschopp@hopitalvs.ch

P. Astoul et al. (eds.), *Thoracoscopy for Pulmonologists*,
DOI 10.1007/978-3-642-38351-9_18, © Springer-Verlag Berlin Heidelberg 2014

Sympatholysis via Thoracoscopy

19

Marc Noppen

19.1 Introduction

Thoracic sympathectomy is defined as the anatomical interruption of the thoracic sympathetic chain. The level of interruption (e.g., T_2, T_3) depends upon the indication for the sympathectomy and the required therapeutic effects (e.g., treatment of essential palmar or axillary hyperhidrosis, treatment of refractory heart rhythm disorders, treatment of chronic pancreatic pain). Anatomically, the interruption can be applied at the preganglionic level; however, current best practice involves ablation by electrocautery ("sympatholysis") or excision/clipping of the sympathetic ganglia (and sometimes part of the chain itself) (Noppen 2004; Tassi et al. 2006).

The current standard approach for thoracic sympathectomy is via thoracoscopy: thoracoscopic sympathectomy combines superior visualization of the upper thoracic ganglia with minimal postoperative morbidity and dysfunction. Open surgical approaches are now obsolete, and percutaneous ablation is not widely used because of a higher risk of early recurrence, postoperative complications, such as pneumothorax, and diffi-

culties in accurately localizing the ganglia (Wilkinson 1984).

Most papers on thoracoscopic sympathectomy, written by surgeons, typically describe a VATS (video-assisted thoracoscopic surgery) technique, which can be defined as a keyhole surgical procedure using single-lung double-lumen ventilation, disposable trocars, unilateral 3-entry port intervention, pleural and sympathetic chain dissection, and often necessitating chest drainage post procedure. However, successful TTS can also be performed using the less invasive "medical" thoracoscopic sympatholysis, often performed by a pulmonologist (Noppen et al. 1996). Recently, various surgical authors (Yim et al. 2000; Yamamoto et al. 2000) have described a less invasive sympathectomy technique (e.g., using 2 or 5 mm diameter (ultra)thin thoracoscopes), which may replace the traditional 10 mm diameter VATS instruments as they appear to offer similar therapeutic results with better esthetic outcomes and lower morbidity (Krasna 2008; Bachmann et al. 2009). This evolution towards a more simplified procedural technique will hopefully lead to the convergence of opinions (pulmonologist and surgeon) on who should perform thoracoscopic sympatholysis in particular and therapeutic thoracoscopy in general. However thoracoscopic sympatholysis is a highly specialized nature and therefore should be categorized in the "red zone" of medical thoracoscopy.

M. Noppen
Interventional Endoscopy Clinic,
University Hospital UZ Brussel, Brussels, Belgium
e-mail: marc.noppen@uzbrussel.be

19.2 Indications and Contraindications

19.2.1 Indications

In the past, sympathectomy was indicated in the treatment of a wide variety of disorders and syndromes (Table 19.1), although for many of these former indications there was little or no objective evidence of efficacy.

Nowadays, thoracoscopic sympathectomy is indicated for a limited number of applications (Table 19.2).

Essential hyperhidrosis, characterized by pathological sweating of the hand and/or armpits, is the main indication for TTS, both in adults (Noppen 2004; Krasna 2008) and children and adolescents (Noppen et al. 1998b;

Table 19.1 Conditions that historically have been treated by sympathectomy

Raynaud's phenomenon	Dysmenorrhea	Glaucoma
Acrocyanosis	Pancreatitis	Perniosis
Buerger's disease	Angina pectoris	Arteriosclerosis
Causalgia	Arrhythmias	Hirschsprung's disease
Migraine	Poliomyelitis	Arthritis
Renal disorders	Hyperhidrosis	Retinitis pigmentosa
Gall bladder disease	Paget's disease of bone	Venous ulcerations
Peptic ulcer	Epilepsy	Constipation

Table 19.2 Current indications for thoracoscopic sympathectomy

1. Universally accepted:
   Essential hyperhidrosis (palmar, axillar, facial)
   Facial blushing/social phobia syndrome
2. In selected cases:
   Raynaud's phenomenon, acrocyanosis, upper limb arterial insufficiency
   Buerger's disease
   Causalgia
   Angina pectoris, long QT syndrome, ventricular and arterial tachycardia
   Chronic pancreatic pain (pancreatic carcinoma, chronic pancreatitis)

Steiner et al. 2008). It is generally believed that patients with essential hyperhidrosis should have completed a trial of nonoperative treatment prior to sympathectomy; these trials include topical agents containing aluminum chloride or hexahydrate, oral agents (anticholinergics, beta-blockers, and antidepressants), locally applied botulinum toxin, iontophoresis, and psychotherapy. However, results of these nonsurgical trials are often disappointing in the long term because of poor efficacy, occurrence of side effects, temporary response, and cost. Recent studies comparing medical to thoracoscopic management have shown that thoracoscopic sympathectomy is superior to medical management in terms of clinical outcome and side effects. Therefore thoracoscopic sympathectomy should be recommended as first-line treatment rather than a "last resort," especially for the typical, severe form of essential palmar and axillary hyperhidrosis (Baumgartner et al. 2009; Ambrogi et al. 2009).

Facial blushing/social phobia (Fig. 19.1) is another possible variant of hypersympathicotony and may also be associated with facial hyperhidrosis. It sometimes presents with extremely disabling effects which has occasionally led to suicide. In these patients, an approach using a combination of medical interventions including daily low-dose anticholinergic (glycopyrrolate), a beta-blocker (propranolol), a central alpha-agonist (clonidine), and an anxiolytic (alprazolam) is often successful (unpublished data). In patients with significant side effects, or when a definitive treatment is requested by the patient, a thoracoscopic sympathectomy can be performed (Neumayer et al. 2005; Drott et al. 1998).

In *Raynaud's phenomenon*, *acrocyanosis*, and *idiopathic thoracic outlet syndrome*, thoracoscopic sympathectomy can provide temporary symptomatic benefit (Di Lorenzo et al. 1998; Sayers et al. 1994). However on occasions the effects can sometimes be longstanding. However, no large-scale controlled studies are available. Nevertheless, numerous case series suggest potential short and intermediate-term benefits as long as patients are carefully selected.

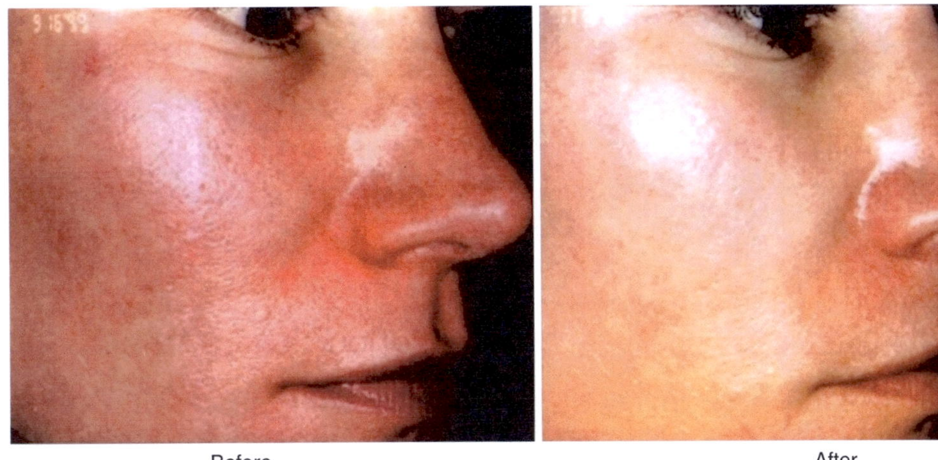

Fig. 19.1 A patient with facial flushing before (*left*) and after (*right*) a T2 thoracoscopic sympatholysis procedure

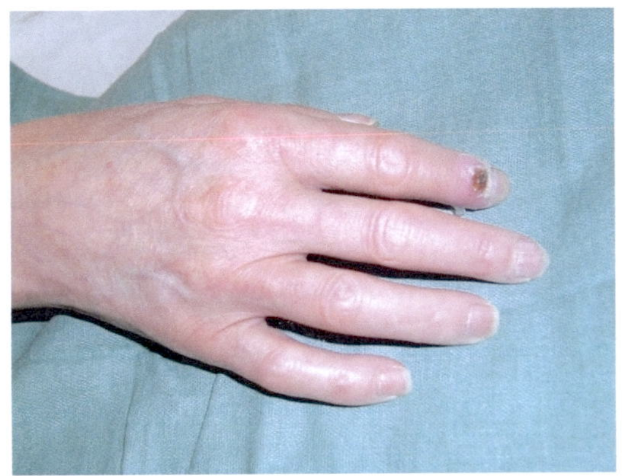

Fig. 19.2 An example of a pre-gangrenous lesion in a patient with Raynaud's disease prior to a T2–T3 thoracoscopic sympatholysis

Thoracoscopic sympathectomy can be considered a reasonable alternative for cases of severe refractory Raynaud's phenomenon (e.g., digital pre-gangrene; Fig. 19.2) as long as patients are well informed and accept a high probability of recurrent disease. However this approach is difficult to justify in cases with less severe disease. Thoracoscopic sympathectomy offers immediate relief in up to 65–90 % of cases; however, the recurrence rates are high, and symptoms will recur in more than half of patients within 1–4 years.

The effects of TTS appear to be very short-lasting in patients with *Buerger's disease*, especially if the subject continues to smoke. However in rare highly selected cases of *upper limb arterial insufficiency* associated with Buerger's disease, we have observed significant symptomatic improvements and significant delay in time to amputation (personal observations).

Thoracoscopic sympathectomy has been – and still is – used in the treatment of *causalgia and reflex sympathetic dystrophy*. The success rates are reported to be above 90 % in selected cases with refractory disease and successful sympathetic block (Mockus et al. 1987). However, the role of the sympathetic nervous system in causalgia and reflex sympathetic dystrophy has recently been questioned. There is little evidence that interrupting the sympathetic supply is more effective in alleviating the pain of causalgia and reflex sympathetic dystrophy when compared to placebo (Schott 1998).

Some series also suggest a potential role of TTS in the treatment of a variety of cardiac disorders, such as severe *angina pectoris* refractory to medical or surgical treatment (Wettervik et al. 1995) and various arrhythmias including *long QT syndrome* (Moss et al. 1985) and *ventricular* and *paroxysmal atrial tachycardia* (Kadowaki and Levett 1986).

Finally, lower sympathetic interruption has been demonstrated to be beneficial in the treatment of chronic *pancreatic pain* with significant pain relief in 64–100 % of patients (Noppen et al. 1998a, b).

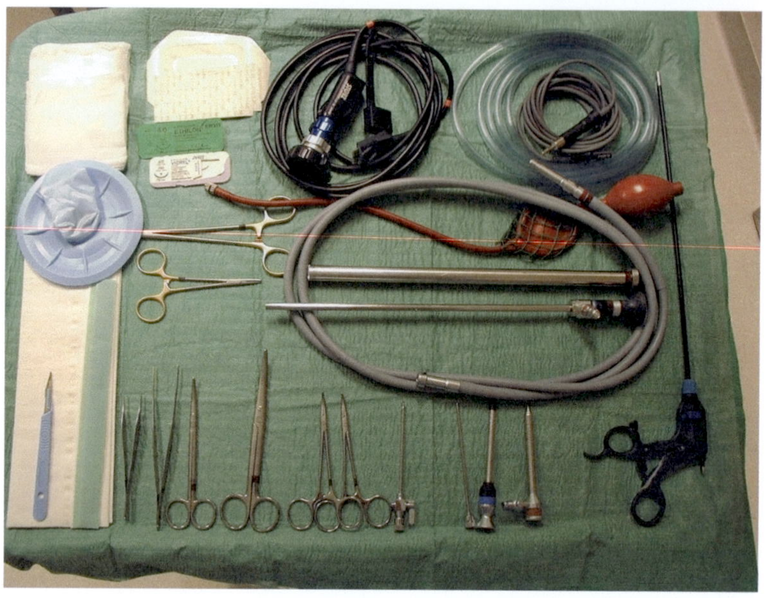

Fig. 19.3 A standard rigid "medical thoracoscopy" set as used for thoracoscopic sympatholysis

All levels of sympathetic interruption can safely be performed by thoracoscopic sympathicolysis when performed by a trained pulmonologist.

19.2.2 Contraindications

Thoracoscopic sympathectomy, like any other thoracoscopic procedure, requires the presence of an open pleural space: small pleural adhesions, which may be encountered apically, especially in elderly patients, can often be easily transected. However the presence of extensive, organized pleural adhesions (e.g., after pleurodesis or as a post infectious sequelae) may compromise thoracoscopic interventions.

Refractory bleeding diathesis is another general contraindication to thoracoscopic sympathectomy.

19.3　Equipment

Although virtually all medical thoracoscopic interventions can safely be performed in a dedicated endoscopy suite (Boutin et al. 1991), we prefer to use a fully equipped operating theater for safety, logistical, and staff reasons. Whereas diagnostic thoracoscopies are often performed under local anaesthesia and intravenous sedation,

interventional "red zone" medical thoracoscopies (e.g., for thoracoscopic sympathicolysis) are usually performed using total intravenous anaesthesia and single-lumen intubation with high-frequency jet ventilation (D'Haese et al. 1996).

With regard to the necessary required equipment, a "simple" medical thoracoscopy set is sufficient (Fig. 19.3). Video assistance is obtained by means of a dedicated video camera and TV display. Sympathetic ablation is easily achieved by means of a coagulation forceps heated by a unipolar electrocoagulation unit. No chest drains are needed.

The total cost of the (multiple-use) medical thoracoscopy equipment and video display is estimated at 10,000 USD. In our institution (with about 100 thoracoscopic interventions per year), the telescopes are renewed every 5 years, and the video camera and imaging and data storage facilities need to be replaced every 5–10 years.

19.4　The Level of Interruption for Thoracoscopic Sympathectomy

Segmental postganglionic fibers synapsing in the paravertebral lower cervical and thoracic sympathetic ganglia (which form the sympathetic chain) provide the sympathetic innervation for a variety of internal organs (the heart, lungs, and intestine

Table 19.3 Level of sympathetic denervation in function of the indication

Indication	Sympathectomy level
Facial blushing and sweating	T_2
Palmar hyperhidrosis	T3
Axillar hyperhidrosis	T4
Upper limb vasospastic disorders; causalgia	T_2–T_3
Cardiac disorders	Lower T_1–T_6 (T_{10})
Pancreatic denervation	T_5–T_{11}

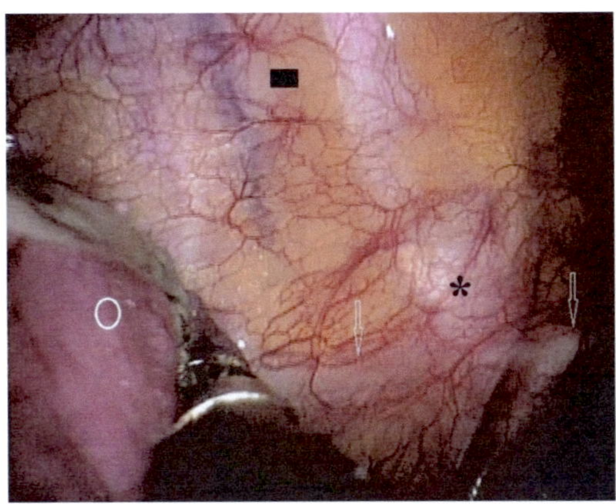

Fig. 19.4 The T3 sympathetic ganglion on the right side (*star*). Successful management of palmar sweating can be obtained by T3 sympathectomy with a lower associated incidence of compensatory sweating. Sympathetic trunk: *white arrow*. Posterior parietal pleura (■) with intercostal vessels on the left and rib on the right. Right upper lobe: O (Courtesy Ph Astoul – Marseille – France)

including the pancreas) and blood vessels and sweat glands of the face and neck, upper limb, and axillary region. Thoracoscopic sympathectomy is performed at the segmental level(s) relevant to the required effect of denervation (Table 19.3). The eighth cervical ganglion and the first thoracic ganglion are often fused together, forming the stellate ganglion; this lies over the neck of the first rib in both hemithoraces. Ablation of the stellate ganglion, which supplies the sympathetic innervation of the face and neck, should be avoided because of the associated risk for developing a Horner's syndrome.

Each rib caudal to the first rib has its corresponding ganglion, although there is a great anatomical variability.

The T_2 ganglion is the primary source of sympathetic innervation of the face and the hands, although more extensive ablation (T_2–T_3, T_2–T_4, even up to T_2–T_6) has been used in the past for the treatment of palmar hyperhidrosis. However, the success rate is identical when only the T2 ganglion is ablated for this condition (Kao 1992; Lin 1992). Limiting the number of levels ablated appears to reduce the extent and severity of side effects, e.g., compensatory hyperhidrosis (Gossot et al. 1997). Our personal experience together with recent published data demonstrates that successful management of palmar sweating can be obtained by T3 sympathectomy (Fig. 19.4), with a lower associated incidence of compensatory sweating (Sciuchetti et al. 2008), and indeed some authors now even "descend" towards T4 for palmar hyperhidrosis (Wolosker et al. 2008).

The division of the sympathetic chain over the caudal part of the first rib, and coagulation down to the second and third ganglion, is effective in relieving facial blushing (and sweating) in the majority of patients (Drott et al. 1998). For the relief of axillary hyperhidrosis, most authors advocate a T_2–T_4 ablation (although contributions can come from T_5). However, current practice which limits the extent of sympathetic denervation to the T4 level appears to offer equal results in controlling sweating with a lesser degree of compensatory sweating (Munia et al. 2008).

For the relief of the various vascular disorders of the upper arms and for causalgia, a T_2–T_3 ablation offers almost complete sympathetic denervation of the forearms and hands (Fig. 19.5).

For the treatment of cardiac disorders, a left-sided or bilateral lower T_1–T_6 denervation (sometimes up to T_{10}) is performed. Finally for the relief of pancreatic pain, coagulation is performed from the 5th to the 11th rib heads.

19.5 The Procedure

The preoperative workup includes a history (with special emphasis on previous pleuropulmonary disorders or interventions) and physical examination. This should then be supported with chest X-ray, ECG, pulmonary function tests, and a

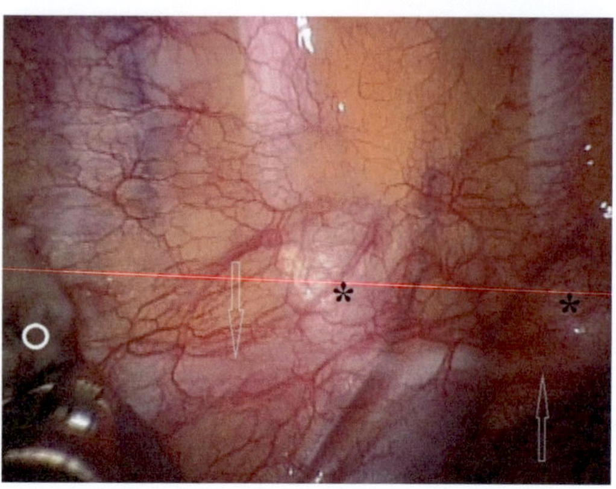

Fig. 19.5 T2 (*star on the right*) and T3 (*star on the middle*) sympathetic ganglion located respectively at the level of the head of the second and third rib. Sympathetic trunk is visible (*white arrows*) on the posterior parietal pleura. For the relief of the various vascular disorders of the upper arms and for causalgia, a T_2–T_3 ablation offers almost complete sympathetic denervation of forearms and hands, *white circle* lung (Courtesy Ph Astoul – Marseille – France)

classical preoperative biochemistry, hematology, and coagulation workup.

Since we perform a one-time bilateral procedure, patients are positioned on the operating table in a supine position with the trunk elevated to 30°. The procedure is performed using total intravenous anaesthesia and single-lumen intubation. Both arms are horizontally spread at 90°. After skin cleaning and sterile wrapping, a right-sided pneumothorax is created using a Küss needle which is introduced in the axillary third intercostal space.

About 1,000–1,500 mL air is insufflated manually into the pleural cavity. Skin incision and blunt dissection is performed, and a 7 mm trocar is placed. A rigid thoracoscope (Richard Wolff, Knitlingen, Germany) is introduced via the trocar, and the pleural space and sympathetic chain are inspected and identified. A second entry point is created about 3 cm anterocephalad from the first trocar. An insulated biopsy forceps, connected to a unipolar coagulation unit, is introduced via the second trocar.

Adhesions, if present, should be transected. The appropriate ganglion(a) is (are) identified and cauterized over the rib head using five to fifteen 60 W bursts. Coagulation is extended

laterally on the rib for 3–4 cm. After removal of the second trocar and skin suture of its entry point, negative suction is applied to the first trocar, while simultaneously switching from high-frequency jet ventilation to manual balloon hyperinflation of the lungs. In this combined maneuver, the trocar is withdrawn and the skin sutured. No drains are left in place. The same procedure is immediately performed on the left hemithorax. Total operating time averages 20 min. After recovery, the patients are transferred to the ward, and discharged some hours later after a control PA chest X-ray.

19.6 Results, Side Effects, and Complications

The majority of the current available evidence which supports sympathectomy (for essential hyperhidrosis) is observational and comes from a variety of retrospective (with some prospective) clinical series as well as comparative studies. Cumulative data from over 6,000 reported patients demonstrates that thoracoscopic sympathectomy is safe, reproducible, and effective and that most (but not all) patients are satisfied with the results of the procedure. However it is difficult to compare the series, and generalization is compromised by a lack of uniform definitions and outcome measures. In addition the operative technique varies widely from study to study, and the optimal technique remains elusive. The lack of uniform outcome measures makes the data difficult to interpret, and standardized metrics of results (objective quantification of sweating, standardized quality of life questionnaires) are required (Henteleff and Kalavrouziotis 2008). Notwithstanding these limitations, the data show that relief of palmar sweating is excellent: immediate success rates are reported from 90 and 100 % and most often reach 95 to 100 %. Long-term success is obtained in 67 to 100 % and most often in over 95 % of cases. Late recurrences are observed in approximately 5 % of cases; in these cases redo interventions are usually successful. Immediate failures most often occur when a parallel neural pathway is present (Kuntz's fiber(s)).

These should be included in the ablation procedure by extending the pleural coagulation laterally over the rib. In addition the procedure will fail if a pleural space cannot be obtained. Late recurrences are probably due to nerve fiber regeneration.

In the past most authors used to perform extended resections/ablations over various segmental levels; however, current evidence suggests that equivalent results on can be obtained by limited sympathetic interruptions to one segmental level ,thus dramatically lowering the incidence, extent, and severity of compensatory hyperhidrosis (which is the major side effect). Compensatory hyperhidrosis is defined as the occurrence of increased sweating after TS, especially at the level of the dermatomes above and below the sympathectomy level; its incidence varies from 0 and 99 % (!) in the published series. However, most authors report rates between 40 and 70 %. Compensatory sweating can occasionally be very severe; therefore some authors propose a temporary sympathetic block prior to the definitive interruption (Miller and Force 2008) and/or prefer clipping instead of resection or cauterization (allowing reversibility in 50 % of cases if severe intractable side effects are encountered) (Sugimura et al. 2009).

Gustatory sweating is reported in 9–64 % of patients: this range is difficult to explain. Development of a temporary or permanent Horner's syndrome occurs in 0–17 % of patients. This suggests that the personal experience and technique of the operator seems to be crucial. Major complications which necessitate additional interventions (e.g., chest tube drainage for persistent pneumothorax, hemothorax, or conversion to thoracotomy) are extremely rare, especially in recent large series. Numerous studies have shown that TS causes measurable but clinically insignificant effects on pulmonary function, cardiac, and autonomic function (Noppen and Vincken 1996a, b, 1997; Noppen et al. 1997a, b).

In summary, modern thoracoscopic thoracic sympathectomy, whether performed by surgeons or pulmonologists, appears to be a highly effective and safe treatment option for patients suffering from essential hyperhidrosis. Whereas success is obtained in 95–100 % of patients, the safety profile seems to increase with increasing operator experience, use of video equipment, extreme care in avoiding the T_1 ganglion (e.g., by careful palpation, radioscopy, or preoperative temperature – or blood flow monitoring if necessary), use of smaller-sized thoracoscopy equipment, and limited and simplified ablation, transection, or clipping procedures instead of extended multilevel dissection and resection techniques (Assalia et al. 2007).

Conclusion

Thoracoscopic sympathectomy is a relatively simple, effective, and safe method for achieving thoracic sympathetic denervation. The procedure can be performed by surgeons and by well-trained pulmonologists, but in the setting of "medical thoracoscopy," it should be categorized as a "red zone" procedure. Over the last decade, the methodology for thoracoscopic sympathectomy has shifted towards a less invasive and more simplified procedure: one-time bilateral electrocautery or clipping with small-diameter medical or surgical thoracoscopy equipment, single-lumen intubation, and general anaesthesia, all performed in a 1-day clinic setting. Excellent and long-lasting results are obtained in essential (palmar and/or axillary and/or facial) hyperhidrosis and facial blushing – with an excellent safety profile. In carefully selected patients, TTS can provide substantial relief in Raynaud's phenomenon, causalgia and reflex sympathetic dystrophy, Buerger's disease and upper limb vascular insufficiency, selected cardiac arrhythmias, long QT syndrome and angina pectoris, and in patients with intractable chronic pancreatic pain.

References

Ambrogi V, Campione E, Mineo D et al (2009) Bilateral thoracoscopic T2 to T3 sympathectomy versus botulinum injection in palmar hyperhidrosis. Ann Thorac Surg 88:238–245

Assalia A, Bahouth H, Ilivitzki A (2007) Thoracoscopic sympathectomy for primary palmar hyperhidrosis: resection versus transaction – a prospective trial. World J Surg 31:1976–1979

Bachmann K, Standl N, Kaifi J (2009) Thoracoscopic sympathectomy for palmar and axillary hyperhidrosis : four-year outcome and quality of life after bilateral 5-mm dual port approach. Surg Endosc 23:1587–1593

Baumgartner FJ, Bertin S, Konecny J (2009) Superiority of thoracoscopic sympathectomy over medical management for the palmoplantar subset of severe hyperhidrosis. Ann Vasc Surg 23:1–7

Boutin C, Viallat JR, Aelony Y (1991) Diagnostic thoracoscopy for pleural effusions. In: Boutin C, Viallat JR, Aelony Y (eds) Practical thoracoscopy. Springer, Berlin, pp 51–64

D'Haese J, Camu F, Noppen M et al (1996) A new approach using total intravenous anaesthesia and high frequency jet ventilation during transthoracic sympathectomy for treatment of essential hyperhidrosis. J Cardiothorac Vasc Anesth 10:767–771

Di Lorenzo N, Sica GS, Sileri P et al (1998) Thoracoscopic sympathectomy for vasospastic diseases. J Soc Laparoendosc Surg 2:249–253

Drott C, Claes G, Olsson-Rex L et al (1998) Successful treatment of facial blushing by endoscopic transthoracic sympathicotony. Br J Dermatol 138:639–643

Gossot D, Toledo L, Fritsch C et al (1997) Thoracoscopic sympathectomy for upper limb hyperhidrosis: looking for the right operation. Ann Thorac Surg 64:975–978

Henteleff HJ, Kalavrouziotis D (2008) Evidence-based review of the surgical management of hyperhidrosis. Thorac Surg Clin 18:209–216

Kadowaki MH, Levett JM (1986) Sympathectomy in the treatment of angina and arrhythmias. Ann Thorac Surg 41:572–578

Kao MC (1992) Laser endoscopic sympathectomy for palmar hyperhidrosis. Lasers Surg Med 12:308–312

Krasna MJ (2008) Thoracoscopic sympathectomy: a standardized approach to therapy for hyperhidrosis. Ann Thorac Surg 85:S764–S767

Lin CC (1992) Extended thoracoscopic T2-sympathectomy in treatment of hyperhidrosis: experience with 130 consecutive cases. J Laparoendosc Surg 2:1–6

Miller DL, Force SD (2008) Temporary thoracoscopic sympathetic block for hyperhidrosis. Ann Thorac Surg 85:1211–1216

Mockus MB, Rutherford RB, Rosales C et al (1987) Sympathectomy for causalgia. Patient selection and long-term results. Arch Surg 122:668–672

Moss AJ, Schwarz PJ, Crampton RS (1985) The long QT syndrome: a prospective international study. Circulation 71:17–22

Munia M, Wolosker N, Kaufmann P et al (2008) Sustained benefit lasting one year from T4 instead of T3-T4 sympathectomy for isolated axillary hyperhidrosis. Clinics 63:771–774

Neumayer C, Panhofer P, Jakesz R et al (2005) Surgical treatment of facial hyperhidrosis and blushing: mid-term results after endoscopic sympathetic block and review of the literature. Eur Surg 37:127–136

Noppen M (2004) Medical thoracoscopy Techniques for thoracic sympathectomy. In: Interventional pulmonary medicine. In: Beamis JF, Mathur PN, Mehta AC (eds) Lung biology in health and disease, vol 189. Marcel Dekker, New York, pp 483–502

Noppen M, Vincken W (1996a) Thoracoscopic sympathicolysis for essential hyperhidrosis: effects on pulmonary function. Eur Respir J 9:1660–1664

Noppen M, Vincken W (1996b) Effects of thoracoscopic upper dorsal sympathicolysis for essential hyperhidrosis on bronchial responsiveness to histamine: implications on the autonomic imbalance theory of asthma. Respirology 3:195–199

Noppen M, Vincken W (1997) Partial pulmonary sympathetic denervation by thoracoscopic D2-D3 sympathicolysis for essential hyperhidrosis: effect on the pulmonary diffusion capacity. Respir Med 91:537–545

Noppen M, Herregodts P, D'Haese J et al (1996) A simplified T2-T3 thoracoscopic sympathicolysis technique for the treatment of essential hyperhidrosis: short term results in 100 patients. J Laparoendosc Surg 6:151–159

Noppen N, Sevens C, Gerlo E et al (1997a) Plasma catecholamine concentrations in essential hyperhidrosis and effects of thoracoscopic D2-D3 sympathicolysis. Eur J Clin Invest 27:202–205

Noppen M, Sevens C, Vincken W (1997b) Effects of non-pharmacological sympathetic sudomotor denervation sweating in humans with essential palmar hyperhidrosis. Clin Biochem 30:171–175

Noppen M, Meysman M, D'Haese J et al (1998a) Thoracoscopic splanchnicolysis for the relief of chronic pancreatic pain. Experience of a group of pulmonologists. Chest 113:528–531

Noppen M, Dab I, D'Haese J et al (1998b) Thoracoscopic T2-T3 sympathicolysis for essential hyperhidrosis in childhood: effects on pulmonary function. Pediatr Pulmonol 26:262–264

Sayers RD, Henner RE, Barrie WW (1994) Transthoracic endoscopic sympathectomy for hyperhidrosis and Raynaud's phenomenon. Eur J Vasc Surg 8:627–631

Schott GD (1998) Interrupting the sympathetic outflow in causalgia and reflex sympathetic dystrophy. A futile procedure for many patients. Br Med J 316:792–793

Sciuchetti JF, Corti F, Ballabio D et al (2008) Results, side effects and complications after thoracoscopic sympathetic block by clamping. Clin Auton Res 18:80–83

Steiner Z, Cohen Z, Kleiner O (2008) Do children tolerate thoracoscopic sympathectomy better than adults? Pediatr Surg Int 24:343–347

Sugimura H, Spratt EH, Compeau CG et al (2009) Thoracoscopic sympathetic clipping for hyperhidrosis: long-term results and reversibility. J Thorac Cardiovasc Surg 137:1370–1378

Tassi GF, Davies RJ, Noppen M (2006) Advanced techniques in medical thoracoscopy. Eur Respir J 28:1051–1059

Wettervik C, Claes G, Drott C et al (1995) Endoscopic transthoracic sympathicotomy for severe angina. Lancet 345:97–98

Wilkinson HA (1984) Radio frequency percutaneous upper thoracic sympathectomy technique and review of indications. N Engl J Med 311:34–36

Wolosker N, Yazbek G, Ishy A et al (2008) Is sympathectomy at T4 level better than at T3 level for treating palmar hyperhidrosis? J Laparoendosc Adv Surg Tech 18:102–106

Yamamoto H, Kanehira A, Kawamura M et al (2000) Needlescopic surgery for palmar hyperhidrosis. J Thorac Cardiovasc Surg 120:276–279

Yim APC, Liu HP, Lee TW et al (2000) 'Needlescopic' video-assisted thoracic surgery for palmar hyperhidrosis. Eur J Cardiothorac Surg 17:697–701

Pericardial Window

20

Paul Van Schil, Bernard Paelinck, Jeroen Hendriks, and Patrick Lauwers

20.1 Introduction

After the introduction of laparoscopic techniques, there was a real revival of thoracoscopy in the 1990s, which was renamed VATS—video-assisted thoracic surgery—using a camera, monitor and video equipment. VATS has been used for a variety of pulmonary, pleural and pericardial disorders, offering superb visualisation of the ipsilateral haemithorax (Van Schil et al. 1996).

Combined procedures are also feasible, and with the advent of robotic techniques, more complex interventions have become possible, e.g. radical thymectomy.

In this chapter the history of pericardiotomy is briefly described, followed by a general overview of pericardial effusions, the surgical approach to the pericardium, the technique of pericardial fenestration by VATS and lastly, the published results for specific indications.

P. Van Schil (✉) • P. Lauwers
Department of Thoracic and Vascular Surgery,
Antwerp University Hospital, Antwerp, Belgium
e-mail: paul.van.schil@uza.be; patrick.lauwers@uza.be

B. Paelinck
Department of Cardiology,
Antwerp University Hospital, Antwerp, Belgium
e-mail: bernard.paelinck@uza.be

J. Hendriks
Department of Surgery,
University Hospital Antwerp, Edegem, Belgium
e-mail: j.hendriks@planetinternet.be

20.2 History of Pericardiotomy

The pericardium, composed of a visceral and parietal layer, was known as an anatomical structure by Hippocrates. It was considered to be an integral part of the heart. For this reason, Shumacker HB proposed that cardiac interventions should also include procedures on the pericardium. In this respect, Francisco Romero is credited as the first cardiac surgeon to perform a pericardiotomy in 1801 (Van Thielen and Van Hee 2008). The patient was a 35-year-old farmer presenting with a pericardial effusion. Using an anterior thoracotomy in the fifth intercostal space, the pericardium was incised. A large volume of stone-coloured fluid was evacuated. Three years after this procedure, the patient only complained of incisional pain. In 1815 Romero presented a memoir on the treatment of thoracic effusions in Paris; however, his approach was found to be too aggressive (Fig. 20.1). Nine years later, Dominique Jean Larrey performed his first pericardiotomy in a 30-year-old former soldier who developed a purulent pericardial effusion after a penetrating wound in the left chest. The procedure was also performed by an anterior thoracotomy, and about 1 l of brown-yellow fluid mixed with blood was evacuated. Moreover, Larrey did some experimental studies which repeated his intervention in several corpses. In this way, he established the scientific basis for the surgical procedure that remains in use today.

P. Astoul et al. (eds.), *Thoracoscopy for Pulmonologists*,
DOI 10.1007/978-3-642-38351-9_20, © Springer-Verlag Berlin Heidelberg 2014

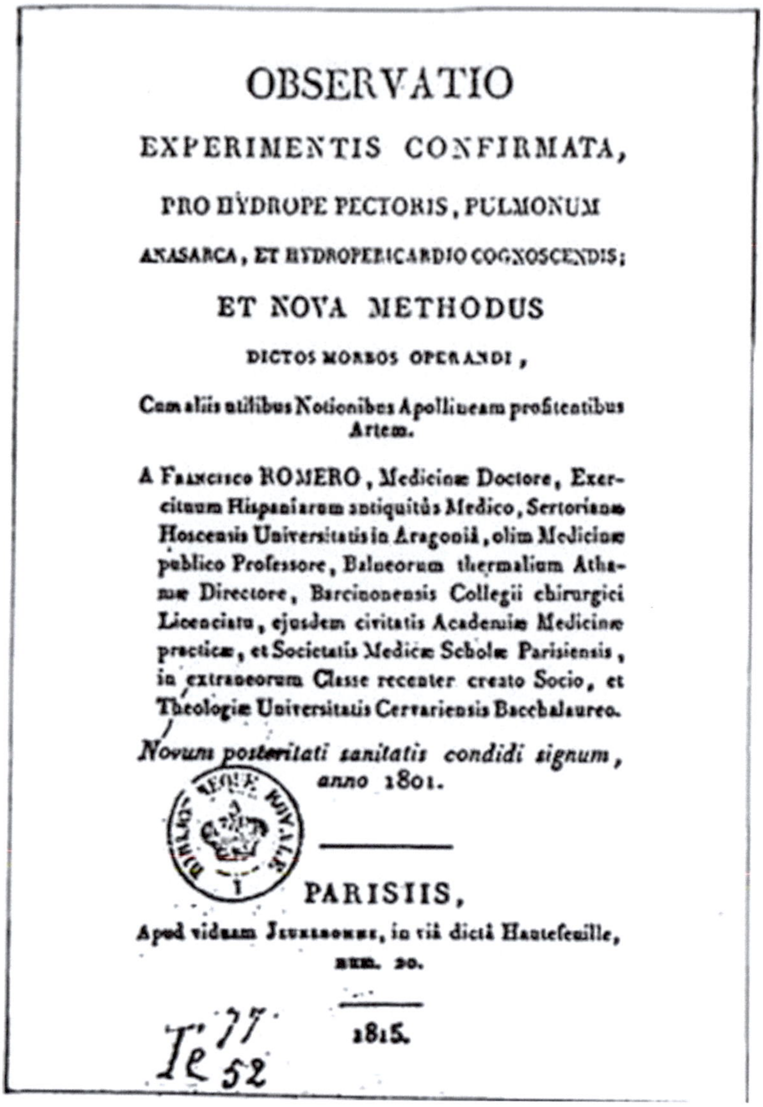

Fig. 20.1 The Memoir of Francisco Romero on the treatment of thoracic effusions as presented in 1815

OBSERVATIO

EXPERIMENTIS CONFIRMATA,

PRO HYDROPE PECTORIS, PULMONUM

ANASARCA, ET HYDROPERICARDIO COGNOSCENDIS;

ET NOVA METHODUS

DICTOS MORBOS OPERANDI,

Cum aliis utilibus Notionibus Apollineam profitentibus Artem.

A Francisco ROMERO, Medicinæ Doctore, Exercituum Hispaniarum antiquitùs Medico, Sertorianæ Hoscensis Universitatis in Aragonii, olim Medicinæ publico Professore, Balneorum thermalium Athamæ Directore, Barcinonensis Collegii chirurgici Licenciata, ejusdem civitatis Academiæ Medicinæ practicæ, et Societatis Medicæ Scholæ Parisiensis, in extraneorum Classe recenter creato Socio, et Theologiæ Universitatis Cervariensis Baccbalaureo.

Novum posteritati sanitatis condidi signum, anno 1801.

PARISIIS,

Apud viduam Jeunehomme, in viâ dictâ Hautefeuille, num. 20.

1815.

20.3 Pericardial Effusions

The pericardium has many physiological functions which mainly prevent overdistension of the cardiac chambers and torsion of the heart by exerting a contact stress (Spodick 1991). However, congenital absence of the pericardium usually does not lead to specific clinical symptoms.

Under normal physiological conditions, only a minimal amount of pericardial fluid is present at the posterior side of the heart. Accumulation of fluid and/or air gives rise to specific conditions which are listed in Table 20.1. An example of air building up inside the pericardium, a so-called pneumopericardium, is provided in Fig. 20.2. A number of disorders may provoke pericardial effusions, and these are summarised in Table 20.2 (Hazelrigg and McGee 1999; Spodick 1991). When the volume of fluid increases in the pericardial space, depending on the amount and rate of accumulation, the pericardial reserve volume is exceeded and the pericardial pressure rises steeply which will ultimately result in cardiac tamponade. This occurs earlier when blood accumulates inside the pericardium and compresses the heart. Symptoms of a pericardial effusion

Table 20.1 Specific conditions in which air and fluid accumulate inside the pericardium

Pneumopericardium (tension)	Air (pneumotamponade)
Hydropericardium	Serous fluid (transudate)
Hydropneumopericardium	Air + serous fluid
Haemopericardium	Blood, clots
Pyopericardium	Purulent effusion
Pyopneumopericardium	Purulent effusion + air
Chylopericardium	Chyle
Lymphopericardium	Lymphatic fluid

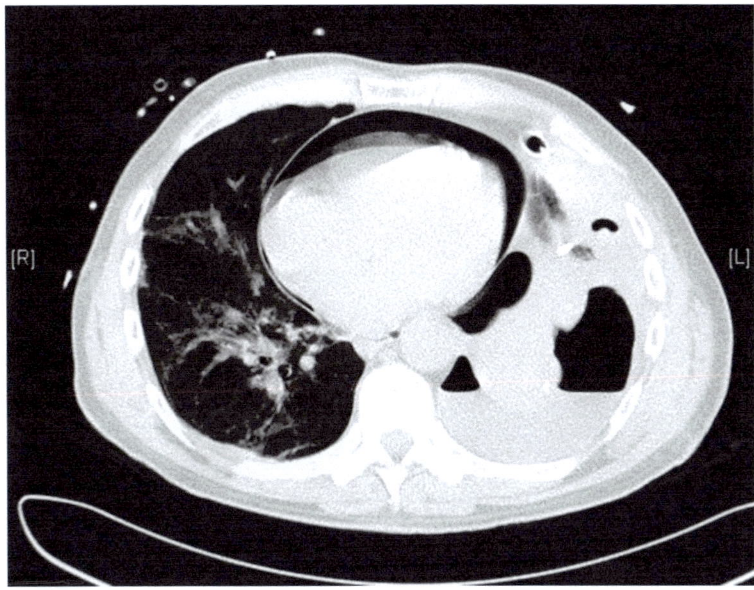

Fig. 20.2 Postoperative pneumopericardium in a patient who underwent a left repeat thoracotomy for recurrent pulmonary metastases

Table 20.2 Disorders associated with pericardial effusions

Infectious	Viral, bacterial, mycotic, parasitic
Traumatic	Penetrating, blunt
Malignant	Primary
	Secondary (lung, breast, lymphoma)
Inflammatory	Connective tissue disorders
	Vasculitis
Metabolic	Renal failure
	Cholesterol pericarditis
Idiopathic/others	Cardiac surgery
	Intrapericardial pneumonectomy
	Post-radiotherapy

include cough, shortness of breath, thoracic pain, malaise, peripheral oedema and symptoms related to the underlying disorder, e.g. cachexia in malignant pericardial effusions.

Chest X-ray usually reveals a clearly enlarged cardiac silhouette, typically with a water bottle configuration (Fig. 20.3). Electrocardiography may show reduced voltage, ST segment elevation and cardiac arrhythmias in cases with associated heart disease. Echocardiography readily provides the correct diagnosis and is able to differentiate between small, moderate and large effusions (Fig. 20.4). CT scan and magnetic resonance imaging may also be helpful to evaluate the pericardial thickness and cardiac function especially in patients with poor echogenic windows (Fig. 20.5). In some cases, the healing process will result in excessive thickening of the pericardium, associated fibrosis and constriction, which may finally give rise to a constrictive pericarditis characterised by a so-called Pantserherz (Fig. 20.5). This results in profound haemodynamic consequences by limiting normal filling of the cardiac cavities.

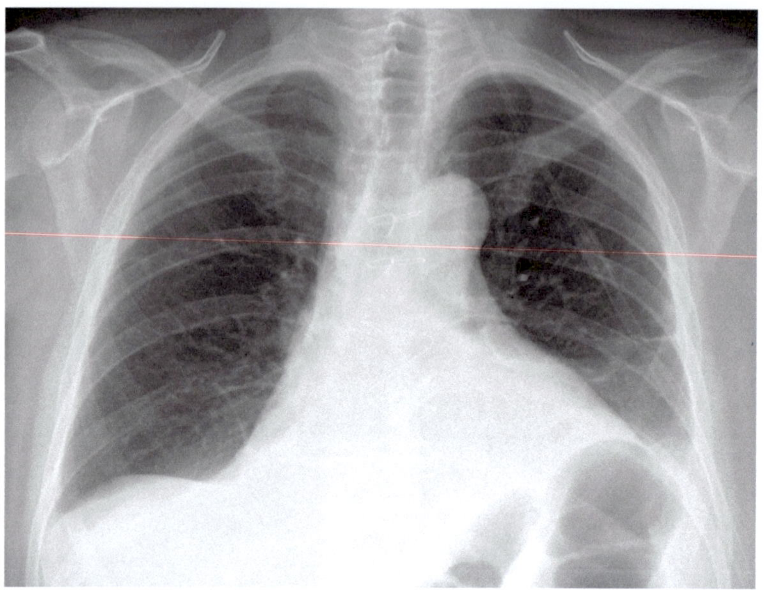

Fig. 20.3 A chest radiograph showing enlarged cardiac shadow due to a pericardial effusion post aortic valve replacement

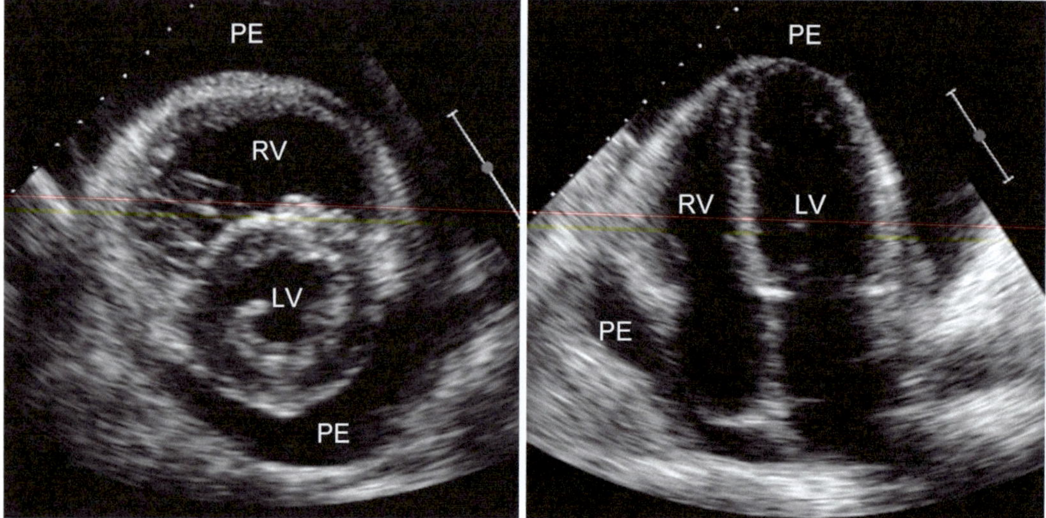

Fig. 20.4 Echocardiographic parasternal short axis (*left panel*) and apical four-chamber view (*right panel*) in a patient with large pericardial effusion (*LV* left ventricle, *RV* right ventricle, *PE* pericardial effusion)

20.4 Surgical Approaches to the Pericardium

Several approaches to the pericardium exist, ranging from minimally invasive to extensive open procedures. These are listed in Table 20.3 together with their specific indication.

During anterior mediastinotomy, it is feasible to open the pericardium for evaluation of tumour extension of a bronchogenic carcinoma and to evaluate the pericardial space (Van Schil et al. 1991). Videopericardioscopy allows extensive intrapericardial inspection, aspiration of fluid and biopsies of different regions (Porte et al. 1999; Demaria et al. 2005). Insertion of a drain and instillation of sclerosing agents are also easily accomplished. In addition, the evaluation of intrapericardial extension of mediastinal or pulmonary neoplasms has been performed by this technique (Pompeo et al. 2007). Recently, a complete endoscopic subxiphoid pericardioscopy has been described allowing diagnostic and therapeutic interventions (Manca et al. 2009).

Video-assisted thoracic surgery or VATS is a more invasive technique requiring general anaesthesia and double-lumen intubation. It can be performed from the left or right side and has several advantages including inspection of the entire haemothorax and evaluation of the visceral, parietal pleura and pericardium. Specific biopsies can be taken including puncture or resection of suspicious pulmonary nodules or mediastinal lesions. Therapeutic procedures such as pericardial fenestration can be performed under direct vision. With the advent of robotic techniques, specific cardiac and thoracic procedures can now be performed by minimally invasive techniques. Extensive cardiac or pericardial interventions, e.g. complete pericardial resection or repair of large, traumatic cardiac injuries, still require sternotomy or thoracotomy depending on the specific procedure.

20.5 Technique of Pericardial Fenestration by VATS

The patient is prepared as for a classical thoracotomy (Fig. 20.6). Our standard technique for most VATS procedures includes general anaesthesia, insertion of a double-lumen endotracheal tube and a thoracic epidural catheter for adequate pain control. Pure local anaesthesia with sedation has been used to perform a pericardial window but experience is rather limited (Katlic 2006). The patient is positioned in the lateral decubitus position on a bean bag and is slightly tilted backwards. In this way, the lung falls away posteriorly thus allowing easier access to the pericardium. The procedure can be performed from the left or right side. If feasible, the right side is chosen as it provides more working space because the largest volume of the heart is on the left side (Fig. 20.7). Usually, the first thoracoport is inserted in the midaxillary line in the 7th intercostal space allowing inspection of the pleural cavity, lung and pericardium. Additional working ports are

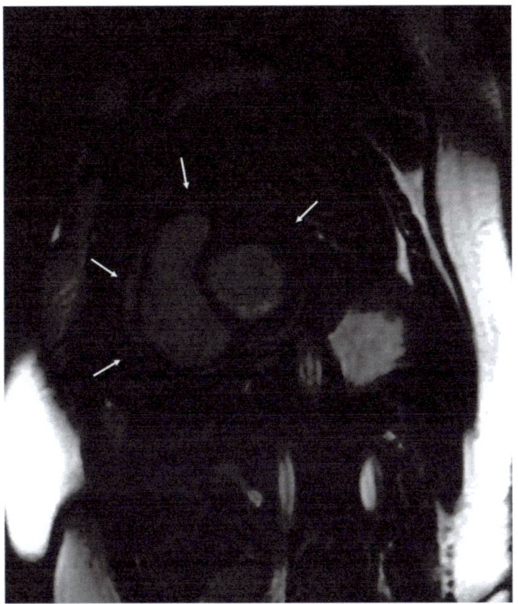

Fig. 20.5 Short-axis magnetic resonance image of the heart in a patient with constrictive pericarditis. The *arrows* indicate thickened pericardium ("Pantserherz")

Table 20.3 Surgical approaches to the pericardium

Technique	Indication
Anterior mediastinotomy with opening of the pericardium	Inspection, diagnosis pericardial + pulmonary disorders
Videopericardioscopy	Inspection, evaluation intrapericardial lesions + biopsy
Subxiphoid approach (surgical)	Drainage, pericardial biopsy, partial pericardial excision, pericardioperitoneal window
Video-assisted thoracic surgery (VATS)	Diagnosis pleural, pulmonary, pericardial disorders; limited therapeutic interventions (pericardiopleural window)
Sternotomy, anterior thoracotomy	Extensive therapeutic procedures (repair heart, complete pericardiectomy)

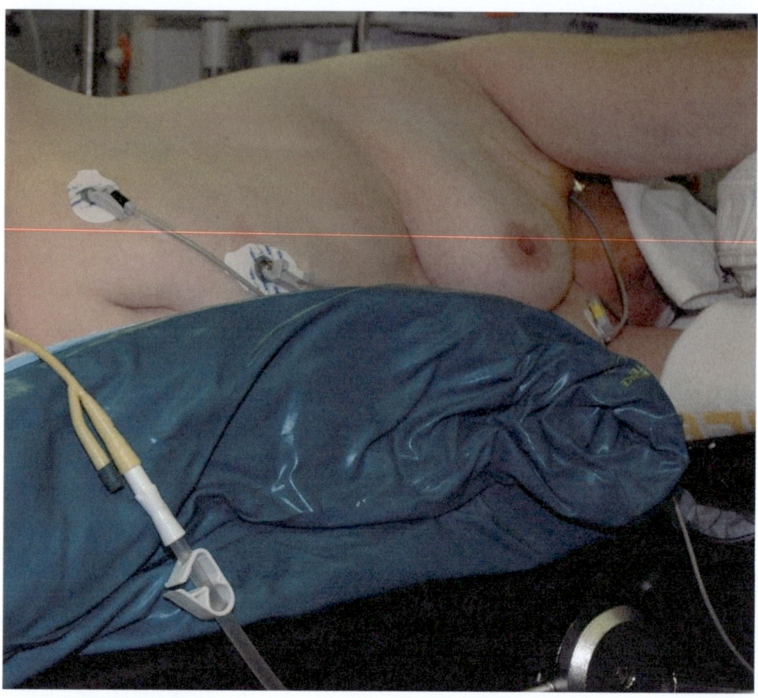

Fig. 20.6 The ideal positioning of the patient on the operating table for a classical VATS procedure

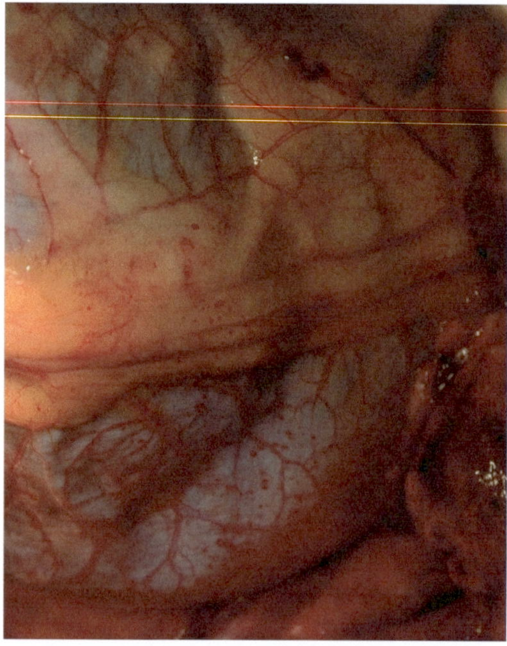

Fig. 20.7 The thoracoscopic view obtained of the right pericardium demonstrating the central route of the phrenic nerve

made anteriorly and posteriorly. A single port technique has been described but access is more limited (Rocco et al. 2006). The pericardium is

grasped and opened with scissors or a diathermy hook. A large pericardial window can be created anterior to the phrenic nerve which should be visualised on its entire length and carefully spared. In cases with a loculated posterior effusion, a fenestration is also performed posterior to the phrenic nerve.

A small-bore drain is inserted in the pericardium, and if there is an associated pleural effusion, a pleural drain is also left behind. They are connected to a thoracic drainage unit with suction of −15 to −20 cm H_2O.

20.6 Specific Indications and Results of Pericardial Fenestration with VATS

The precise treatment of a symptomatic pericardial effusion remains controversial and as there are no prospective randomised studies, no definite guidelines can be given. The principal goals are to obtain a definite cytological or histological diagnosis, to completely drain the pericardial effusion and to prevent its recurrence or development of a constrictive pericarditis (Hazelrigg and

McGee 1999; Veeramachaneni and Battafarano 2007). Most utilised techniques are percutaneous catheter drainage under ultrasound guidance and creation of a subxiphoid pericardiotomy by an open technique. In a retrospective study comparing these two procedures in 246 patients, drainage duration, total drainage volume and duration of follow-up were similar in both groups (McDonald et al. 2003). There was no mortality related to the pericardial intervention, but hospital mortality was high due to the underlying disease—malignancy was present in 32 % of patients. Diagnosis of a malignant disorder was confirmed in 59 % cases investigated by a percutaneous procedure and 62 % in the open group. Symptomatic effusions recurred in 16.5 and 4.6 % of the percutaneous intervention and open procedure groups respectively. Sclerosis did not appear to reduce recurrence rate. So, both techniques can be performed safely, but open drainage resulted in less recurrent effusions although it did not improve the diagnostic accuracy of malignancy.

In haemodynamically unstable patients and those with physiological signs of tamponade, the initial treatment consists of pericardiocentesis and insertion of a small-bore catheter to relieve the effusion and lower the pericardial pressure (Veeramachaneni and Battafarano 2007). In the setting of a high volume output, open drainage is subsequently performed with creation of a pericardioperitoneal window. In stable patients with an effusion of unknown origin, residual effusion or combined pleural and pericardial effusions, an open technique is also preferred as it provides the best chance to obtain a definite histological diagnosis and lower the risk of recurrence.

VATS is particularly useful for patients with combined pleural and pericardial disease and for loculated or recurrent pericardial effusions, especially those located laterally or posteriorly (Geissbühler et al. 1998; Stewart and Sundaresan 2005).

VATS is a very efficient method to create a pleuropericardial window on the left or right side. Additional procedures on the ipsilateral lung, pleura and mediastinum are possible—including biopsies and drainage of a pleural effusion (Nataf et al. 1998). Although Katlic described in 2006 the use of local anaesthesia and sedation for performing VATS procedures including pericardial fenestration, in our institution general anaesthesia is preferred with double-lumen intubation and insertion of a thoracic epidural catheter. This provides a comfortable working space, thus allowing for a correct and complete technical procedure.

In a retrospective comparative study of a subxiphoid approach versus a VATS pericardial window in a total of 71 patients, the operative time and minor morbidity rate were higher with VATS (O'Brien et al. 2005). However, in a multivariate analysis the thoracoscopic approach was a significant independent predictor of freedom from recurrence; so, therefore, VATS appears to provide a better long-term control of the effusion.

In a prospective study of VATS pericardial fenestration, 24 patients were evaluated and 11 had been previously treated (Geissbühler et al. 1998). Inclusion criteria were pericardial effusions requiring diagnosis or relief of symptoms and recurrent effusions after failed percutaneous procedures. Twelve patients had additional pleural pathology identified on chest CT, and talc pleurodesis was performed in six patients. Mean operative time was 45 min. Relief of symptoms was obtained in all patients. After a mean follow-up of 33 months, two recurrences were noted, but none in the patients who were treated by talc pleurodesis. VATS was found to be a safe and effective technique for loculated or recurrent pericardial effusions and those with combined pleural disease.

These findings were confirmed by the more recent study of Georghiou and colleagues who reported, in 2005, their 3-year experience with 18 patients. To create a pericardial window, a VATS approach was used under general anaesthesia with single-lung ventilation. Sixteen procedures were performed on the right side providing a comfortable working environment. Histological diagnosis was readily obtained and there were no complications. VATS is considered to be an effective approach for pericardial drainage and biopsies, creation of a pleuropericardial window and treatment of simultaneous pleural and pulmonary disorders.

Also in the setting of cardiac/thoracic trauma, VATS may be a useful technique for injury evaluation and to create a pericardial window. In a total series of 71 patients with suspected penetrating cardiac injuries, a thoracoscopic pericardial window was successfully completed in 13 patients who sustained stab and gunshot wounds (Navsaria and Nicol 2006). A haemopericardium was present in three patients and two cases proceeded to sternotomy. The mean VATS operative time was only 13.4 min with a hospital stay of 5.4 days. There were no complications related to the procedure.

In conclusion, VATS is a safe and effective technique to create a pericardial window, especially in cases of loculated or recurrent pericardial effusions and in those patients with concomitant pleural or pulmonary disease. General anaesthesia is preferred utilising single-lung ventilation, thus allowing for a technically straightforward procedure with a low risk of recurrence on long-term follow-up.

Acknowledgement The authors wish to thank Mrs. G. Clerx for her excellent editorial assistance, Prof. Dr. R. Van Hee for providing figure 1 and Mrs A. Muys for patiently drawing figure 8.

References

Demaria RG, Piciché M, Battistella P et al (2005) Pericardial exploration by pericardioscopy during a surgical subxyphoid approach. Surg Technol Int 14:241–244

Geissbühler K, Leiser A, Fuhrer J et al (1998) Video-assisted thoracoscopic pericardial fenestration for loculated or recurrent effusions. Eur J Cardiothorac Surg 14:403–408

Hazelrigg SR, McGee MJ (1999) Pericardiectomy. Chapter 15. In: Walker WS (ed) Video-assisted thoracic surgery. Isis Medical Media, Oxford, pp 201–208

Katlic MR (2006) Video-assisted thoracic surgery utilizing local anesthesia and sedation. Eur J Cardiothorac Surg 30:529–532

Manca G, Codecasa R, Valeri A et al (2009) Totally endoscopic subxiphoid pericardioscopy: early steps with a new surgical tool. Surg Endosc 23:444–446

McDonald JM, Meyers BF, Guthrie TJ et al (2003) Comparison of open subxiphoid pericardial drainage with percutaneous catheter drainage for symptomatic pericardial effusion. Ann Thorac Surg 76:811–816

Nataf P, Cacoub P, Regan M et al (1998) Video-thoracoscopic pericardial window in the diagnosis and treatment of pericardial effusions. Am J Cardiol 82:124–126

Navsaria PH, Nicol AJ (2006) Video-assisted thoracoscopic pericardial window for penetrating cardiac trauma. S Afr J Surg 44:18–20

O'Brien PK, Kucharczuk JC, Marshall MB et al (2005) Comparative study of subxiphoid versus video-thoracoscopic pericardial "window". Ann Thorac Surg 80:2013–2019

Pompeo E, Tacconi F, Mineo TC (2007) Flexible video-pericardioscopy in cT4 nonsmall-cell lung cancer with radiologic evidence of proximal vascular invasion. Ann Thorac Surg 83:402–408

Porte HL, Janecki-Delebecq TJ, Finzi L et al (1999) Pericardoscopy for primary management of pericardial effusion in cancer patients. Eur J Cardiothorac Surg 16:287–291

Rocco G, La Rocca A, La Manna C et al (2006) Uniportal video-assisted thoracoscopic surgery pericardial window. J Thorac Cardiovasc Surg 131:921–922

Spodick DH (1991) Pericardial window. Am Heart J 122:1794–1795

Stewart RD, Sundaresan S (2005) Malignant pericardial effusion. Chapter 69. In: Shields TW, LoCicero J III, Ponn RB, Rusch VW (eds) General thoracic surgery, 6th edn. Lippincott Williams & Wilkins, Philadelphia, pp 944–948

Van Schil PE, Knaepen PJ, Brutel de la Rivière A et al (1991) Extended use of diagnostic anterior mediastinotomy: intrapericardial exploration and evaluation of resectability of left-sided bronchogenic carcinoma. Eur J Cardiothorac Surg 5:588–591

Van Schil P, Van Meerbeeck J, Vanmaele R et al (1996) Role of thoracoscopy (VATS) in pleural and pulmonary pathology. Acta Chir Belg 96:23–27

Van Thielen J, Van Hee R (2008) Pericardiotomy: the first cardiac operation. Acta Chir Belg 108:133–138

Veeramachaneni NK, Battafarano RJ (2007) Management of malignant pericardial effusions. Chapter 59. In: Ferguson MK (ed) Difficult decisions in thoracic surgery. An evidence-based approach. Springer, London, pp 482–487

Part V

Complications of Thoracoscopy and Management

The Safety Profile of Medical Thoracoscopy: Expert Advices and Recommendations

Philippe Astoul, GianFranco Tassi, and Jean-Marie Tschopp

Everybody agrees that medical thoracoscopy is a minimally invasive technique which is well tolerated and associated with very few complications—provided the operators are well trained. It has been performed by pulmonologists on continental Europe for more than 100 years. It was an ambulatory procedure during the terrible era of tuberculosis for obtaining lung collapse by cutting pleural adhesions. This was a mainstay of tuberculosis management before antibiotics were invented. This intervention was performed and often repeated on patient.

Over the two decades there have been great improvements in the field of imaging with the invention of videothoracoscopy, thus making thoracoscopy more accessible to chest physicians. Recently the British Thoracic Society recognised that thoracoscopy should no longer be neglected by pulmonologists. This is an evolving view on thoracoscopy as English-speaking physicians once again discover the great potential of this technique.

However, even if complications are very rare, the thoracoscopist must bear them in mind.

P. Astoul (✉)
Division of Thoracic Oncology,
Pleural Diseases, and Interventional Pulmonology,
Hôpital NORD, Marseille, France
e-mail: pastoul@ap-hm.fr

G. Tassi
Division of Pneumology,
Spedali Civili di Brescia, Brescia, Italy
e-mail: gf.tassi@tin.it

J.-M. Tschopp
Département de Médecine Interne
Centre valaisan de pneumologie,
CHCVs, Montana 3963, Switzerland
e-mail: jean-marie.tschopp@hopitalvs.ch

P. Astoul et al. (eds.), *Thoracoscopy for Pulmonologists*,
DOI 10.1007/978-3-642-38351-9_21, © Springer-Verlag Berlin Heidelberg 2014

Complications of Thoracoscopy

22

Francisco Rodríguez-Panadero
and Beatriz Romero Romero

22.1 Introduction

The fear of complications arising from the procedure is often the main quoted reason for the reluctance of many pulmonologists to perform thoracoscopy and for a decline of "medical thoracoscopy" in some countries. In addition there is a trend to transfer pleural investigations to the thoracic surgeon in many centres around the world.

In this chapter we will present the reported incidence of complications, together with our own experience, and we will analyse the possible causes of these complications and provide some methods to prevent or reduce them.

22.2 Complications

When performed by well-trained personnel, thoracoscopy is a safe procedure (see Table 22.1). Oxygen desaturation during thoracoscopy under local anaesthesia is unusual, and – in our experience – the procedure is well tolerated especially when large pleural effusions are drained immediately after insertion of the trocar, thus improving respiratory function. In four studies with 819 patients in total, no fatal cases were reported

(Davidson et al. 1988; Menzies and Charbonneau 1991; Enk and Viskum 1981; De Camp et al. 1973); however, fatal complications can occur (Medford et al. 2009). When talc poudrage is also performed, the complication rate might be expected to rise a little (Froudarakis et al. 2006), especially in patients with a poor performance status (Froudarakis et al. 2010). We report in Table 22.2 the most relevant complications found in our thoracoscopy series; these include talc poudrage for malignant pleural effusions in more than 500 patients, using two different types of talc with small and large particle size.

In order to understand better how to manage thoracoscopic complications, we are separating them into several categories:

22.2.1 Complications of Thoracoscopy Associated with Poor Patient Selection

Most complications can be avoided by proper selection of patients for thoracoscopy (see Table 22.3 and Fig. 22.1). Patients with severe COPD and respiratory insufficiency – with hypoxemia ($PO_2 < 50$ mmHg) and hypercapnia – will not tolerate the induction of a pneumothorax without a further deterioration of the gas exchange, and should be viewed as unsuitable candidates for thoracoscopy. When there is severe contralateral lung or pleural involvement, thoracoscopy is not advisable, unless general anaesthesia and tracheal intubation

F. Rodríguez-Panadero (✉) • B.R. Romero
Unidad Médico-Quirúrgica
de Enfermeda des Respiratorias,
Hospital Universitario Virgen del Rocío, Sevilla, Spain
e-mail: frodriguezpan@gmail.com;
beatrizromero@terra.es

P. Astoul et al. (eds.), *Thoracoscopy for Pulmonologists*,
DOI 10.1007/978-3-642-38351-9_22, © Springer-Verlag Berlin Heidelberg 2014

Table 22.1 Complications of thoracoscopy as reported in four series

Viskum and Enk (1981)

> Revision of 2,298 reported procedures in 15 (general) series
>
>> Subcutaneous emphysema: 1.3 %
>>
>> Empyema: 2 %
>>
>> (Significant) bleeding: 2.3 %
>>
>> Air embolism: 0.2 %
>>
>> Death due to the technique: 0.09 %

Viallat et al. (1996) (360 patients undergoing talc poudrage)

> Subcutaneous emphysema: 0.6 %
>
> Empyema: 2.5 %

Ribas et al. (2001) (614 patients undergoing talc poudrage)

> Empyema: 2.7 %
>
> Re-expansion pulmonary oedema: 2.2 %
>
> Respiratory failure: 1.3 %
>
> Air leak: 0.5 %
>
> Postoperative bleeding: 0.4 %

Colt (2005) (52 prospective procedures)

> Major adverse event: 1.92 % (1/52) [This was a patient with severe dyspnea, advanced scleroderma and recurrent pleural effusion who underwent a thoracoscopy for drainage and assessment of lung expansibility. A severely trapped lung was observed, so pleurodesis was not performed. Symptoms resolved after drainage with a small-bore chest tube]
>
> No procedure-related deaths or intraoperative accidents
>
> No patient required immediate open-chest surgery
>
> There were no episodes of procedure-related sepsis, prolonged intubation or prolonged air leak requiring re-intervention or thoracotomy
>
> Thoracoscopy was never aborted due to failure of entry into the pleural space (extended thoracoscopy was performed in two patients with empyema)
>
> Minor adverse events: 19.2 % (10/52) including talc-related fever in 7 subjects. This adverse rate decreased to 5.7 % (3/52) if talc-related fever removed from the analysis [These included wound infection at a chest tube insertion site (1), fever (1) and a small clinically insignificant pneumothorax after chest tube removal]

Table 22.2 Complications of thoracoscopy in patients with malignant pleural effusion undergoing talc poudrage using two different types of talc (personal experience)

Complications	Patients ($N=512$)	Small-particle talc ($N=232$) Death <10 days $N=26/232$ (11 %)	Large-particle talc ($N=280$) Death <10 days $N=5/280$ (1.8 %)
Transient dyspnea after talc	50 (9.8 %)	31 (13.4 %)	19 (6.8 %)
Acute pain after talc	44 (8.6 %)	28 (12 %)	16 (5.7 %)
Subcutaneous emphysema	20 (3.9 %)	16 (6.9 %)	4 (1.4 %)
Neoplastic invasion of the thoracoscopy tract	14 (2.7 %)	12 (5.2 %)	2 (0.7 %)
Pulmonary embolism	12 (2.3 %)	9 (3.9 %)	3 (1 %)
Empyema	9 (1.9 %)	4 (1.7 %)	5 (1.8 %)
Bleeding (requiring blood transfusion)	2 (0.4 %)	1 (0.5 %)	1 (0.4 %)
Acute respiratory distress	1 (0.2 %)	1 (0.5 %)	–

Small talc (Spanish talc): particles with a mean diameter $=9.8$ μm (0.5–42). Large-particle talc (Steritalc®): particles with mean diameter $=24.5$ μm (1.1–74)

are used. Patients with unstable cardiovascular status should not undergo thoracoscopy: any patient with a history of cardiovascular disease – especially those with unstable angina or recent history of myocardial infarction – should be carefully evaluated before undertaking a thoracoscopy. Cough, fever and infection are relative contraindications to thoracoscopy, and definitive treatment or optimisation of these pre-existing conditions should be considered before a procedure is scheduled. Thoracoscopy is not feasible in the setting of tight adhesions between the visceral and the parietal pleura. In cases of localised pleural adhesions, it might be possible to create a pleural space by extended thoracoscopy using digital dissection in the pleural cavity (Janssen and Boutin 1992). However, this technique should be performed only by experienced thoracoscopists. Medical thoracoscopy is not safe in advanced pulmonary fibrosis; after induction of pneumothorax in these cases, severe acute hypoxemia might occur, and re-expansion of the lung can be difficult due to the loss of elasticity of the pulmonary tissue. In addition, biopsy of the lung parenchyma in pulmonary fibrosis may result in prolonged air leakage. Biopsy should also be avoided in hydatid cyst disease, arterio-venous malformations and other highly vascularised lesions.

22.2.1.1 Pain and Anxiety

Pain and anxiety are frequent during the procedure – especially when the thoracoscopy is performed under local anaesthesia, even if talc poudrage is not performed. Although medical thoracoscopy is safe and relatively simple, this depends on the experience of the physician. In addition the operator needs to understand the cavity anatomy from the thoracoscopic point of view (which is not always the same as the conventional anatomy, as there is a limited field of vision compared with open thoracotomy or autopsy). The presence of multiple loculations can also make the exploration difficult. The technique should be explained clearly to the patient, especially when the procedure is going to be

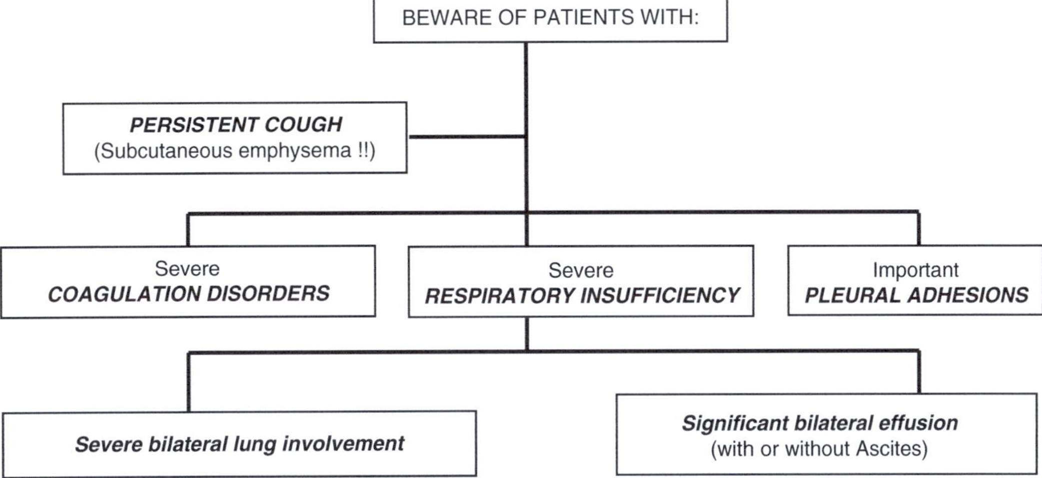

Table 22.3 Patient selection criteria for thoracoscopy is critical, in order to prevent complications. In patient A, a contralateral lesion is seen in the lung parenchyma, and medical thoracoscopy (using conscious sedation and spontaneous ventilation) would be problematic. Patient B has a bilateral pleural effusion, and therapeutic thoracentesis in one side should be performed before attempting thoracoscopy on the contralateral side

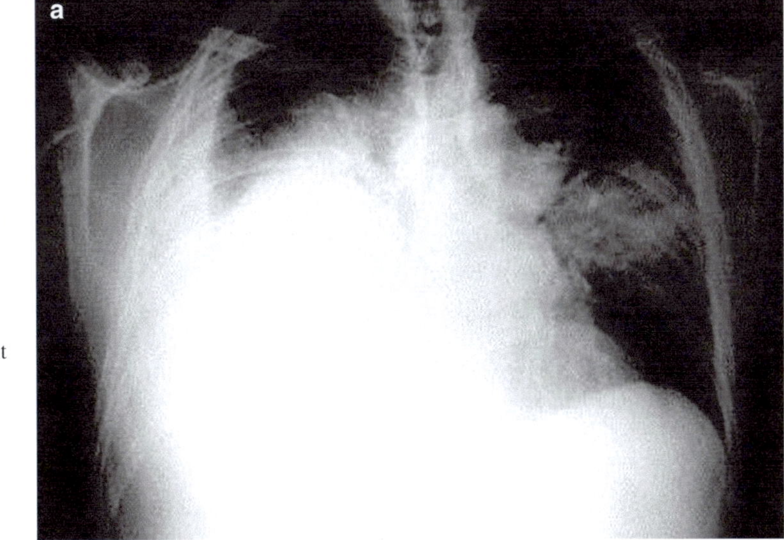

Fig. 22.1 Patient *A* – a contralateral lesion is seen in the lung parenchyma, and medical thoracoscopy (under conscious sedation and spontaneous ventilation) would be problematic. Patient *B* – a patient with bilateral pleural effusions. In this scenario a therapeutic thoracentesis is required on one side prior to attempting thoracoscopy on the contralateral side

Fig. 22.1 (continued)

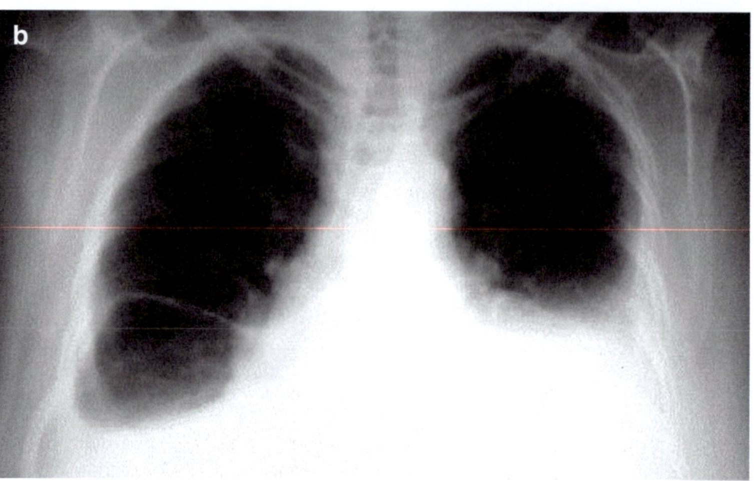

done under local anaesthesia, as this will allay the patients' fears and make them more confident and relaxed during the exploration. The role of preoperative medication has not been subjected to randomised studies: we routinely administer 0.4–0.8 mg atropine (intramuscular or subcutaneous) prior to the procedure, to prevent vasovagal reactions. Intravenous midazolam can be very useful, especially in young patients. Sedation during the procedure can be performed using incremental dosages of a narcotic (morphine, pethidine or fentanyl) and a benzodiazepine, and agents to antagonise both morphine and benzodiazepine should be available. A number of considerations should be taken into account when choosing the anaesthetic technique:

- Mental status of the patient (patients afraid of any medical procedure should be offered general anaesthesia; children and mentally retarded patients should be treated under general anaesthesia).
- Suspected duration and type of thoracoscopy: when a procedure is suspected to be long or painful (e.g. multiloculated empyema), general anaesthesia is preferred. Procedures with two or more ports of entry, or those including chemical pleurodesis, are potentially more painful, and generous amounts of opiates may be required. We titrate intravenous pethidine while keeping the patient awake – and have obtained good results in more than 500 local anaesthesia procedures undergoing talc poudrage.

22.2.1.2 Acute Respiratory Insufficiency or Heart Failure

A posteroanterior and lateral chest X-ray film is mandatory in order to evaluate the most convenient port of entry, to exclude the presence of contralateral pulmonary lesions (that could lead to acute respiratory insufficiency at the time of inducing the pneumothorax for thoracoscopy) and to evaluate the size and shape of the pleural effusion. Electrocardiogram, coagulation and blood gas analysis are also necessary.

22.2.1.3 Other Complications Associated with Patient Selection

Great care is required with patients who are in a very poor clinical condition, hypoproteinemic or with diffuse neoplastic infiltration of the chest wall (Rodriguez Panadero 1995). In addition, medical thoracoscopy should be deferred in patients with an uncontrolled cough, because the exploration is likely to be difficult and results in more complications especially subcutaneous emphysema. Preoperative preparation of patients with obstructive lung disease should include chest physiotherapy, bronchodilators, antibiotics and corticosteroids.

In order to prevent pulmonary embolism, especially in patients with malignant pleural effusions treated with talc pleurodesis, we advise prophylactic heparin throughout the whole hospital stay.

22.2.2 Complications Associated with the Thoracoscopy Technique

22.2.2.1 Laceration of the Lung During Insertion of the Trocar

Some authors advocate the creation of a pneumothorax a few hours or even the day before the thoracoscopy. This technique may help reduce blood flow in the periphery of the lung, and may prevent damage to the lung after the introduction of the thoracoscopy instruments. However, direct introduction of a blunt trocar into the thoracic wall without prior induction of pneumothorax is, in our experience, safe and effective especially if there is enough pleural fluid. A previously induced pneumothorax can be useful to assess for pleural lesions and lung collapsibility in advance of a thoracoscopy, but a contrast CT scan, which is strongly recommended in the evaluation of every undiagnosed exudative pleural effusion, can also be very useful. Ultrasound examination can be also very helpful to identify loculations in the pleural cavity and to locate the best entry site for thoracoscopy (Tsai and Yang 2003; Medford 2010). The trocar should always be inserted perpendicular to the chest wall with a rotating/corkscrewing motion (see Fig. 22.2). It is safer to locate the tip over the border of the inferior rib at the chosen port of entry, in order to prevent damage to the intercostal vessels and nerves. Rarely the introduction of the trocar can be troublesome especially in cases of pleural adhesions. When the physician is not sure about the presence of tight adhesions between the lung and the chest wall at the chosen site of entry, a digital dissection and direct exploration of the port of entry with the telescope may be of help.

22.2.2.2 Bleeding

Patients with pancytopenia or coagulation disorders can be at risk, and no invasive procedure should be performed if the platelets are below $60,000/\text{mm}^3$. To perform a safe biopsy in patients on anticoagulant medication, the INR should be <2.0. Aspirin may prolong bleeding time, but is not an absolute contraindication for biopsies. Clopidogrel or other antiplatelet agents might be more problematic and should be discontinued before thoracoscopy. In order to prevent inadvertent biopsy from vascular structures, a perfect knowledge of the anatomy is mandatory. The operator should never take biopsies inside the fissures of the lung (because large vessels are close to the surface in these zones), and special care is also required when sampling areas near the internal mammary artery and vein (anterior mediastinal pleura). Although these structures can be easily identified by expert thoracoscopists, the vessels may sometimes be covered by tumour or fibrin, and in this scenario inadvertently sampled,

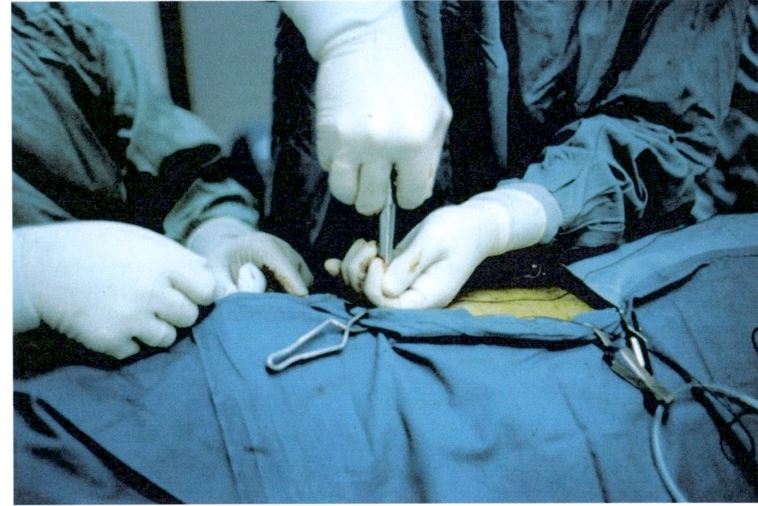

Fig. 22.2 Recommended technique for insertion of the trocar at thoracoscopy: – Apply firm pressure over the trocar with a rotating motion – Always keep the trocar vertical (perpendicular to the chest wall) – Use your other hand as a "brake", to prevent laceration of the underlying lung with the trocar (by a sudden loss of resistance when the trocar passes through the pleura)

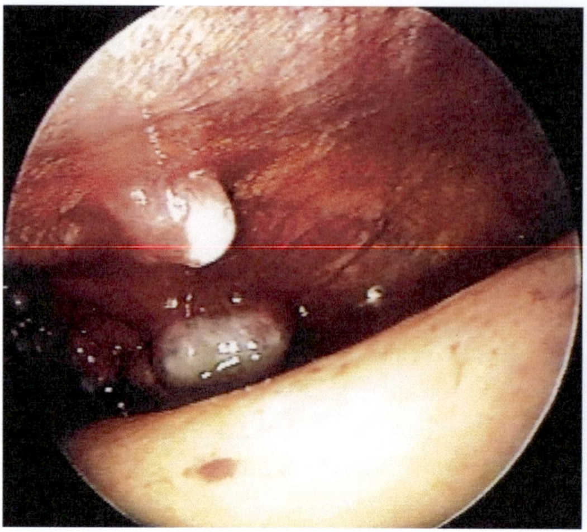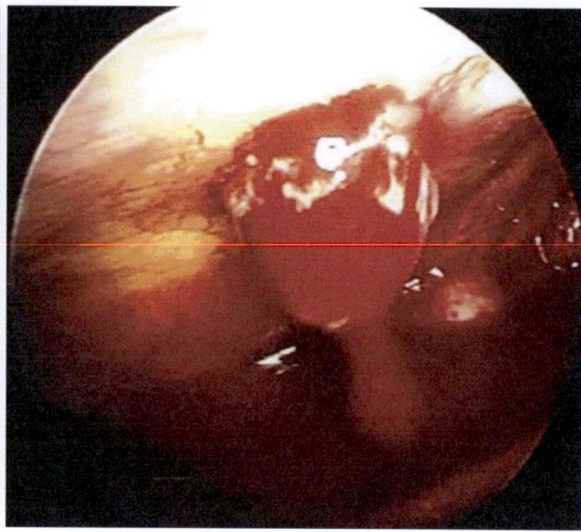

Fig. 22.3 Recommendations in case of pleural bleeding: – Compress with the (closed) biopsy forceps – Electrocautery can be very useful and should always be available – Local instillation of adrenaline is seldom needed – Local instillation of tranexamic acid can help to stop the bleeding (see text)

with fatal consequences if emergency surgery is not immediately available.

In cases of excessive bleeding after biopsy (see Fig. 22.3), we would recommend compressing with the forceps and the local application of tranexamic acid (antifibrinolytic agent) which, in our experience, can help to stop the haemorrhage, both in thoracoscopy and bronchoscopy (Marquez-Martın et al. 2010). However, we would advise that electrocautery is always available.

22.2.2.3 Infection

Although routine prophylactic antibiotics are not necessary, they should be used in neutropenic patients. Deep antiseptic cleaning of the chest wall is mandatory, and very strict care of the drain and the chest wound is essential. The likelihood of occurrence of empyema is higher in neutropenic patients and in those with prolonged chest drains: we never leave the drain for more than 5 days after thoracoscopy; this includes cases where talc poudrage was performed.

22.2.2.4 Neoplastic Invasion of the Thoracoscopy Tract

This complication is frequently seen in mesothelioma but can also be found in long-term surviving patients with pleural metastatic carcinoma. To prevent tract invasion by mesothelioma, the

application of local radiation therapy to the scar 10–14 days after thoracoscopy is recommended (21 Gy over 3 fractions).

22.2.3 Complications Associated with Lung Re-expansion

A chest drain should be inserted in every case at the end of the procedure, and this is then connected to a water-seal system; gentle step-by-step suction is applied, and the drain is kept in place until complete re-expansion of the lung has been achieved.

22.2.3.1 Pulmonary Re-expansion Oedema

This can occur if suction is too strong, especially in patients with an associated trapped lung. In order to prevent this complication, careful and graded suction should be applied, especially when a pleurodesis procedure has been performed. We usually leave the drain connected to water-seal without suction for at least 3 h following the pleurodesis procedure and then gradually apply increasing suction. Pulmonary oedema can occur when expanding the lung in pneumothorax and malignant effusions, even without the application of a sclerosant agent. Although oedema usually appears on the ipsilateral hemithorax, it has been reported on the contralateral side in rare cases (Chang et al. 2009; Heller and Grathwohl 2000). Mahfood and co-workers reported three cases where the oedema was contralateral, with fatal outcomes in two cases (Mahfood et al. 1988). The mechanism for this complication is not fully understood; however, a rapid re-expansion, especially if the lung was collapsed for several weeks, may play an important role, as pointed out by several authors (Nakamura et al. 1994) and supported by our experience. It also appears that a high production of IL-8 and other pro-inflammatory cytokines has a role in the development of this complication (Sakao et al. 2001).

22.2.3.2 Prolonged Air Leak

In our experience, this most frequently happens in neoplastic patients who have undergone prior chemotherapy. In those cases, necrotic tumour nodules can be seen on the surface of the lung, and it is postulated that some of these nodules could eventually rupture during lung re-expansion. If this occurs, suction must be stopped immediately, and the drain left only on water-seal (without suction) until the air leaking stops.

22.2.3.3 Subcutaneous Emphysema

This complication is frequently associated with prolonged air leak and may require specific surgical measures in some cases, especially if there is any compromise to the upper airways. It can also be observed in patients who have persistent uncontrolled coughing during thoracoscopy exploration. If this occurs, the trocar should be left open, so that high intrathoracic pressures are prevented. Manual compression over the area surrounding the port of entry and the trocar may prevent the subcutaneous spreading of air.

22.2.4 Complications Associated to Pleurodesis

22.2.4.1 Acute Respiratory Distress or Pneumonitis

This has been described in some cases of talc pleurodesis (Rinaldo et al. 1983; Bouchama et al. 1984; Rehse et al. 1999). The precise pathophysiological mechanism responsible for this severe complication is still unclear, but it appears that a high dose of talc might play a significant role in some cases. There is some concern about the systemic absorption of the sclerosing agents, and this is suspected for almost all of the soluble agents that are instilled into the pleural space and for talc with very small particles (<10 µm). Thus, the size of talc particles used for pleurodesis appears to be critical (Maskell et al. 2004). Talc is thought to persist in the pleura for a long time, thus accounting – at least in part – for its better pleurodesis results. However, there are some reports where talc particles have been deposited in distant organs after intrapleural application, both in animals (Campos et al. 1997; Werebe et al. 1999) and humans (Milanez de Campos et al. 1997). In a study on experimental talc slurry pleurodesis in rabbits, Kennedy and co-workers found prominent perivascular infiltrates with mononuclear inflammation in the underlying lung, and they speculated that some mediators might spread through the pulmonary circulation (Kennedy et al. 1995). It seems that the size of particles might play an important role in the process (Ferrer et al. 2001; Navarro Jiménez et al. 2005), and two recent European multicenter studies carried out in patients with recurrent malignant pleural effusions ($n=558$) and recurrent primary spontaneous pneumothoraces ($n=418$) investigating the safety of talc poudrage using large-size particle talc (with a median diameter of 25.6 µm) found no cases of acute respiratory distress (Janssen et al. 2007; Bridevaux et al. 2011).

It is our belief that acute respiratory complications arise more frequently in patients who are sick at the time of thoracoscopy. Therefore, a careful evaluation of the performance status of those patients prior to thoracoscopy and planned pleurodesis is mandatory.

22.2.4.2 Possible Activation of the Systemic Coagulation Cascade After Pleurodesis

Agrenius and co-workers reported an increase in the coagulation pathway and an associated inhibition of fibrinolytic activity in the pleural space after instillation of quinacrine as a sclerosing agent (Agrenius et al. 1989, 1991). We also demonstrated similar effects after talc pleurodesis in

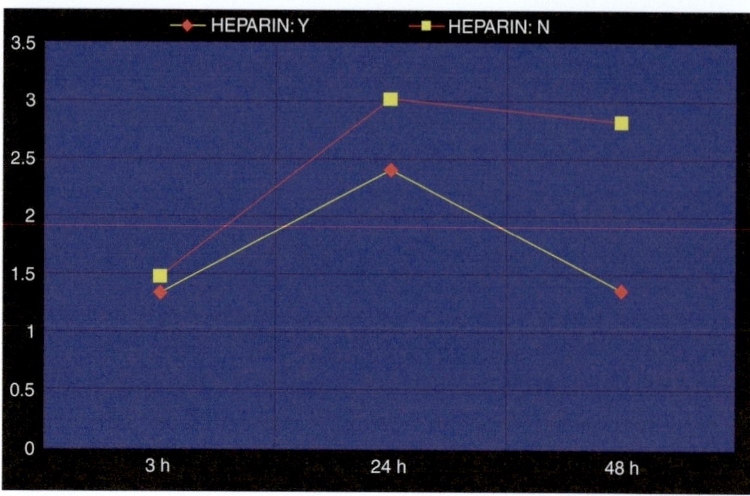

Fig. 22.4 Increment of thrombin-antithrombin complex (TAT) vs. D-dimer (coagulation/fibrinolysis balance) in the plasma of patients post thoracoscopic talc pleurodesis ("poudrage"). Administration of subcutaneous low-molecular prophylactic heparin can help to prevent deep-vein thrombosis and pulmonary embolism in patients (Taken from Rodriguez-Panadero and Antony 1997)

our patients (Rodriguez-Panadero et al. 1995). We were subsequently concerned about the possible systemic implications of the pleural coagulation/fibrinolysis imbalance involved in the pleurodesis process itself. Prompted by this concern and our findings of several cases of massive pulmonary embolism after talc pleurodesis, we performed a preliminary study on levels of simultaneous pleural/plasma markers for coagulation and fibrinolysis and found that there is an activation of the systemic coagulation after talc poudrage (Rodriguez-Panadero et al. 1995). Moreover, this effect can be partially controlled with prophylactic heparin (Rodriguez-Panadero and Antony 1997) (see Fig. 22.4). The relevance of this finding in clinical practice remains unclear, but some early deaths (less than 30 days) following pleurodesis procedures (up to 43 % in the series of Seaton and co-workers) (Seaton et al. 1995) may be in part related to an undetected pulmonary embolism, and to advanced neoplastic disease, as it is commonly believed.

To summarise this chapter, according to Boutin (1999), complications can best be prevented by observing the following rules:

1. Postpone thoracoscopy for several days if the patient is coughing.
2. Measure blood gases, and monitor cardiac signs by simultaneous ECG during the procedure.
3. Give supplementary oxygen to the patient during thoracoscopy.
4. Avoid taking biopsy samples from the internal parts of the fissures or from the mediastinum.
5. Coagulate and ensure haemostasis if haemorrhage exceeds 20 ml.
6. Insert a chest tube (at least until the lung expands) to prevent subcutaneous emphysema.
7. Start physiotherapy on the day of thoracoscopy to exercise the diaphragm and to avoid accumulation of secretions and bronchial obstruction.
8. To prevent invasion in cases of mesothelioma, administer radiation therapy of 7 Gy/day for 3 days to the trocar site on postoperative day 10.

References

Agrenius V, Chmielewska J, Widström O et al (1989) Pleural fibrinolytic activity is decreased in inflammation as demonstrated in quinacrine pleurodesis treatment of malignant pleural effusion. Am Rev Respir Dis 140:1381–1385

Agrenius V, Chmielewska J, Widström O et al (1991) Increased coagulation activity of the pleura after tube drainage and quinacrine instillation in malignant pleural effusion. Eur Respir J 4:1135–1139

Bouchama A, Chastre J, Gaudichet A et al (1984) Acute pneumonitis with bilateral pleural effusion after talc pleurodesis. Chest 86:795–797

Boutin C (1999) Methods and indications of pleuroscopy or medical thoracoscopy. Pneumology 12:16–19

Bridevaux PO, Tschopp JM, Cardillo G et al (2011) Short-term safety of thoracoscopic talc pleurodesis for recurrent primary spontaneous pneumothorax: a prospective European multicentre study. Eur Respir J 38:770–773

Campos JR, Werebe EC, Vargas FS et al (1997) Respiratory failure due to insufflated talc. Lancet 349:251–252

Chang CY, Hung MH, Chang HC et al (2009) Delayed onset of contralateral pulmonary edema following reexpansion pulmonary edema of a collapsed lung after video-assisted thoracoscopic surgery. Acta Anaesthesiol Taiwan 47:87–91

Davidson AC, George RJ, Sheldon CD et al (1988) Thoracoscopy: assessment of a physician service and comparison of a flexible bronchoscope used as a thoracoscope with a rigid thoracoscope. Thorax 43:327–332

De Camp PT, Moseley PW, Scott ML et al (1973) Diagnostic thoracoscopy. Ann Thorac Surg 16:79–84

Enk B, Viskum K (1981) Diagnostic thoracoscopy. Eur J Respir Dis 62:344–351

Ferrer J, Villarino MA, Tura JM (2001) Talc preparations used for pleurodesis vary markedly from one preparation to another. Chest 119:1901–1905

Froudarakis ME, Klimathianaki M, Pougounias M (2006) Systemic inflammatory reaction after thoracoscopic talc poudrage. Chest 129:356–361

Froudarakis ME, Pataka A, Makris D et al (2010) Respiratory muscle strength and lung function in patients undergoing medical thoracoscopy. Respiration 80:220–227

Heller BJ, Grathwohl MK (2000) Contralateral reexpansion pulmonary edema. South Med J 93:828–831

Janssen JP, Boutin C (1992) Extended thoracoscopy: a biopsy method to be used in case of pleural adhesions. Eur Respir J 5:763–766

Janssen JP, Collier G, Astoul P et al (2007) Safety of pleurodesis with talc poudrage in malignant pleural effusion: a prospective cohort study. Lancet 369:1535–1539

Kennedy L, Harley RA, Sahn SA et al (1995) Talc slurry pleurodesis: pleural fluid and histologic analysis. Chest 107:1707–1712

Lee P, Colt HG (2005) Rigid and semirigid pleuroscopy: the future is bright. Respirology 10:418–425. (Review)

Mahfood S, Hix WR, Aaron BL et al (1988) Reexpansion pulmonary edema. Ann Thorac Surg 45:340–345

Marquez-Martın E, Gonzalez Vergara D, Martin-Juan J et al (2010) Endobronchial administration of tranexamic acid for controlling pulmonary bleeding. A pilot study. J Bronchol Intervent Pulmonol 17:122–125

Maskell NA, Lee YC, Gleeson FV et al (2004) Randomized trials describing lung inflammation after pleurodesis with talc of varying particle size. Am J Respir Crit Care Med 170:377–382

Medford AR (2010) Additional cost benefits of chest physician-operated thoracic ultrasound (TUS) prior to medical thoracoscopy (MT). Respir Med 104: 1077–1078

Medford AR, Agrawal S, Free CM et al (2009) A local anaesthetic video-assisted thoracoscopy service: pro-spective performance analysis in a UK tertiary respiratory centre. Lung Cancer 66:355–358

Menzies R, Charbonneau M (1991) Thoracoscopy for the diagnosis of pleural disease. Ann Intern Med 114:271–276

Milanez de Campos JR, Campos Werebe E, Vargas FS et al (1997) Respiratory failure due to insufflated talc. Lancet 349:251–252

Nakamura H, Ishizaka A, Sawafuji M et al (1994) Elevated levels of interleukin-8 and leukotriene B4 in pulmonary edema fluid of a patient with reexpansion pulmonary edema. Am J Respir Crit Care Med 149:1037–1040

Navarro Jiménez C, Gómez Izquierdo L, Sánchez Gutiérrez C et al (2005) Análisis morfométrico y min-eralógico de 14 muestras de talco usado para pleurode-sis en distintos países de Europa y América. Neumosur 17:197–202

Rehse DH, Aye RW, Florence MG (1999) Respiratory failure following talc pleurodesis. Am J Surg 177: 437–440

Ribas J, Jiménez MJ, Barberà JA et al (2001) Gas exchange and pulmonary hemodynamics during lung resection in patients at increased risk: relationship with preopera-tive exercise testing. Chest 120:852-859

Rinaldo JE, Owens GR, Rogers RM (1983) Adult respiratory distress syndrome following intrapleu-ral instillation of talc. J Thorac Cardiovasc Surg 85: 523–526

Rodriguez Panadero F (1995) Lung cancer and ipsilateral pleural effusion. Ann Oncol 6:S25–S27

Rodriguez-Panadero F, Antony VB (1997) Pleurodesis: state of the art. Eur Respir J 10:1648–1654

Rodriguez-Panadero F, Segado A, Torres I et al (1995) Thoracoscopy and talc poudrage induce an activation of the systemic coagulation system. Am J Respir Crit Care Med 151:A357

Sakao Y, Kajikawa O, Martin TR et al (2001) Association of IL-8 and MCP-1 with the development of reexpan-sion pulmonary edema in rabbits. Ann Thorac Surg 71:1825–1832

Seaton KG, Patz EF Jr, Goodman PC (1995) Palliative treatment of malignant pleural effusions: value of small-bore catheter thoracostomy and doxycycline sclerotherapy. Am J Roentgenol 164:589–591

Tsai TH, Yang PC (2003) Ultrasound in the diagnosis and management of pleural disease. Curr Opin Pulm Med 9:282–290

Viallat JR, Rey F, Astoul P et al (1996) Thoracoscopic talc poudrage pleurodesis for malignant effusions. A review of 360 cases. Chest 110:1387–1393

Viskum K, Enk B (1981) Complications of thoracoscopy. Poumon Cœur 37:25–28. (Review)

Werebe EC, Pazetti R, Milanez de Campos JR et al (1999) Systemic distribution of talc after intrapleural admin-istration in rats. Chest 115:190–193

Julius Janssen

23.1 Proper Selection of Patients and Indications

Thoracoscopy is a safe procedure, provided that it is performed for an accepted indication in a well-selected patient. In this paragraph, we will discuss selection of patients and indications.

23.1.1 Selection of Patients

The most common indication for diagnostic thoracoscopy is a patient with undiagnosed exudative pleural effusion. Because metastatic cancer is often suspected in these cases, the majority of patients are over 60 years. This in turn means that there is often associated comorbidity and a decreased performance status. Thoracoscopy, in general, should only be performed if the life expectancy is more than 3 months and the performance status is adequate (Karnofsky index at least 70 %, ECOG scale at least 3).

It is not easy to assess the optimal timing for thoracoscopic intervention in a patient with (suspected) malignant pleural effusion. The volume of an early detected effusion may be too small to cause dyspnea. In a palliative setting, most physicians tend to postpone treatment until symptoms are impairing the patient's quality of life. Waiting too long without performing a thoracoscopic intervention in the setting of a malignant pleural effusion may be detrimental to the patient, as in the later stages of malignant pleural effusion the success rate achieved by pleurodesis is inferior; this is often explained by the incomplete re-expansion of the lung after removal of pleural fluid. Patients with a pleural effusion due to malignant disease benefit from early pleurodesis, as has been demonstrated recently (Steger et al. 2007). In their study, the most favorable outcome after talc pleurodesis was seen in women whose lungs were fully expandable, in patients whose Karnofsky index exceeded 60 %, in patients whose body mass index was greater than 25 kg/m^2, and in patients with benign disease.

An absolute contraindication to thoracoscopy exists in patients where no pleural space can be created. This occurs if no air enters the pleural cavity after penetration of the parietal pleura, and hence no pneumothorax can be created. In experienced hands, it is possible to perform a so-called extended thoracoscopy. In this case, the incision is enlarged to 3–4 cm, and the thoracoscopist introduces his/her finger into the intercostal space and palpates the area beyond the parietal pleura. If the parietal and visceral pleura are attached by small adhesions, these can be manually broken by rotation of the finger (Janssen and Boutin 1992). In this scenario, a small pleural space can be created, which in most cases is sufficient to take a pleural biopsy.

J. Janssen
Department of Pulmonary Diseases,
Canisius Wilhelmina Hospital, Nijmegen,
The Netherlands
e-mail: j.janssen@cwz.nl

P. Astoul et al. (eds.), *Thoracoscopy for Pulmonologists*,
DOI 10.1007/978-3-642-38351-9_23, © Springer-Verlag Berlin Heidelberg 2014

Other absolute contraindications for thoracoscopy include respiratory insufficiency, bleeding disorders, and end-stage fibrosis. In the case of an end-stage lung fibrosis, the induction of a pneumothorax is dangerous, because re-expansion can be difficult, and there is a risk of persistent air leakage due to a bronchopleural fistula and respiratory insufficiency.

Relative contraindications for thoracoscopy arc poor gcncral health status, fever, uncontrolled cough, unstable cardiovascular status, and hypoxemia. If any of these contraindications exist/persist, then the indication for thoracoscopy should be reevaluated, and the procedure should be postponed until the problem has been solved.

23.1.2 Selection of Indications

Thoracoscopy can be performed for a wide selection of diagnostic and therapeutic procedures. In general, thoracoscopy is a safe procedure in experienced hands. The less-experienced thoracoscopist should restrict their practice to cases with a minimal risk of complications. The best indication for thoracoscopy with limited risk (the best indication when you start a thoracoscopy service) is a large pleural effusion in an otherwise healthy patient. For diagnostic biopsy of pleural disease, CT-guided biopsy and ultrasound-guided biopsy are safe procedures with a high diagnostic yield (Rahman and Gleeson 2008). In debilitated patients, CT- or ultrasound-guided biopsy may serve as an alternative to thoracoscopy, especially in cases with a small pleural effusion, when no lung re-expansion or pleurodesis is necessary.

23.2 Preparation of Staff and Equipment

The team should include a pulmonary physician qualified to perform thoracoscopy, an assisting nurse (sterile), and one nurse to monitor the patient, the oxygenation, and the ventilatory and cardiac parameters. An extra nurse (non-sterile) should also be available to provide additional support, for example, if equipment and/or medication is required. However, this is not mandatory.

A well-equipped and up-to-date resuscitation trolley should be close to hand. This trolley should contain equipment for defibrillation and intubation.

23.3 Preparation of the Patient

Before thoracoscopy, the patient should be well informed about the procedure. A patient with recent heart issues or a suspected unstable cardiovascular status should be seen by a cardiologist before the thoracoscopy is performed. Adult patients without hypoxemia, COPD, and cardiovascular problems can undergo a diagnostic thoracoscopy under local anesthesia, without the attendance of an anesthesiologist.

23.4 Safety Measures During Thoracoscopy

The trocar can be safely introduced in the intercostal space if a pneumothorax exists or has been introduced before the thoracoscopy procedure. If the pneumothorax is introduced on the operation table using blunt scissors to dissect the intercostal tissues, a pneumothorax is created after opening the parietal pleura. In this case, the hissing sound of air entering the pleural cavity is heard. If not, there may be adhesions between the parietal and visceral pleura, and the lung cannot collapse. In this case, the trocar should not be introduced blindly. An extended thoracoscopy (Janssen and Boutin 1992) may be performed to separate the parietal and the visceral pleura manually. Alternatively, thoracic ultrasound may help to determine if the port of entry has been well chosen. In cases with a small pleural effusion, thoracic ultrasound may be performed before the thoracoscopy procedure, to determine the optimal port of entry.

It is not recommended to use force when the trocar is introduced. When there are adhesions of the lung to the chest wall, the forced introduction of the trocar may lead to damage to the lung and consequently persistent air leak and bleeding. Severe hemorrhage is rare, as the vessels in the periphery of the lung are mostly small. If the thoracoscopist is in doubt about the safe introduction of the trocar, it is sometimes useful to choose another port of entry, where more pleural fluid is present.

23.5 Prevention of Post-thoracoscopy Complications

Severe complications after thoracoscopy are rare. Procedure-related mortality is below 0.02 %. The most common complication is fever, which occurs in 2.6 % of patients, and may start a few hours after the procedure. The post-thoracoscopy fever is moderate, rarely over 39 °C, and in general resolves within 1 day.

Empyema is rare and can be avoided by a careful maintenance of sterile conditions during the thoracoscopy. Some centers give routine antibiotics during chest tube drainage.

Subcutaneous emphysema can be prevented by optimal cough prevention and treatment before, during, and after the procedure; proper drain placement; and making small incisions (as small as possible) to prevent leakage of false air.

Re-expansion edema is also very rare, especially after removal of pleural fluid in elderly patients. In cases with a very large effusion, some centers advise the removal of the pleural fluid in aliquots of a maximum of 2 l/24 h, to prevent re-expansion edema. However, this practice is subject to discussion. In our center, the pleural fluid is removed in one session, even if the amount is larger than 2 l. In this case, however, no suction is performed on the chest tube for the first 24 h.

References

Janssen JP, Boutin C (1992) Extended thoracoscopy: a biopsy method to be used in case of pleural adhesions. Eur Respir J 5:763–766

Rahman NM, Gleeson FV (2008) Image-guided pleural biopsy. Curr Opin Pulm Med 14:331–336

Steger V, Mika U, Toomes H et al (2007) Who gains most? A 10-year experience with 611 thoracoscopic talc pleurodeses. Ann Thorac Surg 83:1940–1945

Part VI

Future in the Field of Thoracoscopy

Future Developments in Medical Thoracoscopy

24

Philippe Astoul, GianFranco Tassi, and Jean-Marie Tschopp

Progress in medical thoracoscopy, as discussed in the following chapters, will be centered on instrument development, new diagnostic methods, and associated clinical research.

The miniaturization of instruments is an ongoing process. After the initial pioneering application of small instruments in laparoscopy, their use has become more commonplace in all areas of endoscopy. This represents a further evolution towards minimal invasiveness which is the current vogue in medicine.

Following the extensive use of autofluorescence in bronchoscopy, its use has been extended to the assessment of pleural pathologies. Although still in development, initial results are encouraging. Autofluorescence may improve the diagnostic accuracy of thoracoscopy by facilitating the identification of early neoplastic processes, and, in benign disease such as primary spontaneous pneumothorax, it may allow for visualization of abnormal areas at the visceral lung surface. Improvements in instruments include the development of the flexi-rigid thoracoscope which, through its compatibility with various existing video processors, allows the integration of equipment for both thoracoscopy and bronchoscopy. This may make thoracoscopy available to a greater number of pulmonologists.

In real terms, however, the future of thoracoscopy will be safeguarded by quality clinical research. This will promote increased knowledge which, in the long term, will improve patient care.

P. Astoul (✉)
Division of Thoracic Oncology,
Pleural Diseases, and Interventional Pulmonology,
Hôpital NORD, Marseille, France
e-mail: pastoul@ap-hm.fr

G. Tassi
Division of Pneumology,
Spedali Civili di Brescia, Brescia, Italy
e-mail: gf.tassi@tin.it

J.-M. Tschopp
Département de Médecine Interne
Centre valaisan de pneumologie,
CHCVs, Montana 3963, Switzerland
e-mail: jean-marie.tschopp@hopitalvs.ch

P. Astoul et al. (eds.), *Thoracoscopy for Pulmonologists*,
DOI 10.1007/978-3-642-38351-9_24, © Springer-Verlag Berlin Heidelberg 2014

Minithoracoscopy

25

GianFranco Tassi and Gian Pietro Marchetti

25.1 Introduction

The use of small-calibre instruments, termed minithoracoscopy, allows for a minimally invasive procedure and is part of the overall evolution in medicine towards the reduction of trauma caused by diagnostic and therapeutic procedures.

Small-calibre instruments have been designed with this objective in mind and are now identified as miniendoscopes if the diameter ranges from 2 to 5 mm or microendoscopes if the diameter is 2 mm or less (Tu and Advincula 2008).

These types of instruments have been used for a number of years for diagnostic and therapeutic purposes in specialized surgical and medical centres, principally in the field of laparoscopy (Schneider et al. 2001). Indeed, as far back as 10 years ago, it was stated that "In most cases undergoing laparoscopy for diagnostic purposes 2 mm microlaparoscopy yields sufficient information to abandon the conventional 10 mm technique" (Haeusler et al. 1996).

Their use is now widespread in surgical endoscopy such as in abdominal interventions (El-Dhuwaib et al. 2004; Lee et al. 2004; Mamazza et al. 2001), urological (Gill 2001), gynaecological (Bruhat and Goldchmit 1998), and endocrine surgery (Gagner and Inabnet 2001), and in the field of paediatrics (Freud 2000).

G. Tassi (✉) • G.P. Marchetti
Division of Pneumology,
Spedali Civili di Brescia, Brescia, Italy
e-mail: gf.tassi@tin.it; marchetti.giampietro@libero.it

Small-calibre instruments are now routinely used for cholecystectomy and appendectomy but also in laparoscopic fundoplication, inguinal herniorrhaphy, splenectomy, resection of thyroid nodules, parathyroidectomy, oophorectomy, hysterectomy, division of adhesions, and foetoscopy.

Despite these published advances, the uptake of miniendoscopes has been less impressive in thoracic medicine as evidenced by the doubts expressed in the Chest editorial (Yim and Izzat 1998) "Is Less Better?"

25.2 Thoracoscopy with Small-Calibre Instruments in Thoracic Pathology

The use of small-calibre endoscopic instruments in the treatment of thoracic diseases is still somewhat limited both in the surgical and medical setting (Table 25.1) when compared to laparoscopy.

25.2.1 Experience

Small-calibre thoracoscopes were first proposed more than 30 years ago (Ash and Manfredi 1974); however, due to the limited technology of the instrumentation, there was minimal uptake of the procedure. The idea resurfaced again in the 1990s when some thoracic surgeons used small-calibre instruments both for diagnostic (d'Alessandro 1997; Malthaner and Inculet

P. Astoul et al. (eds.), *Thoracoscopy for Pulmonologists*,
DOI 10.1007/978-3-642-38351-9_25, © Springer-Verlag Berlin Heidelberg 2014

Table 25.1 Medical (M) and surgical (S) thoracoscopy with small endoscopes (micro/needle thoracoscopes [micro] and minithoracoscopes [mini])

Author	Year	Patients	Endoscope	Indication
Ash (M)	1974	11	Micro	Pleural effusion diagnosis
d'Alessandro (S)	1997	2	Micro	Pleural disease diagnosis
Nezu (S)	1997	34	Micro	Video assistance in pneumothorax surgery
Malthaner (S)	1998	3	Mini	Pleural effusion diagnosis
Nakamoto (S)	1998	31	Micro/mini	Video assistance in preoperative diagnosis
Yim (S)	2000	38	Micro	Sympathectomy for palmar hyperhidrosis
Yoon (S)	2000	130	Mini	Video assistance in pneumothorax surgery
Lazopoulos (S)	2002	54	Micro	Pleural and lung disease diagnosis
Lin (S)	2002	102	Micro	Sympathectomy for palmar hyperhidrosis
Ikeda (S)	2003	35	Mini	Video assistance in partial lung resection
Chen (S)	2003	28	Mini	Video assistance in pneumothorax surgery
Tassi (M)	2003	30	Mini	Pleural effusion diagnosis
Janssen (M)	2003	9	Micro/mini	Pleural effusion diagnosis
Chen (S)	2006	142	Mini	Video assistance in pneumothorax surgery
Sihoe (S)	2007	31	Mini	Sympathectomy for palmar hyperhidrosis
Kim (S)	2008	65	Micro	Video assistance for lung biopsies

1998; Nakamoto et al. 1998) and therapeutic purposes (Nezu et al. 1997). There was confusion regarding the precise terminology, since some called the technique "microthoracoscopy" (d'Alessandro 1997) and others called it "minithoracoscopy" (Malthaner and Inculet 1998) or "mini thoracoscopy" or "mini-VAT" (video-assisted thoracoscopy using a miniaturized endoscope) (Nakamoto et al. 1998).

Even in the subsequent decade, experience has remained limited and predominantly surgical (Yim et al. 2000; Yoon et al. 2000; Lazopoulos et al. 2002; Ikeda et al. 2003; Chen et al. 2003; Lin and Chou 2004; Sihoe et al. 2007; Kim et al. 2008), although there have been some medical applications (Tassi and Marchetti 2003; Janssen et al. 2003). The terminology has expanded to include "needle video-thoracoscopic surgery" (NVTS) (Chen et al. 2003) or "needlescopic VATS" (Sihoe et al. 2007).

Some therapeutic applications have now become standard practice, such as for palmar hyperhidrosis (Yim et al. 2000; Lin and Chou 2004; Sihoe et al. 2007) and pneumothorax (Yoon et al. 2000; Chen et al. 2003, 2006).

The current standard treatment for palmar hyperhidrosis is thoracoscopic sympathotomy or sympathectomy, making thoracotomy obsolete. In this type of intervention, the use of small-calibre instruments became commonplace. This is because the small surgical window did necessary the use of miniendoscopes with a narrow field of vision.

In the treatment of pneumothorax, the use of small-calibre endoscopes has become more common, both in the examination of the pleural cavity and video assistance for bullectomy (Yoon et al. 2000) but also for treatment in general. Chen stated (Chen et al. 2003) that "…needle-scopic VATS can be a satisfactory alternative to conventional VATS in treating primary spontaneous pneumothorax…" given that the results and incidence of recurrence were comparable, and moreover needlescopic VATS gave better cosmetic results and less residual chest pain. He also suggested the instillation of a pleurodesis agent such as minocycline to reduce recurrence (Chen et al. 2006).

Thoracoscopy with small-calibre endoscopes has also been used in various other applications such as video assistance in stapler lung biopsies for interstitial lung disease and lung nodules (Kim et al. 2008). It has also been applied for the management of traumatic pneumothorax, pericardial windows, and minor intrapleural bleeding, all of which are historically treated with a large-calibre thoracoscope (Lazopoulos et al. 2002).

In the field of medical thoracoscopy, the experience with small-calibre endoscopes is more limited. In 2003, we published our initial case

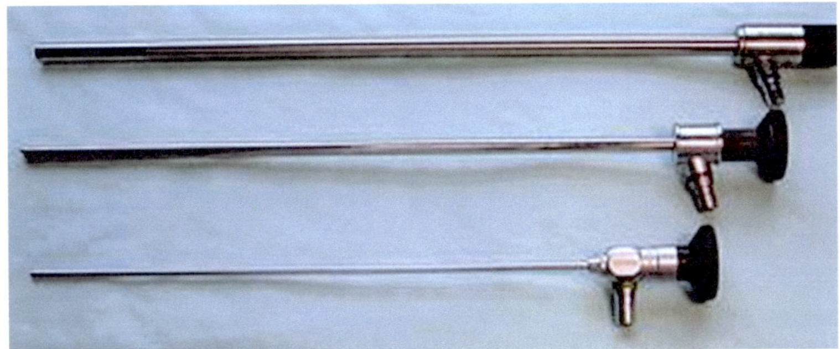

Fig. 25.1 From top to bottom, 10, 5, and 3 mm 0° telescopes

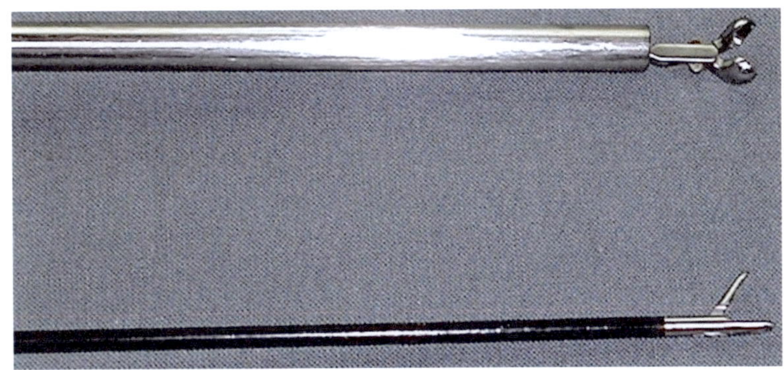

Fig. 25.2 Seven millimeter (*above*) and 3 mm (*below*) forceps with the same 7 mm opening

study (Tassi and Marchetti 2003) using a 3 mm thoracoscope for diagnostic thoracoscopy in pleural effusions. This technique allowed for pleural biopsies and a diagnostic yield of 93.4 %, which was similar to that of standard thoracoscopy. Janssen (Janssen et al. 2003) compared the results obtained from a 7 mm thoracoscope with those from two types of small-calibre endoscopes (3.5 and 2 mm). The diagnostic yield from the 7 and 3.5 mm instruments was 100 %, whereas the yield from the 2 mm endoscope was 40 %.

25.2.2 Instruments

As noted above, small-calibre endoscopes are defined as *miniendoscopes* if their diameter is 2–5 mm (Fig. 25.1) and *microendoscopes* or *needlescopes* if the diameter is 2 mm or less (Tu and Advincula 2008).

Essential requirements to carry out an adequate thoracoscopy include acceptable illumination of the cavity to be examined and sufficiently high definition images. These aspects are directly linked to the size of the instrument, and if inadequate, then examination and identification become difficult.

With *minithoracoscopes*, as with larger-calibre traditional thoracoscopes, light is transmitted by means of the classical Hopkins rod-lens system which gives good visibility and sufficient depth of light penetration. Although the quality is slightly inferior to that obtained by standard thoracoscopy, it is sufficient for the examination of the pleural cavity and for performing adequate biopsies especially when taken with forceps of ~3 mm (Fig. 25.2).

With *microendoscopes* and *needlescopes*, light is generally transmitted through fibre-optic bundles, though recent developments have seen needlescopes produced which use the Hopkins system (Figs. 25.3 and 25.4).

Although the visibility is adequate, the definition is not always optimal. Due to the small calibre, the temperature of the instrument can change quickly with each introduction and extraction, thus subjecting the optic to frequent misting. In addition, since the optic and accessory instruments are flexible, they can at times oscillate and

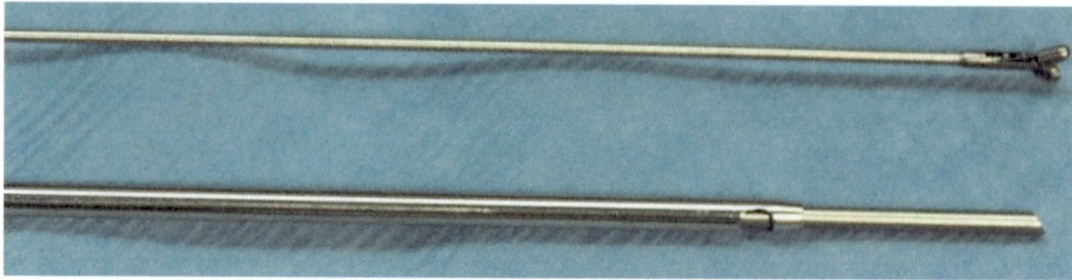

Fig. 25.3 Typical instruments used in needlescopic thoracoscopy: 2 mm forceps (*above*) and 2 mm needle thoracoscope (*below*)

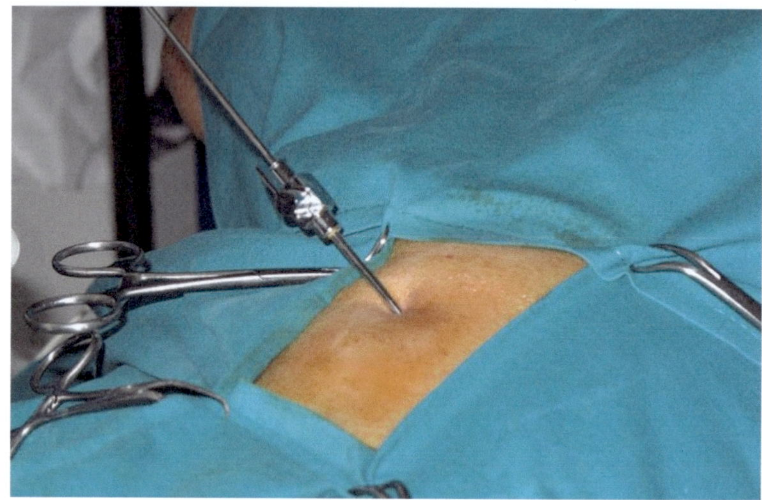

Fig. 25.4 Two millimeter thoracoscope introduced into the pleural cavity through a Boutin thoracocentesis needle

make it more difficult to control a manoeuvre which requires precision.

Biopsies taken with forceps of ~2 mm are often inadequate because of their small size.

A large variety of accessory instruments is now available both for minithoracoscopy and for micro/needlethoracoscopy: forceps, scissors, blunt probe, biopsy punch, grasps, aspiration/irrigation cannulae, etc. All these instruments, together with small endoscopes, are very fragile and should be handled with great care. It should be stressed that their use requires both ability and experience in standard thoracoscopy. The technological advances which have enabled the creation of these instruments could further improve their diagnostic sensitivity and, in turn, extend their application.

25.3 Minithoracoscopy

Minithoracoscopy is currently defined as endoscopy using small instruments with a diameter from 2 mm up to 5 mm. It is more appropriate in medical thoracoscopy, since it permits good

visualization of the pleural cavity and if required, biopsy.

In our opinion, minithoracoscopy was never considered to be a substitute for traditional medical thoracoscopy, which, over the years, has demonstrated efficacy and reliability and, in addition, has dedicated optics, forceps, and accessory instruments. It was considered to be a complementary diagnostic approach, which is minimally invasive, safe, and cost-effective and, in certain cases, may be seen as a substitute for the traditional intervention.

25.3.1 Instruments and Technique

The instruments comprise two metal 3.8 mm trocars with a pointed stylet, a 3.3 mm optic which is 25 cm in length (Karl Storz Endoskope, Tuttlingen, Germany), and a 3 mm rotating biopsy forceps (available in different shapes). In addition, 3 mm scissors, needles, and small rigid catheters for aspiration are available. All instruments are multi-use and autoclavable (121 °C per 15 min).

Important differences between minithoracoscopy and standard thoracoscopy are summarized in Table 25.2.

The exam is carried out under local anaesthesia or deep sedation, as in medical thoracoscopy, with administration of small doses of midazolam (2 mg immediately before the exam with subsequent administration up to a maximum of 10 mg). Alternatively, propofol can be given in continuous infusion or via bolus injections of 20–30 mg if necessary.

The patient is placed in the lateral decubitus position, healthy side down, and after a small incision in the skin with a scalpel, the trocar is introduced into the pleural cavity where fluid accumulation, as defined by pleural ultrasound, is maximal.

After aspirating the liquid and allowing the free entry of air into the pleural cavity, examination of the space can proceed. Biopsies are performed through a second port of entry, normally positioned in the adjacent intercostal space (Fig. 25.5). They are carried out under direct visual control on endoscopically significant lesions (i.e. nodules with a neoplastic aspect, localized thickening, diaphragmatic and visceral alterations) or, in the setting of normal appearing pleura, at different locations on the parietal pleura.

It is also possible to use coagulating forceps to perform biopsies of the visceral pleura or lung. Other instruments can also be introduced through the second trocar. These include catheters for fluid aspiration or instillation of saline or thrombolytic agents. In addition, the second trocar will allow the use of electroscalpels to resect difficult adhesions or needles to aspirate pathological material.

At the end of the examination, a small drain (8 F) is placed and removed some hours later, once x-ray has demonstrated the complete re-expansion of the lung.

Table 25.2 Comparison of thoracoscopy instruments

Instruments	Standard thoracoscopy	Minithoracoscopy
Trocar Ø	8 mm	3.8 mm
Optic Ø	7 mm	3.3 mm
Optics	0°–25°–50°–90°	0°–30°–45°
Optics length	300 mm	250 mm
Forceps opening/Ø	7/5 mm	7/3.3 mm
Electrical coagulation	Yes	Yes
Multi-usable	Yes	Yes
Accessory instruments	Forceps, aspirator, scissors	Forceps, aspirator, scissors
Autoclavable	Yes	Yes

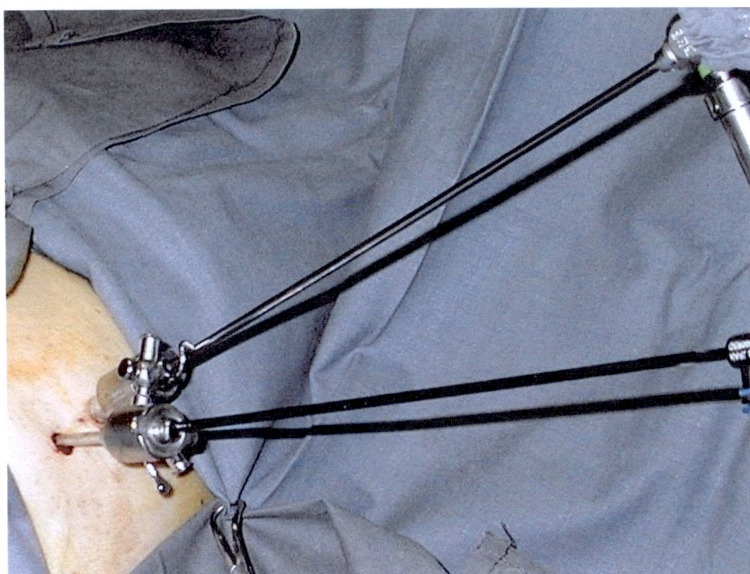

Fig. 25.5 Forceps (*below*) and optic (*above*) during minithoracoscopy

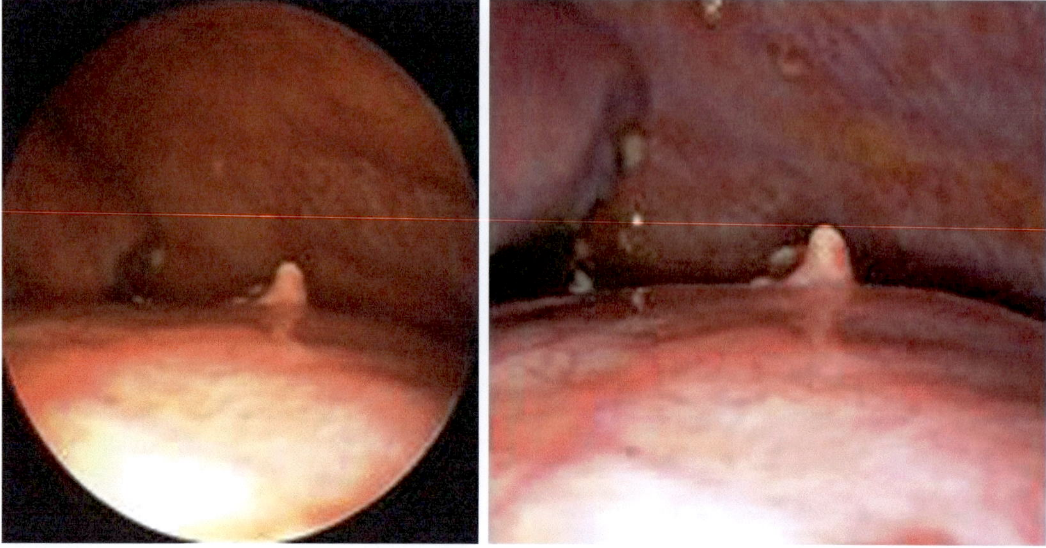

Fig. 25.6 Nodule on the diaphragm observed using minithoracoscopy (*left*) and standard thoracoscopy (*right*)

25.3.2 Indications and Results

The main indications for minithoracoscopy are:
- Endoscopy of a small loculated effusion
- Evaluation for drainage of a loculated empyema
- Complete endoscopic examination of the pleural cavity
- Pre-standard thoracoscopic evaluation in complex cases

Absolute contraindications to the procedure are identical to those defined for standard thoracoscopy (Boutin and Astoul 1998; Colt 1998), particularly cardiac and respiratory insufficiency and coagulation disorders.

In our practice, we initially performed minithoracoscopy for loculated effusions and advanced over time to more extensive effusions on which standard thoracoscopy could also be performed. The technique is particularly helpful in the elderly, patients of small stature or narrow intercostal spaces. In these situations, as has been noted by others (Janssen et al. 2003), the use of small-calibre endoscopes is especially helpful. On the other hand, massive effusions should be avoided, especially those cases which require pleurodesis, as this necessitates a large-calibre drain post-procedure.

Another interesting application of minithoracoscopy is to evaluate the accessibility of the pleural cavity in cases where adhesions are suspected, and once their presence is excluded, standard thoracoscopy can safely be carried out.

No substantial difference in the quality of vision has been found between minithoracoscopy and the standard technique (Figs. 25.6 and 25.7).

Performing biopsies was found to be simple and efficacious in almost all cases. (The span of the forceps is 7 mm, which is the same as the standard forceps, although they are not as wide and thus can only obtain a smaller quantity of tissue; average histological sample$=0.5\times1$ cm.) The pleural biopsy yield (91 %) is comparable to the standard technique. However, the removal of adhesions is more difficult than with a larger-calibre instrument.

The time taken for the exam is, on average, 20 % longer, and it is necessary to convert to the standard procedure in only a few cases. Pain experienced by patients under local anaesthesia is minor – both during and after the exam – and the exam is overall well tolerated. In some cases, pulmonary biopsies are performed with 40 W coagulating forceps. The majority of biopsies produce sufficient material for diagnosis, but others samples are adversely affected by

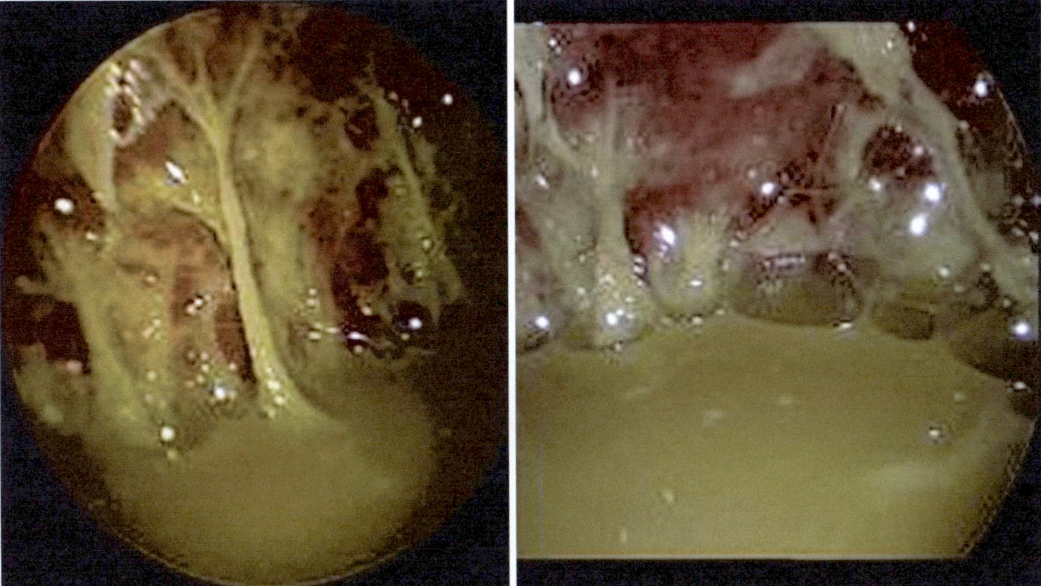

Fig. 25.7 Purulent material in the pleural cavity observed using minithoracoscopy (*left*) and standard thoracoscopy (*right*)

coagulation of the tissue. In cases with fibrinous infectious pleurisy, the removal of fibrin is satisfactory, and it is possible to perform a pleural biopsy.

25.3.3 Overall Evaluation of the Method

The overall evaluation of minithoracoscopy should take into account the advantages and limitations of the method (Table 25.3).

The main advantage of minithoracoscopy over the standard approach is the better tolerance of the patient to an instrument of 3.3 mm diameter compared to one of 7 mm. Sutures are not necessary and the cosmetic result is excellent. The examination is easier to perform in patients with a small hemithorax or restricted intercostal space, and the trocars can be moved more comfortably with less pain. It is also possible to examine small loculated effusions which are less accessible to the standard technique. The slight reduction in the field of vision can be resolved by alternating the introduction of the optic in the second trocar, thereby increasing the field of view.

Table 25.3 Advantages and limitations of minithoracoscopy

Advantages	Limitations
Good visibility	Small size of biopsies
Reliable instruments	Fragile instruments
Easy manoeuvrability	No drains >8 F
Less pain during and after the examination	Necessity of experience in standard thoracoscopy
Less local anaesthesia required	Conversion required in some cases
No stitches required	Possible inadequacy of lung biopsy
Better cosmetic results	20 % more time required

The small biopsy size does not really create a limitation; it is possible to obtain adequate tissue even with a 3 mm forceps, facilitated by the rotating tip of the forceps. However, some limitations were encountered, in particular in cases of mesothelioma where neoplastic tissue may be hard and smooth. The presence of nodules and granulations does not create difficulties.

The results from cases of tuberculous pleuritis are extremely good, to the point where we would propose that minithoracoscopy should be the investigation of choice if this pathology is suspected. Closed pleural needle biopsy has significant diagnostic limitations. There is an increasing frequency of pleural tuberculosis where healthy tissue is interspersed with significant lesions; hence, biopsy under visual control is preferable.

The manoeuvrability of the optic inside the pleural cavity is excellent. Normally a single operator using both hands is able to coordinate instrument movement to orientate their view towards the area of interest. In some cases, the presence of two operators is advisable; both will need to have experience in standard thoracoscopy. The optic is fragile, and care should be taken to avoid breaking it.

It is important to highlight the role of pleural ultrasound in thoracic pathology. Its great advantage, apart from the safety profile, is that it is the only method which provides an examination in "real time", i.e. it enables the study of a pleural effusion during the respiratory cycle and in different anatomical positions. A great deal of information can be gathered from ultrasound which will assist the minithoracoscopic approach. In our experience, a carefully performed ultrasound scan with the patient on the endoscopic bed in the thoracoscopy position has enabled the procedure to be performed successfully even in the presence of adhesions and small effusions. The combination of ultrasound and minithoracoscopy has reduced the number of "unfeasible" exams to 1 %, whereas previously it had been 5 %. The trocar can be introduced even in cases with a complete absence of effusion but with the presence of the "gliding sign" – the movement of the parietal and visceral lines during respiratory movements.

The development of minioptics has resulted in improved versatility. It is possible to introduce both a 3 mm optic and 3 mm forceps through a 7 mm trocar or, alternatively, the optic and an aspiration catheter. This enables pulmonary biopsy without the need for a second port of entry using coagulating forceps on the lung under visual control. With such a range of instruments and some experience, it is possible to have two instruments working inside the pleural cavity: one through a 7 mm trocar and another through a second 3 mm port. There is a clear advantage to

positioning a drain under visual control and aspirating the smallest liquid collections from difficult to reach recesses. On occasion, the minioptic can be introduced through the chest drain to check its position or function. There are a high number of conversions from mini- to standard thoracoscopy; this is currently running at 18 % in our service. However, we do not believe that this represents a limitation of the procedure. In most cases, we had planned to convert to standard thoracoscopy after the initial inspection. In addition, the procedure was converted to standard thoracoscopy if it was apparent that careful lavage or pleurodesis was required and a large-bore drain would be needed.

Minithoracoscopy can be considered complementary to the standard method, and in some cases, it may substitute for it completely. In our opinion, its most important indications are in the setting of small pleural effusions and cases of suspected tuberculous pleuritis where it has demonstrated to be reliable and a high diagnostic yield and should replace the now redundant pleural needle biopsy.

References

Ash SR, Manfredi F (1974) Directed biopsy using a small endoscope: thoracoscopy and peritoneoscopy simplified. N Engl J Med 291:1398–1399

Boutin C, Astoul P (1998) Diagnostic thoracoscopy. Clin Chest Med 19:295–309

Bruhat MA, Goldchmit R (1998) Minilaparoscopy in gynecology. Eur J Obstet Gynecol Reprod Biol 76:207–210

Chen JS, Hsu HH, Kuo SW et al (2003) Needlescopic versus conventional video-assisted thoracic surgery for primary spontaneous pneumothorax: a comparative study. Ann Thorac Surg 75:1080–1085

Chen JS, Hsu HH, Chen RJ et al (2006) Additional minocycline pleurodesis after thoracoscopic surgery for primary spontaneous pneumothorax. Am J Respir Crit Care Med 173:548–554

Colt HG (1998) Therapeutic thoracoscopy. Clin Chest Med 19:383–394

d'Alessandro AA (1997) Microthoracoscopy. At the cutting edge of thoracic surgery. J Laparoendosc Adv Surg Tech A 7:313–318

El-Dhuwaib Y, Hamade AM, Issa ME et al (2004) An "all 5-mm ports" selective approach to laparoscopic cholecistectomy, appendectomy, and anti-reflux surgery. Surg Laparosc Endosc Percutan Tech 14:141–144

Freud E (2000) Minimally invasive surgery in childhood: current status. Isr Med Assoc J 2:377–381

Gagner M, Inabnet WB 3rd (2001) Endoscopic thyroidectomy for solitary thyroid nodules. Thyroid 11:161–163

Gill IS (2001) Needlescopic urology: current status. Urol Clin North Am 28:71–83

Haeusler G, Lehner R, Hanzal E et al (1996) Diagnostic accuracy of 2 mm microlaparoscopy. Acta Obstet Gynecol Scand 75:672–675

Ikeda W, Miyoshi S, Seki N et al (2003) Needlescopic operation for partial lung resection. Ann Thorac Surg 75:599–601

Janssen JP, Thunnissen F, Visser F (2003) Comparison of the 2.0 mm and the 3.5 mm minithoracoscopy set to standard equipment for medical thoracoscopy. Eur Respir J Suppl 45:S451

Kim HK, Jo WM, Jung JH et al (2008) Needlescopic lung biopsy for interstitial lung disease and indeterminate pulmonary nodules: a report on 65 cases. Ann Thorac Surg 86:1098–1103

Lazopoulos G, Kotoulas C, Kokotsakis J et al (2002) Diagnostic mini-video assisted thoracic surgery. Effectiveness and accuracy of new generation 2.0 mm instruments. Surg Endosc 16:1793–1795

Lee P et al (2004) An audit of medical thoracoscopy and talc poudrage for pneumothorax prevention in advanced COPD. Chest 125:1315–1320

Lin TS, Chou MC (2004) Treatment of palmar hyperhidrosis using needlescopic T2 sympathetic block by clipping: analysis of 102 cases. Int Surg 89:198–201

Malthaner RA, Inculet RI (1998) Minithoracoscopy for pleural effusions. Can Respir J 5:253–254

Mamazza J, Schlachta CM, Seshadri PA et al (2001) Needlescopic surgery. A logical evolution from conventional laparoscopic surgery. Surg Endosc 15:1208–1212

Nakamoto K, Maeda M, Okamoto T et al (1998) Preoperative diagnosis with video- assisted thoracoscopy with miniaturized endoscopes in general thoracic surgery. A preliminary study. Chest 114:1749–1755

Nezu K, Kushibe K, Tojo T et al (1997) Thoracoscopic wedge resection of blebs under local anesthesia with sedation for treatment of spontaneous pneumothorax. Chest 111:230–235

Schneider AR, Eickhoff A, Arnold JC et al (2001) Diagnostic laparoscopy. Endoscopy 33:55–59

Sihoe ADL, Manlulu AV, Lee TW et al (2007) Preemptive local anesthesia for needlescopic video-assisted thoracicsurgery: a randomized controlled trial. Eur J Cardiothorac Surg 31:103–108

Tassi G, Marchetti G (2003) Minithoracoscopy: a less invasive approach to thoracoscopy. Chest 124:1975–1977

Tu FF, Advincula AP (2008) Miniaturizing the laparoscope: current applications of micro- and minilaparoscopy. Int J Gynaecol Obstet 100:94–98

Yim APC, Izzat MB (1998) Is less better? Chest 113:270–271

Yim APC, Liu HP, Lee TW et al (2000) 'Needlescopic' video-assisted thoracic surgery for palmar hyperhidrosis. Eur J Cardiothor Surg 17:697–701

Yoon YH, Kim KH, Han JW et al (2000) Management of persistent or recurrent pneumothorax with a two millimeter mini-video-thoracoscope. J Korean Med Sci 15:507–509

Autofluorescence and Thoracoscopy

Miltiadis G. Chrysanthidis

26.1 Introduction

Based on research published by Boutin (Boutin et al. 1981), medical thoracoscopy established a definitive diagnosis in 97 % of 1,000 consecutive patients presenting with a pleural effusion. Most series in the last 25 years (Loddenkemper and Boutin 1993; Colt 1999; Blanc et al. 2002; Maskell and Butland 2003; Lee and Light 2004) have reported the diagnostic sensitivity of thoracoscopy in the setting of malignant pleural effusions to be greater than 90 % with an associated specificity of 100 %. In addition, studies on the role of thoracoscopy for staging lung carcinoma or malignant mesothelioma have yielded encouraging results (Harris et al. 1995).

The endoscopic appearance of the pleural lesions observed at medical thoracoscopy is suggestive of malignancy in 86 % of cases (Boutin et al. 1991). Features suggestive of malignancy include nodules, polypoid lesions, masses, malignant thickening of the pleura or localised "candle wax drops". However, some tumours may resemble features associated with non-specific inflammation, and conversely, certain inflammatory lesions can mimic tumours. Even mesothelioma, which usually has a characteristic grapelike nodular appearance, can appear on gross inspection as inflammation. In some patients, the studying of the pleural surfaces with tumour can be subtle (Heffner and Klein 2008), and it should be noted that white-light inspection of the pleura may fail to detect pleural metastases. Finally coexisting benign lesions may misdirect biopsy sampling towards non-malignant lesions (Heffner 2008). Therefore, despite thoracoscopy some cases still remain undiagnosed and understaged or patients might experience biopsy-related complications.

Fluorescence techniques have been proposed to improve the diagnostic accuracy of thoracoscopy. The effectiveness of this technology has been proven: both for accurate detection of early malignant or invasive lesions and directing appropriate sampling during bronchoscopy. In addition, fluorescence thoracoscopy may be helpful for delineating tumour margins and precise staging of intrathoracic abnormalities. In benign pleural diseases, fluorescence thoracoscopy has an important role to play in the management of patients with primary spontaneous pneumothorax.

Furthermore, evolving clinical research has provided significant data on the implementation of newer modalities for the improved detection of peripheral lung cancer. Various technologies have been utilised including microcatheter fluorescence thoracoscopy, virally detected fluorescent imaging for endoscopic staging and viruses carrying fluorescent protein transgene

M.G. Chrysanthidis
Department of Pulmonology,
Sismanoglio Hospital, Athens, Greece
e-mail: m.chrysanthidis@otenet.gr

P. Astoul et al. (eds.), *Thoracoscopy for Pulmonologists*,
DOI 10.1007/978-3-642-38351-9_26, © Springer-Verlag Berlin Heidelberg 2014

237

for the intraoperative localisation of lymph node metastases in patients with mesothelioma and other thoracic malignancies.

26.2 Fluorescence Techniques in Respiratory Endoscopy

Fluorescence endoscopy is based on the physical phenomenon of light remission of certain wavelengths from an object, when light of a shorter wavelength is directed to it. This was first reported by Stokes in 1852 and the possible effects on body tissue were described in the early 1900s (Stübel 1911). Later findings, in 1933 (Sutro and Burman 1933) and in 1944 (Herley 1944), documented that the fluorescence reaction of a tumour to ultraviolet light had distinct characteristics compared to healthy tissue.

Fluorescence illumination techniques have been primarily developed for urology. Flat neoplastic lesions such as dysplasia, carcinoma in situ or small papillary tumours of the bladder may be difficult to diagnose because they can grow in normal or in areas with non-specific inflammation. A significantly higher detection rate is achieved with fluorescence endoscopy compared to conventional white light. Therefore, fluorescence has subsequently become a diagnostic tool in gastroenterology, otolaryngology and gynaecology, where it is used to diagnose premalignant and malignant tumours, particularly flat mucosal lesions. Neurosurgeons also use fluorescence for the intraoperative detection of malignant gliomas, while in the field of dermatology, great efforts have been made to diagnose and demarcate lesions, for example, basal cell carcinoma (Gahlen et al. 2000).

Substances responsible for fluorescence are called fluorophores and include tryptophan, collagen and elastin (Barenboim 1969), porphyrin and intracellular nicotinamide adenine nucleotide – NADH, riboflavin and flavin coenzymes (Andersson-Engels et al. 1997; Aubin 1979). In contrast, the fluorescence intensity is decreased by lactic acid (Andersson-Engels et al. 1992), which is actively produced by the tumour cells due to its increased absorption of glucose, known as the Warburg effect (Adachi et al. 1999).

Fluorescence diagnosis can be classified into two groups:

26.2.1 Photodynamic Diagnosis (PDD)

Photodynamic diagnosis (PDD) using exogenous fluorophores or fluorophore precursors, such as haematoporphyrin derivatives [HpD], provides a tumour-localising property due to the preferential retention of the fluorophore by malignant tissue (Lipson et al. 1961; Profio and Doiron 1977; Hayata et al. 1982; Kato et al. 1990). Photodynamic methods using HpD have been rather unsuccessful as a result of poor sensitivity and reported complications, mainly cutaneous photosensitivity. Later studies proposed the replacement of HpD by 5-aminolaevulinic acid [ALA] (Kennedy and Pottier 1992) and aminolaevulinic esters (Kloek et al. 1998) with better results (Pichler et al. 1998). The application of δ-ALA was reported to have a high sensitivity for detection of dysplasia and carcinoma in situ (Kriegmair et al. 1994), but the specificity remained low due to the non-specific uptake of the fluorophore in normal and inflamed mucosa, even when administered by inhalation (Baumgartner et al. 1996).

ALA, the natural precursor of the haem pathway, administered either systemically or locally, overloads the last step in haem biosynthesis of tumour cells via failed negative feedback mechanisms and reduced enzymatic activities. The final result is the increased accumulation of protoporphyrin IX (Pp-IX), a metabolite of ALA. ALA-induced Pp-IX photosensitisation has several advantages: (*a*) ALA, Pp-IX and other intermediates are rapidly eliminated from humans, thus minimising the risk of skin phototoxicity; (*b*) ALA can be applied locally and major side effects can be expected to be less compared to systemic administration; and (*c*) the fluorescence ratio between the tumour and surrounding healthy tissue is superior to that of other photosensitisers (Prosst et al. 2002).

26.2.2 Autofluorescence Diagnosis (AFD)

Autofluorescence diagnosis (AFD) using methods which reflect the variations in the biochemistry of the tissue detects the endogenous fluorophores of tissues and includes the emission signal from the tissue itself. The wavelength and intensity of the emitted light depend on the concentration of the fluorophores, on their maximal absorption and remission and on the characteristics of the light source. A reduction in the level of autofluorescence light within malignant and premalignant areas is a result of epithelial thickening, redox changes in the tumour cells matrix and reduced fluorophore concentration. The implementation of AFD methods in respiratory endoscopy was supported by evidence of a strong correlation between abnormal fluorescence and the histological findings of angiogenic dysplasia (Keith et al. 2000). The increase in the microvasculature in dysplastic lesions may cause a decrease in autofluorescence, because haemoglobin absorbs the excitation light. Malignant areas may be distinguished from normal tissue by a noticeable reduction in autofluorescence even when there is a complete absence of porphyrins that selectively concentrate in tumours (Staël et al. 1996; Lam et al. 1990).

Autofluorescence systems, incorporating the most recent advances in optical technology to provide accurate imaging, have been widely introduced into clinical practice for the early detection of lung cancer during bronchoscopy (Nakhosteen and Khavankar 2000; Sutedja et al. 2001; Moro-Sibilot et al. 2002; Häussinger et al. 2005).

26.3 Fluorescence and Autofluorescence Thoracoscopy in Exudative Pleural Effusions

26.3.1 Thoracoscopic Fluorescence Diagnosis (TFD) of Pleural Malignancies

The diagnosis of pleural malignancies using fluorescence was first attempted in an experimental animal setting in the Department of Surgery of Ruprecht-Karls University of Heidelberg, Germany (Prosst et al. 2002). The goal was to achieve optimum diagnostic results, approximating 100 % sensitivity, by precise assessment of disseminated intrathoracic tumour spread at the time of video-assisted thoracic surgery (VATS). Thoracoscopy was combined with photodynamic

diagnosis (PDD) as it was known that there was almost specific accumulation of administered photosensitisers in malignant cells. Human lung adenocarcinoma cells were initially cultivated in nude mice and then inoculated in 38 female nude rats, resulting in disseminated carcinosis in the whole pleural cavity. After 5–7 weeks of tumour growth, a pleural lavage was performed either with 1.5 or 3.0 % 5-aminolaevulinic acid (ALA) solution. Unlike earlier generations of photosensitisers such as Photofrin which were already fluorescent at the time of application, ALA requires endogenous metabolism to protoporphyrin IX (Pp-IX) before it can fluoresce. Pp-IX becomes a fluorescent agent when stimulated by light of a defined wavelength within its absorption spectrum. The emission wavelength is within the visible light spectrum at 635 nm (red light). The positive red fluorescence of Pp-IX is even detectable in macroscopically invisible tumour foci and can indicate lesions which would be missed when illuminated with conventional white light only (Gahlen et al. 2000).

The researchers had chosen photosensitisation intervals of 2, 4 and 6 h post ALA application. Conventional white-light VATS followed by TFD was performed using the D-Light® system (Karl Storz, Germany) so that the two possible illumination modes – conventional white-light mode and a specific blue-light (380–440 nm) mode for Pp-IX fluorescence excitation – could be easily switched at any time using a footswitch or directly by a button on the modified CCD camera (Tricam) head. The fluorescence intensities of tumours and surrounding healthy tissue in the pleural cavity were measured by spectrometry, and all tumours identified either by conventional white light or by fluorescence were subsequently removed for histological examination.

In all animal groups except one (with a 2-h photosensitisation period with 1.5 % ALA interval), TFD enabled the detection of tumour foci which would have been missed if examined by conventional VATS alone. Lesions, indicative of the diagnostic value of TFD and associated with an increase in sensitivity, were mainly observed after 6 h of photosensitisation using 3.0 % ALA solution. Photosensitisation for an interval of 4 h gave slightly poorer results, while the 2-h photosensitisation interval further decreased sensitivity.

Only three of the macroscopically visible neoplasms showed no fluorescence under blue light, leading to false negative results. On the other hand, four macroscopically visible lesions, which showed no fluorescence, were histologically benign, leading to true negative results.

The spectrometry studies yielded an increasing absolute fluorescence intensity and tumour/normal tissue ratio with longer photosensitisation time in malignancies of the parietal pleura. The best fluorescence contrast obtained between neoplasms and surrounding tumour-free tissue – providing 11 times higher fluorescence intensity in tumour – was achieved after 6 h of photosensitisation with both ALA concentrations.

In conclusion, thoracoscopic fluorescence diagnosis detects an additional 30 % of pleural malignant lesions compared with conventional white-light VATS alone. It is a feasible technique for improving the preoperative diagnosis and staging in patients with intrathoracic malignancies (Prosst et al. 2002).

26.3.2 Autofluorescence Videothoracoscopy in Exudative Pleural Effusions

26.3.2.1 The Preliminary Results

The preliminary results from the implementation of autofluorescence videothoracoscopy (AFVT) in 24 patients, who had presented with an exudative pleural effusion and/or abnormal pleural findings on CT scans, were first published in 2005 (Chrysanthidis and Janssen 2005). With the exception of the imaging device, the AFVT system utilised the same medical thoracoscopy equipment as white-light thoracoscopy (WLT). AFVTs were performed under local anaesthesia [spontaneous breathing patients, premedication with 0.25–0.5 mg atropine and 10 mg morphine] in the endoscopy suite of the Pulmonary Department in Canisius Wilhelmina Ziekenhuis – CWZ Hospital in Nijmegen, the Netherlands. Firstly all pleural fluid was removed. The entire pleural cavity was thoroughly evaluated using conventional WLT and subsequent mapping of areas of abnormal pleura. The pleural space was

then reinspected with AFVT, and the change in colour of the areas of abnormal pleura was assessed. Furthermore, the pleural cavity was inspected with AFVT for areas of abnormal pleura which were not observed during WLT inspection. Finally biopsies of areas of abnormal pleura were taken for histological analysis.

The device used in this study, performed under *Dr Julius Janssen*'s supervision, was the Diagnostic Auto-Fluorescence Endoscopy (DAFE®) system, developed by Richard Wolf Corporation (Knittligen, Germany). The autofluorescence excitation in DAFE® is achieved by means of a 300 W xenon lamp in the violet-blue range (390–460 nm), while the photodetection system relies on one charge-coupled device (CCD) camera and a dual detection range (a green region of 500–590 nm wavelength and a red region of 600–700 nm wavelength), as at least two spectral domains are necessary for efficient contrast enhancement. During further development and associated technical evolution of the DAFE® system, it was discovered that the excitation wavelength yielding the highest sensitivity and specificity was above 400 nm with a peak value near 405 nm.

Normal areas in the pleural surface appeared white or white-pink in both WLT and AFVT (Fig. 26.1). Areas with fat on the pleural layer appeared yellow under the conventional mode but orange under the autofluorescence mode. In all cases with histologically proven malignant pleural disease – including nine patients with metastatic pleural carcinomas and seven cases with mesotheliomas – the colour of the affected area of the pleura changed from white-pink to red under AFVT (Figs. 26.2, 26.3, and 26.4). Therefore, the sensitivity of AFVT for detecting malignant lesions on the pleural surface was 100 %. On the other hand, the specificity of AFVT was found to be 75 %, as in two out of eight cases with chronic pleuritis, a colour change from white-pink to orange-red was found. In addition, in the remaining six patients there was no difference in pleural surface colour between WLT and AFVT. The researchers proposed that the positive predictive value (PPV) was a more realistic parameter for the evaluation of AFVT as

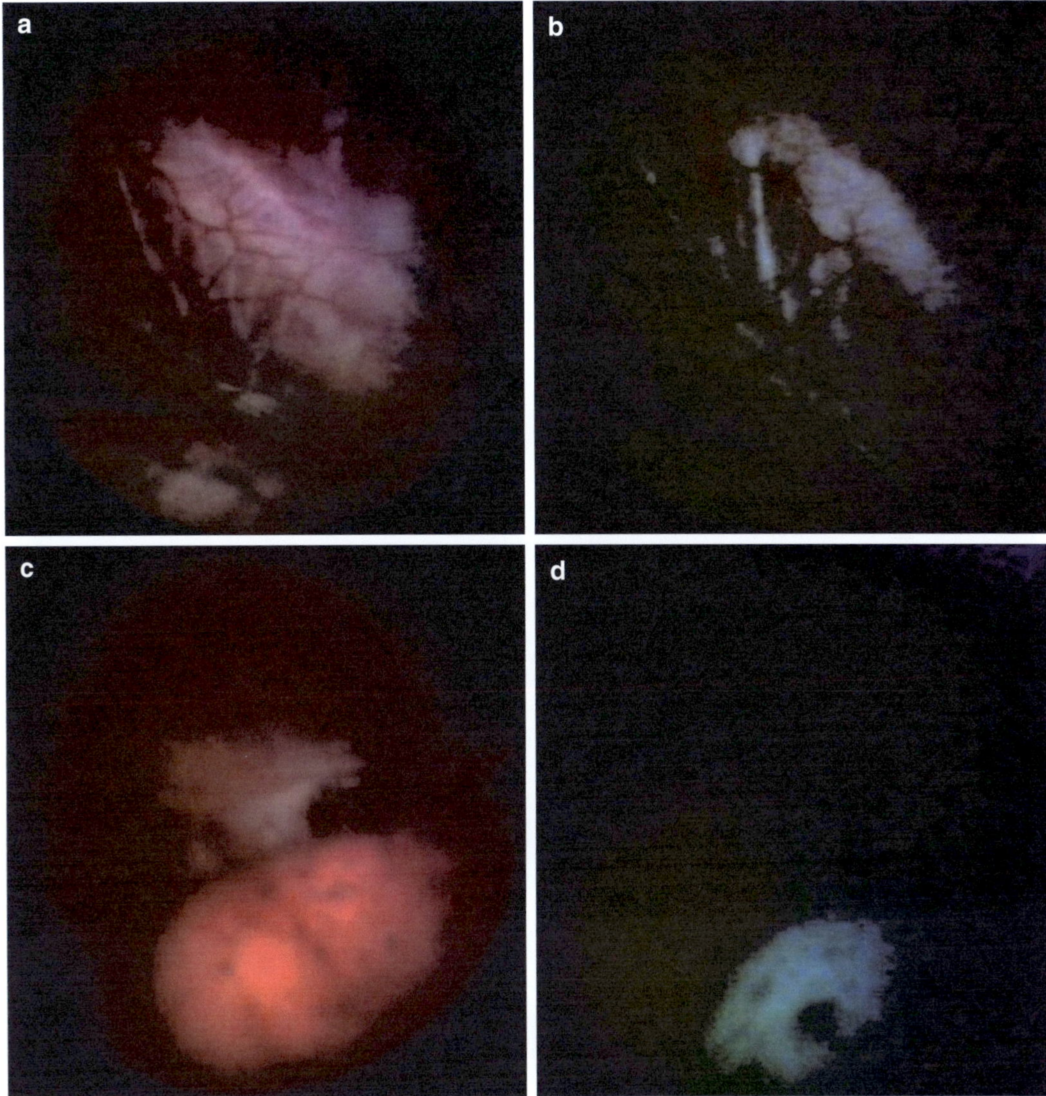

Fig. 26.1 Normal parietal (**a**, **b**) and visceral (**c**, **d**) pleura as shown by white-light thoracoscopy (WLT) and autofluorescence thoracoscopy (AT), respectively

a diagnostic method. PPV, defined as the probability that a positive result under AFVT represents an existing lesion, was calculated as the ratio of true positive results over the overall (true and false) positive results under AFVT and in this study was calculated to be 92 %.

The study of Chrysanthidis and Janssen had two important limitations: (*a*) patients had extended pleural disease at the time of medical thoracoscopy was done and therefore it was easy to diagnose malignancy with WLT-guided biopsies alone. However, the findings using blue-light mode were more obvious, and the same malignant lesions were more precisely mapped during AFVT; (*b*) biopsies were obtained from a rather restricted number of sites on the pleural space, and it was practically impossible to have specimens from the entire pleural surface with the goal of obtaining a reliable value of false negatives to precisely estimate the sensitivity of the method (e.g. the ability to find a lesion if there was one).

26.3.2.2 The Initial Experience

The initial experience of performing AFVT, using the same DAFE® fluorescence endoscopy system, was also recently published (Belák et al. 2007). According to the researchers, the tissue autofluorescence response originates mostly from the subepithelial tissue, and local hypertrophy "obstructs" the penetration of the blue-violet light into the tissue. As a response to the decreased intensity of the excitation light, the intensity of the autofluorescence emission is also decreased.

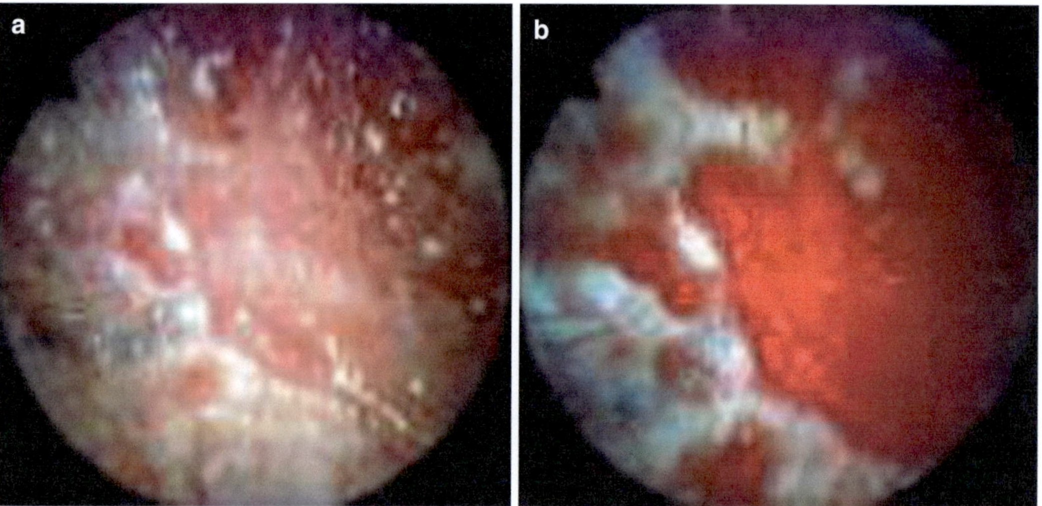

Fig. 26.2 Breast cancer metastasis to the parietal pleura as shown by (**a**) white-light thoracoscopy (WLT) and (**b**) autofluorescence thoracoscopy (AFT). During WLT the colour of the malignant tissue is light pink. During AFT the malignant tissue is deep red, whereas the normal tissue has turned white. The line between the normal and malignant tissue is well demarcated (From Chrysanthidis and Janssen (2005))

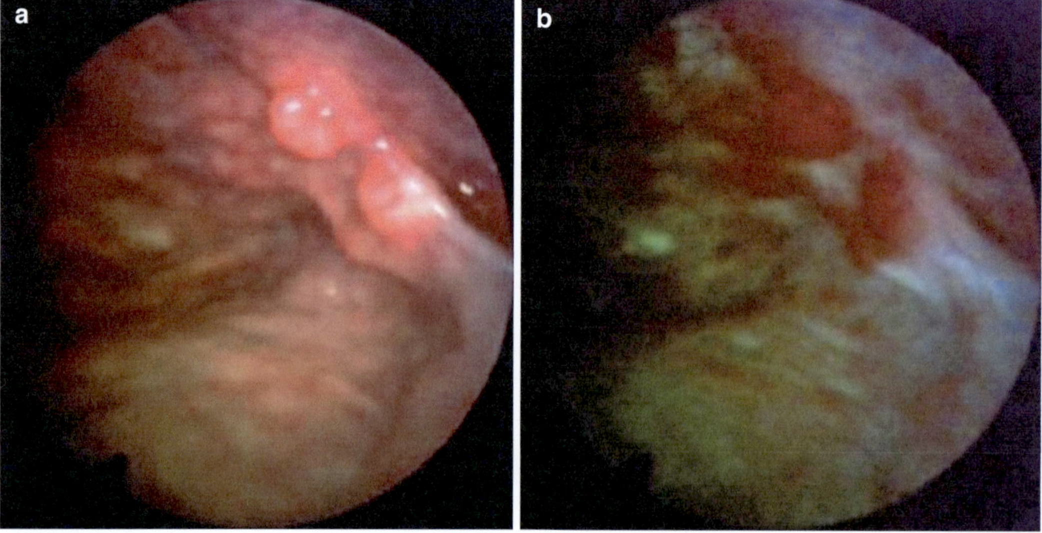

Fig. 26.3 Malignant pleural mesothelioma detected in occupational asbestos-exposed patient by white-light source (**a, c**) and autofluorescence thoracoscopy (**b, d**) (true positive) (Courtesy D Fielding, Department of Thoracic Medicine, Royal Brisbane and womens' Hospital, Brisbane, Queensland, Australia)

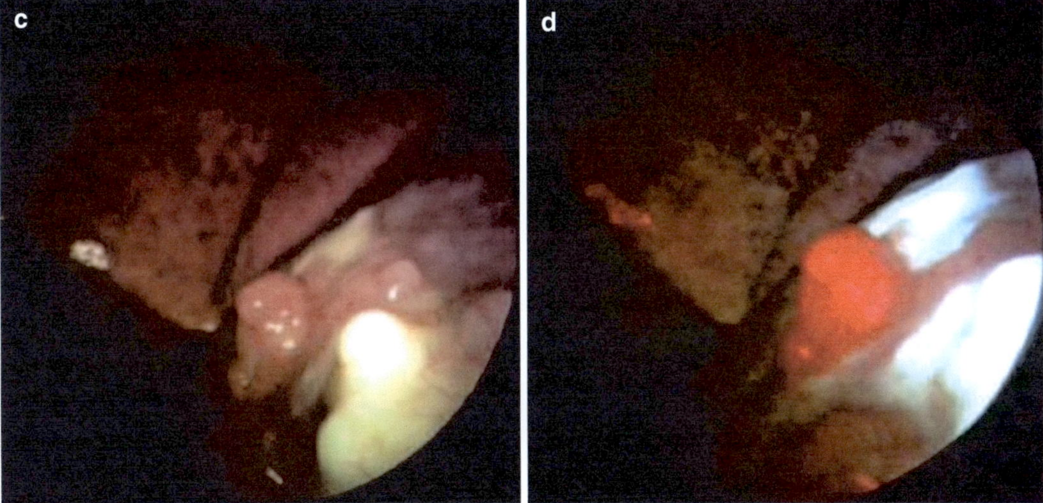

Fig. 26.3 (continued)

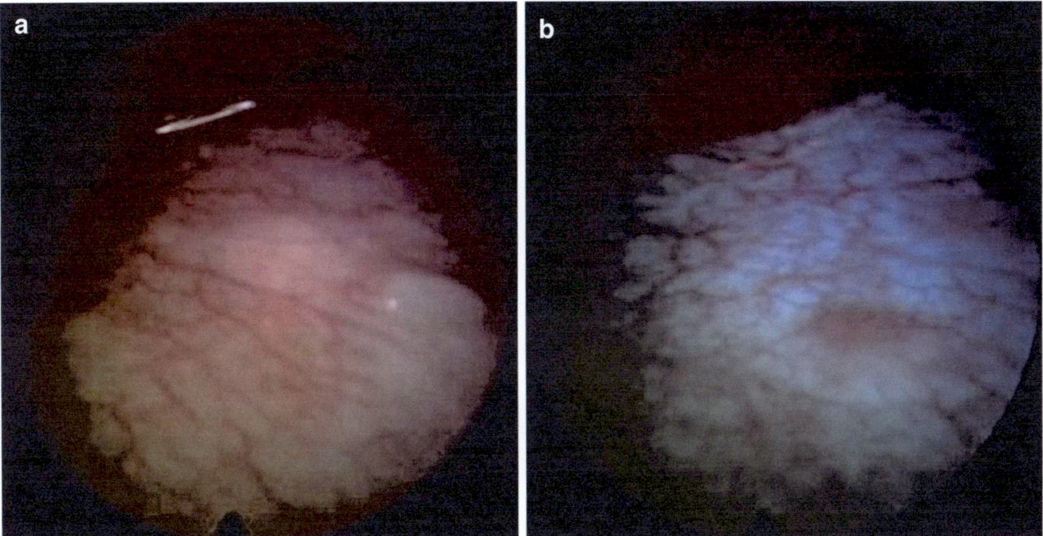

Fig. 26.4 Malignant pleural mesothelioma. True negative on the diaphragm assessed by white-light source (**a**) and autofluorescence thoracoscopy (**b**)

The resulting indirect autofluorescence image represents the following: (*a*) healthy tissue with physiologic concentration of collagen and elastic fibres presenting with a white-green colour; (*b*) a low-density blue colour from deeper layer (1–2 mm) tissue with increased concentration of haemoglobin or inflammatory infiltrates; (*c*) a black or grey colour from tissue with increased superficial concentration of haemoglobin [e.g. stained with blood tissues], as well as superficially localised vessels; and (*d*) a vivid high-density blue foci from tissue with a roughened surface due to hyperplastic inflammatory processes (pachypleuritis, adhesions) and malignant or dysplastic processes.

The AFVT technique is reported to be more precise in locating pleural disorders. In another group of 43 patients who underwent AFVT in 1 year – from March 2007 to March 2008 – a malignant diagnosis was made in 30 cases with 9 cases of inflammatory pleural disease and 4 cases of diffuse lung impairment.

Both these autofluorescence videothoracoscopy studies have provided initial or preliminary results. The authors underline the necessity of conducting further studies using AFVT in order to clarify the real, precise value of this method in clinical practice and to include more cases with earlier stage malignant pleural disease.

26.3.3 Fluorescence Detection of Pleural Malignancies Using 5-ALA

In 2006, a feasibility study of the impact of 5-aminolaevulinic acid (ALA)-mediated fluorescence diagnosis (FD) on the diagnostic workup and staging of various malignancies during VATS was published by researchers from the Netherlands Cancer Institute/Antoni van Leeuwenhoek Hospital and the Laser Center in Academic Medical Center of University of Amsterdam (Baas et al. 2006).

The theoretical basis of the study was focused on the known metabolic pathway of 5-ALA into haemoglobin, where the rate-limiting step is the presence of ferrochelatase. The expression of this enzyme, required in the final stage of transformation of 5-ALA to haemoglobin, is found to be decreased in malignant and inflamed cells, leading to an accumulation of Pp-IX, which has photodynamic properties. The increase in concentration of intracellular Pp-IX and the associated differences in pharmacokinetics between abnormal cells and normal cells facilitate the use of 5-ALA for diagnostic or therapeutic purposes. 5-ALA can be administered systemically (per os or intravenous) or locally into the pleural space and has relatively few side effects – skin photosensitivity for 24–36 h and a transient rise of liver enzymes.

For the purposes of FD (PDD), 5-ALA was administered with ample amounts of water 3–4 h prior to thoracoscopy. Three dosage groups were defined: 1,500 mg for patients with a weight less than 60 kg, 2,000 mg for patients 60–80 kg and 2,500 mg for patients with a weight more than 80 kg. Fluorescence images were obtained using the D-Light® autofluorescence system (Karl Storz – Tuttlingen, Germany), and both illumination and observation of the tissue of interest were achieved with a rigid endoscope integrated with a long-pass filter (cut-off wavelength at 470 nm). The camera had a white-light mode and a blue-light mode, in which the integration time could be increased to correct the relative low intensity of the fluorescent light. An additional low-pass filter (>550 nm) was placed between the endoscope and the camera to further increase the contrast of the images.

From January 2003 to January 2005, 25 patients with a non-diagnosed pleural effusion were included in the analyses. All these patients underwent FD thoracoscopy under general anaesthesia. A final diagnosis was obtained in 24 patients. The definitive diagnosis included 15 cases of malignant mesothelioma, 5 cases of metastases (bronchoalveolar, tongue, mammary, oesophagus and malignancy of unknown origin), 3 cases of plaques with or without inflammatory changes and 1 case of empyema. The undiagnosed case was conformed as a mesothelioma after 6 months of follow-up.

In total, 111 biopsy specimens were obtained from parietal, visceral and diaphragmatic pleura during the examination, and an impressive classification into three equal groups was subsequently formed: (*a*) both FD and white-light imaging (WLI) results were positive in 37 biopsies, 7 of which were found to be false positives; (*b*) FD and WLI results were negative in 37 biopsies, 13 of which were proven false negatives; and (*c*) in the remaining 37 biopsies, there was a discrepancy between observations with WLI and FD. In 26 of the discrepant biopsies, fluorescence detection was positive and white light was negative, with 19 true positive and 7 false positive results. FD was negative in 8 biopsies, the majority of which were taken from a patient with desmoplastic mesothelioma. WLI results were positive over FD in 11 biopsies, with 8 true positive and 3 false positive results.

A detailed analysis of the findings in the 37 biopsies specimens with discrepancies between WLI and FD imaging results showed that there was no overall diagnostic improvement obtained by using FD. Therefore, the researchers demonstrated only a limited benefit of 5-ALA fluorescence for the individual patient. However, for the staging of mesothelioma, it was clear that in four patients, FD upstaged the patient due to improved visualisation of lesions on the visceral pleura which could not be seen using WLI alone, and it was felt that the whole staging process was facilitated by the fluorescence thoracoscopy.

In the future, higher doses of 5-ALA could be administered for imaging if local photodynamic therapy is also indicated for the treatment of the identified tumours (Stanzel et al. 2000; Baas et al. 2006). To date, this option has not been investigated due to the limited access of the thoracoscope in the chest cavity and the diffuse growth of pleural malignancies.

26.4 Fluorescein-Enhanced Autofluorescence Thoracoscopy in Primary Spontaneous Pneumothorax

Marc Noppen and colleagues performed the first prospective, controlled study of in vivo visualisation of abnormal lung regions which may play an important role in the pathophysiology of primary spontaneous pneumothorax (PSP). This study used fluorescein-enhanced autofluorescence thoracoscopy (FEAT) compared to white-light thoracoscopy (WLT) in patients with PSP and in normal control subjects (Noppen et al. 2006).

FEAT was conceptualised to try to visualise abnormal areas at the visceral lung surface and identify sites of potential air leakage. The idea of using a "dye" to make air leaks visible during thoracoscopy was first discussed by *C. Boutin* in his reference book "Practical Thoracoscopy" (Boutin et al. 1991). However, the results of fluorescein inhalation in the setting of white-light illumination for detecting air leaks were disappointing (Boutin C and M Noppen – unpublished observations). Illumination with blue light, taking advantage of the physical fluorescence properties of fluorescein, appeared to dramatically increase its sensitivity.

Sodium fluorescein is a relatively low-molecular-weight, highly water-soluble compound, which when exposed to light of wavelength 465–490 nm [blue light, corresponding to the wavelength used by the DAFE® system] emits light at a wavelength of 520–530 nm [green-yellow light, also detectable by the DAFE® system]. During 30 years of clinical use in the diagnosis and treatment of retinal vascular disorders, the intravenous injection of fluorescein has been shown to be safe. Inhalation of fluorescein had not been reported in controlled series prior to 2004, when the same researchers administered a fluorescein aerosol to a patient with PSP, followed by WLT and FEAT (Noppen et al. 2004). This first case report demonstrated several areas of subpleural fluorescein accumulation not detected by normal WLT. In the subsequent study, all subjects inhaled an aerosolised 10 % fluorescein solution for approximately 10 min under normal tide volume conditions. The fluorescein aerosol was delivered via a pressure-driven nebuliser, attached to a mask. All patients underwent total intravenous anaesthesia, with single-lumen intubation and high-frequency jet ventilation via an endotracheal tube.

During a 6-month period, 12 consecutive patients presented with recurrent and/or persistent (air leak for more than 4 days) PSP. These patients were suitable for thoracoscopic treatment and were enrolled in the study. In addition, 17 control subjects were recruited during the same period. These subjects were referred for bilateral thoracoscopic sympathicolysis for the treatment of essential hyperhidrosis (16 cases) or idiopathic pathologic flushing/social phobia syndrome (1 case). PSP lungs showed significantly more abnormalities at WLT when compared with normal lungs, including the presence of emphysema-like changes (ELCs) like blebs and/or bullae. FEAT showed low-grade anthracotic lesions in the majority of normal lungs. However, in contrast high-grade lesions with extensive subpleural fluorescein accumulation and fluorescein leakage were exclusively found in patients presenting with PSP. It is important to note that these high-grade lesions, which may be considered as possible sites where air leakage can originate, were not necessarily associated with blebs or bullae or other associated abnormalities visible at WLT. These findings suggest that the observed high-grade FEAT phenomena, limited to PSP lungs only, may be proof that PSP patients suffer from a more extensive disease process of parenchymal inflammation and destruction than previously thought. It also confirms that ELC rupture is not necessary for every case of PSP. Finally these finding have major therapeutic implications relating to the definitive treatment of the ELC, as in many cases abnormalities were found distant from the blebs and bullae, which were previously thought to be the primary culprits of air leakage in PSP.

Nevertheless, the pathophysiological significance of these observations remains to be further explored and analysed, while it is important to acknowledge the limitations inherent to this technique: (*a*) the FEAT data can only be obtained in a semiquantitative fashion, because the fluorescence measurements are planar measurements with the light intensity dependent on the local concentrations of fluorophore and on the depth of penetration of the fluorophore in the lung tissue; (*b*) the semiquantitative scoring is entirely unblinded, as the thoracoscopist was fully aware of whether the patient had suffered from a PSP or was a control subject, and this highlights the need for improved score blinding and a more objective method of fluorescence measurement in the future; and (*c*) the kinetics of inhaled fluorescein with respect to absorption in the bloodstream, interstitium or cells are unknown. Therefore, the hypothesis that high-grade lesions, exclusively seen in PSP and not in normal lungs, may be the result of the accumulation of inhaled fluorescein aerosol in certain pulmonary areas due to local air trapping, which needs to be further studied. Alternatively, fluorescein may accumulate in areas that receive more rather than less ventilation. However, the study of the wash-in and wash-out phases of fluorescein administration in a patient or an animal model would help clarify the true meaning of the fluorescein accumulation.

The use of FEAT in patients with PSP demonstrated the existence of actual fluorophore leakage through the visceral pleura. This can be explained by the presence of pleural porosity (e.g. the presence of pleural pores with a width of several microns) in the absence of blebs, bullae or other abnormalities observed at white-light thoracoscopic inspection. The exact nature of the pleural porosity is also unknown but may be associated with the loss of surface mesothelial cells, thinning and rupture of the basement membrane and/or downregulation of junctional proteins. It is possible that an interplay between peripheral airway and airspace inflammation (that may be enhanced by smoking), mechanical factors (such as more negative surrounding pressures and increased mechanical stretching of the lung apices in ectomorphic individuals) and differentiation in collagen quality may lead to the structural changes defined as "pleural porosity".

26.5 Newer Fluorescence Techniques in Endoscopic Diagnosis, Staging and Therapy

Fluorescence techniques are continuously evolving and have already been implemented in several areas of clinical practice. In addition the technique may be combined with different methods for diagnosis and therapy in the future. In this chapter, we attempt to show brief characteristics of some of the most important research activities on the field of fluorescence diagnosis, staging and therapy in respiratory endoscopy.

26.5.1 Near-Infrared Thoracoscopy of Tumoural Protease Activity for Improved Detection of Peripheral Lung Cancer

Researchers from the Centre for Molecular Imaging Research in Massachusetts General Hospital, Boston, USA, have recently attempted to evaluate the ability to use activated probes targeting proteases which are overexpressed in many tumour types, in order to improve the visualisation of parenchymal-surface lung tumours during thoracoscopy (Figueiredo et al. 2006).

Direct visualisation of the pleural space and lung surface at the time of video-assisted thoracoscopic surgery (VATS) offers a higher spatial resolution than non-invasive cross-sectional imaging modalities, such as CT or MRI. Therefore, micrometastatic disease not identified by these modalities may, in some cases, be seen directly. In addition the luminescence of tumours, especially small foci, is often similar to the adjacent lung parenchyma. The basic objective of the study was to determine the possibility of providing adjuncts to VATS, which could result in better visualisation of tumours and would be beneficial in increasing the sensitivity of lesion detection as well as allowing for a shorter procedure duration by decreasing the time needed to adequately inspect the pleural space and identify areas that require sampling and removal.

Activatable fluorescent imaging agents typically increase their fluorescence intensity after target interaction: when initially injected, they are optically silent, but after interaction with enzymes that are overexpressed in tumours, they become brightly fluorescent. Because of their low initial fluorescence, which results in lower background signal, higher target to background ratios (TBR) can be achieved when compared to other fluorescent agents, allowing easier detection of tumour foci. Additionally, compared to fluorophores, which are often of low molecular weight, the activatable agents remain at their target for longer periods of time, allowing detection of the probe during long procedures. Many of the activatable agents fluoresce in the near-infrared region (NIR) of the electromagnetic spectrum, and this results in several advantages: (*a*) deeper penetration of NIR signal when compared to visible light, allowing the visualisation of pathology below the surface, and (*b*) a simultaneous acquisition of full-colour white-light images, as seen during conventional thoracoscopy, combining with NIR images, thus provide information on molecular activity. These can be overlaid onto the white-light anatomical images to guide the surgeon during a procedure. Two different near-infrared fluorescent activatable "smart" imaging probes were used in this study, which differed in the attached fluorochrome and in peak absorption

and emission wavelengths – one probe with a peak absorption of 680 nm and peak emission of 700 nm [ProSense 680] and another activatable probe with peak absorption of 750 nm and peak emission of 780 nm [ProSense 750].

Twenty-four hours prior to imaging, 15 female nude mice were randomly separated in three groups – the first five received intravenous administration of 2 nmol/mouse ProSense 680, five animals received intravenous administration of 2 nmol/mouse ProSense 750, and the remaining five mice – control subjects – did not receive any probe injection. A specific imaging microcatheter was also adapted to aid selective intubation under visual guidance and to perform thoracoscopy. Briefly, the catheter had an outer diameter of 0.8 mm and consisted of 10,000 ordered fibres, surrounded by a group of 14 bundles of illumination fibres. Visible light was separated from NIR light through a 670 nm dichroic mirror, while the NIR light was additionally passed through a sharp cut-off bandpass filter. The two components were recorded separately but simultaneously onto white-light or NIR video cameras, thus allowing display and video capture of full-colour spectrum white-light images adjacent to the NIR images, which, based upon probe fluorescence, reflected the protease tissue activity.

To compare the effect of wavelength on detection, both wavelength imaging "smart" probes reported upon the same target: proteases that cleave lysine–lysine bonds. In vivo, cathepsin B is the major contributor to this probe cleavage. Many primary lung tumours contain significantly higher levels of cathepsin B protein and express higher levels of cathepsin B activity than the adjacent lung parenchyma. These high levels correlate to a worse prognosis. In lung tumours not overexpressing cathepsin B directly or from a host response, the benefits of probe activation in tumour detection will likely be diminished. An additional confounding factor is where there is protease overexpression in areas of inflammation, which may increase the background signal. In focal cases, such as some inflammatory pulmonary nodules that express high levels of cathepsin B, false positive results may occur. The probes at both wavelengths gave similar results with respect to TBRs, showing that either wavelength probe combination could be used with equivalent efficacy.

At both wavelength pairs evaluated (680/700 and 750/780 nm excitation/emission), the intrinsic luminosity differences between the tumour and normal lung in uninjected animals were low. In mice receiving protease probes, tumours were significantly more fluorescent than adjacent lung and TBR increased by approximately ninefold. Confirmatory fluorescence microscopy and immunohistochemistry were similar and revealed that normal lung had very low levels when compared to tumours of cathepsin B and probe fluorescence.

In conclusion, protease-sensitive imaging probes selective for cathepsin B, imaged with NIR microcatheters, significantly increase the TBR, making small peripheral lung tumours more easily apparent. Such an approach may be a useful adjunct in staging or restaging patients with lung cancer in order to find minimal disease in the pleural and subpleural space.

26.5.2 Virally Directed Fluorescent Imaging (VFI)

A few years before the above study was undertaken, a group of researchers from the Memorial Sloan-Kettering Cancer Centre in New York, USA, started investigating methods for improving fluorescent imaging during endoscopic procedures (including thoracoscopy) by using a herpes viral vector. Intense research activities resulted in several publications, which determined the feasibility of the proposed technology in the endoscopic staging of pleural and other malignancies, in facilitation of minimally invasive oncological surgery, in intraoperative localisation of lymph node metastases and in localisation of metastatic pleural cancer.

Virally directed fluorescent imaging in all these studies was focused on NV1066: a genetically modified, replication-competent, attenuated

herpes simplex HSV-1 oncolytic virus, which had been previously shown to be highly specific for infection of tumour cells while sparing normal cells and was also effective against multiple tumour types, including lung cancer. NV1066 carries a transgene for an enhanced green fluorescent protein (GFP), which is constitutively expressed 2–6 h following viral entry into cells.

26.5.2.1 Virally Directed Fluorescent Imaging (VFI) Can Facilitate Endoscopic Staging

The first study (Adusumilli et al. 2006a) was conducted to determine the feasibility of a GFP-guided imaging method in the intraoperative detection of small tumour nodules. Human cancer cell lines were infected with NV1066 at several multiplicities of infection, and green fluorescent protein was expressed, producing a significantly higher fluorescence obtained from normal cells. One single dose of the viral vector spread within and across the pleural cavity and selectively infected tumour nodules and spared the normal tissue. The tumour nodules undetected by conventional thoracoscopy were identified by GFP fluorescence.

The initial conclusion was that virally directed fluorescent imaging (VFI) has the potential to enhance the intraoperative detection of endocavitary tumour nodules.

26.5.2.2 Real-Time Diagnostic Imaging of Tumours/Metastases by Use of a Replication-Competent Herpes Vector to Facilitate Minimally Invasive Oncological Surgery

Systemic delivery of the herpes viral vector NV1066 with cancer-selective infection and replication was used to precisely differentiate between normal and malignant tissue with the aim to facilitate minimally invasive oncological surgery (Adusumilli et al. 2006b).

Minimally invasive surgical techniques are currently guided by conventional visual inspection, and the optical imaging is limited by the strong absorbance and scattering of light by the surrounding tissues. Previous attempts to use gene therapy to enhance visualisation had been limited by the efficiency of tumour cell transduction in vivo. In this study a total of 111 human cancer cell lines from 16 different primary organs were used. Animal models were created in athymic mice, 8–10 weeks old, in which pleural models were developed by injection of mesothelioma cells into the thoracic cavity. Micro- and macroscopic lymph node metastases developed 3–8 weeks following intrathoracic tumour cell inoculation.

The pleural cavity of all animals was systematically examined by conventional and fluorescence thoracoscopy, using a dedicated endoscopic system developed by Olympus America, Inc. The objective was to permit the detection of GFP. This system was equipped with an interchangeable excitation filter set at 470 ± 20 nm to accommodate the minor excitation peak of GFP at 475 nm and an emission filter fixed at 500 nm to accommodate the emission peak of GFP at 509 nm. GFP images were taken with minimal illumination to illustrate the surrounding organs. Each mouse was individually and systematically examined for the presence of metastatic disease as determined by the presence or absence of green fluorescence.

A single dose of NV1066 instilled into the thoracic cavity was found to spread, infect and express green fluorescence in tumour tissue, while the normal lung and heart tissue were spared. Fluorescent expression facilitated clear identification of tumour nodules in between the lobar fissures, on the diaphragm and on the pleural surface. NV1066-guided fluorescence enhanced the identification of microscopic nodules that were not evident with standard examination.

Injection of the viral vector into the primary tumour resulted in dissemination of virus to metastatic sites to allow identification of metastatic disease with thoracoscopic examination. A single dose of NV1066 injected into the primary breast tumour resulted in the infection and fluorescence of multiple metastatic lung tumours. In addition, disease in the axillary and mediastinal lymph nodes was also found. Splenic metastases from pleural mesothelioma were identified after administration of NV1066 into the pleural cavity, and similarly, systemic injection of NV1066 clearly delineated adrenal and renal metastases in a primary lung cancer model. The administration of NV1066 into the primary tumour also resulted in spread via lymphatics, revealing metastases in both the regional stations and in distant nodes. In a model for advanced malignant pleural mesothelioma, the intrathoracic administration of NV1066 led to selective infection and fluorescence of otherwise inconspicuous nodal metastases in the para-aortic region as well as adrenal metastases.

This study presented a unique approach to the challenge of accurately defining the extent and margins of macroscopic disease and the identification of microscopic tumour foci thus allowing optimal resection and staging. The development of a real-time intraoperative detection system that is sensitive and specific for tumour will probably improve surgical performance and expand the applicability of minimally invasive oncological surgery while improving tumour visualisation and ensuring the completeness of tumour resection and in turn reducing the risk of locoregional recurrence.

26.5.2.3 Intraoperative Localisation of Lymph Node Metastases with a Replication-Competent Herpes Simplex Virus in Malignant Mesothelioma

Another study from the Memorial Sloan-Kettering Cancer Centre in New York, USA, (Adusumilli et al. 2006c) investigated the potential to identify lymph node metastases intraoperatively in patients with malignant pleural mesothelioma (MPM) by using herpes (NV1066)-guided cancer cell-specific expression of green fluorescent protein (GFP).

The rationale for conducting clinical research in this area is based on the accumulated data that accurate localisation of lymph node metastases in patients with MPM is necessary to improve selection of resectable for surgical intervention. 20–30 % of patients undergo exploratory thoracotomy without resection often due to the failure of computed tomographic (CT) and magnetic resonance imaging (MRI) scans to predict mediastinal nodal metastases and locally advanced disease. Even positron emission tomographic (PET) scans have failed to reliably identify mediastinal nodal metastases. Therefore, endoscopic techniques (mediastinoscopy, thoracoscopy and laparoscopy) have emerged as valuable diagnostic procedures for assessing patients with MPM who are considered candidates for surgical-based therapy. The development of a real-time in vivo technique which may enhance the accurate detection of metastatic lymph nodes is thought to be essential to further increase the sensitivity and specificity of the above endoscopic methods.

After administration of NV1066, which has been shown to infect and express GFP in more than 18 thoracic malignancies, human mesothelioma cancer cells were assessed for cancer cell-specific infection, GFP expression, viral replication and cytotoxicity. Fluorescence thoracoscopy, laparoscopy and stereomicroscopy were used to localise lymph node metastases which were later confirmed by means of immunohistochemistry.

In vitro, the viral vector NV1066 infected, replicated and expressed green fluorescent protein in all cancer cells, even when infected at a low ratio of one viral plaque-forming unit per 100 tumour cells. In vivo, NV1066, injected into primary tumours, was able to locate and infect lymph node metastases and producing GFP which was visualised by means of fluorescent imaging. Histological assessment confirmed lymphatic metastases, and immunohistochemistry proved viral presence in regions expressing GFP. One limitation of this work was that data to further define the predicted value of the proposed technique was lacking.

The technology presented in the final publication holds promise for improved care for malignant pleural mesothelioma and other malignancies. Pilot studies conducted by the same researchers have obtained similar levels of fluorescence lymphatic detection in lung cancer, as well as in oesophageal malignancies.

26.5.2.4 Minimally Invasive Localisation of Metastatic Pleural Cancer by Oncolytic Herpes Simplex Viral Therapy

The oncolytic properties of the herpes simplex virus NV1066 and associated clinical applications have also been studied (Stiles et al. 2006). The purpose of these studies was to determine whether this viral vector is cytotoxic to lung cancer and whether enhanced green fluorescent protein (EGFP) is a detectable marker of viral infection in vitro and in vivo. In addition, the researchers investigated whether EGFP expression in infected cells can be used to localise the virus and to identify small metastatic tumour foci (less than 1 mm) in vivo by means of endoscopic systems equipped with fluorescent filters.

NV1066 replicated and expressed EGFP in infected cells and killed tumour cells in vitro, while in vivo, the treatment with intrapleural NV1066 decreased pleural disease burden, as measured by chest wall nodule counts and organ weights in experimental animal models. EGFP was easily visualised by fluorescence thoracoscopy in tumour deposits, including microscopic foci.

NV1066 has significant oncolytic activity against a human non-small-cell lung cancer (NSCLC) cell line and is effective in limiting the progression of metastatic disease in an in vivo orthotopic model.

In the future, by incorporating fluorescent filters into endoscopic devices and systems, a minimally invasive technique for diagnosing small metastatic pleural deposits and localisation of viral therapy for thoracic malignancies may be developed using the EGFP marker gene inserted into oncolytic herpes simplex viruses.

Acknowledgement The author is grateful to Dr Julius P. Janssen for his invaluable support in learning, performing and critically evaluating medical thoracoscopy, as well as several aspects of interventional pulmonology.

References

Adachi R, Utsui T, Furusawa K (1999) Development of the autofluorescence endoscope imaging system. Diagn Ther Endosc 5:65–70

Adusumilli PS, Eisenberg DP, Stiles BM et al (2006a) Virally-directed fluorescent imaging (VFI) can facilitate endoscopic staging. J Surg Endosc 20:628–35

Adusumilli PS, Stiles BM, Chan M-K et al (2006b) Real-time diagnostic imaging of tumours and metastases by use of a replication-competent herpes vector to facilitate minimally invasive oncological surgery. FASEB J 20:726–28

Adusumilli PS, Eisenberg DP, Stiles BM et al (2006c) Intraoperative localisation of lymph node metastases with a replication-competent herpes simplex virus. J Thorac Cardiovasc Surg 132:1179–88

Andersson-Engels S, Berg R, Svanberg S (1992) Effects of optical constants on time-gated transillumination of tissue and tissue-like media. J Photochem Photobiol B 16:155–67

Andersson-Engels S, Klinterberg C, Svanberg K et al (1997) In vivo fluorescence imaging for tissue diagnostics. Phys Med Biol 42:815–24

Aubin JE (1979) Autofluorescence of viable cultured mammalian cells. J Histochem Cytochem 27:36–43

Baas P, Triesscheijn M, Burgers S et al (2006) Fluorescence detection of pleural malignancies using 5-aminolaevulinic acid. Chest 129:718–24

Barenboim GM (1969) Luminescence of biopolymers and cells. Plenum Press, New York, pp 64–75

Baumgartner R, Huber RM, Schulz H et al (1996) Inhalation of 5-aminolevulinic acid: a new technique for fluorescence detection of early stage lung cancer. J Photochem Photobiol B 36:169–74

Belák J, Kudlák M, Cavarga I et al (2007) Autofluorescence videothoracoscopy – our initial experience. Rozhl Chir 86:558–61

Blanc F-X, Atassi K, Bignon J et al (2002) Diagnostic value of medical thoracoscopy in pleural disease. Chest 121:1677–83

Boutin C, Viallat JR, Cargnino P et al (1981) Thoracoscopy in malignant pleural effusions. Am Rev Respir Dis 124:588–592

Boutin C, Viallat JR, Aelony Y (1991) Diagnostic thoracoscopy for pleural effusions. In: Boutin C, Viallat JR, Aelony Y (eds) Practical thoracoscopy. Springer, Berlin, pp 51–64

Chrysanthidis MG, Janssen JP (2005) Autofluorescence videothoracoscopy in exudative pleural effusions: preliminary results. Eur Respir J 26:989–992

Colt HG (1999) Thoracoscopy: window to the pleural space. Chest 116:1409–15

Figueiredo J-L, Alencar H, Weissleder R et al (2006) Near infrared thoracoscopy of tumoural protease activity for improved detection of peripheral lung cancer. Int J Cancer 118:2672–7

Gahlen J, Prosst RL, Herfarth C et al (2000) Blue light illumination for minimally-invasive fluorescence detection of tumours: technology, clinical experience and future perspectives. Minim Invasive Ther Allied Technol 9:119–24

Harris RJ, Kavuru MS, Rice TW et al (1995) The diagnostic and therapeutic utility of thoracoscopy: a review. Chest 108:828–41

Häussinger K, Becker H, Stanzel F et al (2005) Autofluorescence bronchoscopy with white light bronchoscopy compared with white light bronchoscopy alone for the detection of precancerous lesions: a European randomised controlled multicentre trial. Thorax 60:496–503

Hayata Y, Kato H, Konaka C et al (1982) Fiberoptic bronchoscopic laser photoradiation for tumour localisation in lung cancer. Chest 82:10–14

Heffner JE (2008) Diagnosis and management of malignant pleural effusions. Respirology 13:5–20

Heffner JE, Klein JS (2008) Recent advances in the diagnosis and management of malignant pleural effusions. Mayo Clin Proc 83:235–50

Herley L (1944) Studies in selective differentiation of tissue by means of ultraviolet light. Cancer Res 227–31

Kato H, Imaizumi T, Aisawa K et al (1990) Photodynamic diagnosis in respiratory tract malignancy using an excimer dye laser system. J Photochem Photobiol B 6:189–96

Keith RL, Miller YE, Gemmill RM et al (2000) Angiogenic squamous dysplasia in bronchi of individuals at high risk of lung cancer. Clin Cancer Res 6:1616–25

Kennedy J, Pottier R (1992) Endogenous protoporhyrin IX, a clinically useful photosensitiser for photodynamic therapy. J Photochem Photobiol B 14:275–92

Kloek J, Akkermans W, Beijersbergen-van-Henegouven GM (1998) Derivatives of 5-aminolevulinic acid for photodynamic therapy: enzymatic conversion into protoporphyrin. Photochem Photobiol 67:150–154

Kriegmair M, Baumgartner R, Knuechel R et al (1994) Fluorescence photodetection of neoplastic urothelial lesions following intravesical instillation of 5-aminolevulinic acid. Urology 44:836–841

Lam S, Hang J, Palcic B (1990) Detection of lung cancer by ratio fluorometry with and without Photofrin II. SPIE Opt Fibers Med 1201:561–568

Lee YC, Light RW (2004) Management of malignant pleural effusions. Respirology 9:148–156

Lipson RL, Blades EG, Olsen A (1961) Haematoporphyrin derivative: a new aid for endoscopy detection of malignant disease. J Thorac Cardiovasc Surg 42:623–9

Loddenkemper R, Boutin C (1993) Thoracoscopy: present diagnostic and therapeutic indications. Eur Respir J 6:1544–55

Maskell NA, Butland RJA (2003) BTS guidelines for the investigation of a unilateral pleural effusion in adults. Thorax 58(Suppl II):ii8–ii17

Moro-Sibilot D, Jeanmart M, Lantuejoul S et al (2002) Cigarette smoking, preinvasive bronchial lesions and autofluorescence bronchoscopy. Chest 122:1902–8

Nakhosteen JA, Khavankar B (2000) Autofluorescence bronchoscopy: the laser imaging fluorescence bronchoscope. In: Bolliger CT, Mathur PN (eds) Interventional bronchoscopy. Karger, Basel, pp 236–242

Noppen M, Stratakos G, Verbank S et al (2004) Fluorescein-enhanced autofluorescence thoracoscopy in primary spontaneous pneumothorax. Am J Respir Crit Care Med 170:680–2

Noppen M, Dekeukeleire T, Hanon S et al (2006) Fluorescein-enhanced autofluorescence thoracoscopy in patients with primary spontaneous pneumothorax and normal subjects. Am J Respir Crit Care Med 174:26–30

Pichler J, Stepp H, Baumgartner R et al (1998) Fluoreszenztumorlokalisation nach Application von 5-Aminolävulin-säure. Anwendung in der Pulmologie. Lazer-medizin 13:151

Profio AE, Doiron DR (1977) A feasibility study of the use of bronchoscopy for localisation of small lung tumours. Phys Med Biol 22:949–57

Prosst RL, Winkler S, Boehm E et al (2002) Thoracoscopic fluorescence diagnosis (TFD) of pleural malignancies: experimental studies. Thorax 57:1005–9

Staël V, Holstein C, Nilsson AMK et al (1996) Detection of adenocarcinoma in Barrett's oesophagus by means of laser induced fluorescence. Gut 39:711–6

Stanzel F, Häussinger K, Geiger D (2000) Photodynamic therapy in pneumology. Pneumologie 54:269–77

Stiles BM, Adusumilli PS, Bhargava A et al (2006) Minimally invasive localisation of oncolytic herpes simplex viral therapy of metastatic pleural cancer. Cancer Gene Ther 13:53–64

Stübel H (1911) Die Fluoreszence tierischer Gewebe im ultravioletten Licht. Pflügers Arch Physiol 142:1

Sutedja G, Venmans BJ, Smit EF et al (2001) Fluorescence bronchoscopy for early detection of lung cancer. A clinical perspective. Lung Cancer 34:157–68

Sutro CJ, Burman MS (1933) Examination of pathologic tissue by filtered ultraviolet radiation. Arch Pathol 16:346–9

Flexi-Rigid Thoracoscopy

27

Teruomi Miyazawa and Atsuko Ishida

27.1 Introduction

In routine clinical practice, pulmonologists are frequently required to evaluate patients with pleural effusions. For diagnosis, conventional methods such as thoracentesis and closed pleural biopsy are often performed first. However, approximately 20–25 % of pleural effusions remain undiagnosed (Boutin et al. 1993; Loddenkemper 1998) and medical thoracoscopy should then be performed.

From the time that thoracoscopy was introduced in 1910 by Jacobaeus (Jacobaeus 1910), the rigid thoracoscope has primarily been utilized to examine the pleural space (Boutin et al. 1993; Loddenkemper 1998; Boutin and Astoul 1998; Colt 1995a, b; Blanc et al. 2002). With the advent of fiber-optic technology, however, flexible bronchoscopes were employed for thoracoscopy (Davidson et al. 1988; Robinson and Gleeson 1995; Tsukamoto et al. 1991). These scopes contained working channels, making it possible to perform suction and biopsy under direct observation. Due to the relative difficulty in controlling these scopes – because of their inherent flexibility – a thoracofiberscope with a

T. Miyazawa (✉) • A. Ishida
Division of Respiratory and Infectious Diseases,
Department of Internal Medicine,
St Marianna University School of Medicine,
Kawasaki, Japan
e-mail: miyazawat@marianna-u.ac.jp;
atsuko-i@do3.enjoy.ne.jp

rigid shaft and a bidirectional flexible tip, also known as a pleuroscope or semirigid thoracoscope, was developed (McLean et al. 1998). The latest model, the flexi-rigid thoracoscope, has a large working channel, allowing for larger biopsy samples (Ernst et al. 2002; Lee and Colt 2005; Munavvar et al. 2007; Ishida et al. 2004). In this chapter we describe the flexi-rigid thoracoscopy under local anaesthesia as used in the investigation of pleural effusions.

27.2 Indications

The major clinical utility of the flexi-rigid thoracoscopy is thoracoscopic pleural biopsy and pleurodesis. Indications for thoracoscopic pleural biopsy include diagnosis of pleural effusions which remain unclassified after biochemical, bacteriological, and cytological analysis, and mutation analysis of the epidermal growth factor receptor (EGFR) gene in lung cancer. Pleurodesis, primarily with talc, is performed to control malignant pleural effusion.

27.3 Contraindication

As procedures are performed under local anaesthesia, the main contraindications to flexi-rigid thoracoscopy include lack of pleural space due to adhesions, uncontrolled cough, inadequate lung function parameters, uncorrectable bleeding tendency, and severe heart failure.

P. Astoul et al. (eds.), *Thoracoscopy for Pulmonologists*,
DOI 10.1007/978-3-642-38351-9_27, © Springer-Verlag Berlin Heidelberg 2014

27.4 Equipment

The equipment used for flexi-rigid thoracoscopy is shown in Fig. 27.1. The flexi-rigid thoracoscopy (LTF-260 or LTF-160; Olympus; Tokyo, Japan) is 53 cm (LTF-260) and 52 cm (LTF-160) in total length, with the 27-cm insertion portion. The proximal 22 cm is rigid and the distal 5 cm is flexible. The external diameter of the insertion portion is 6.9 mm (LTF-260) and 7.0 mm

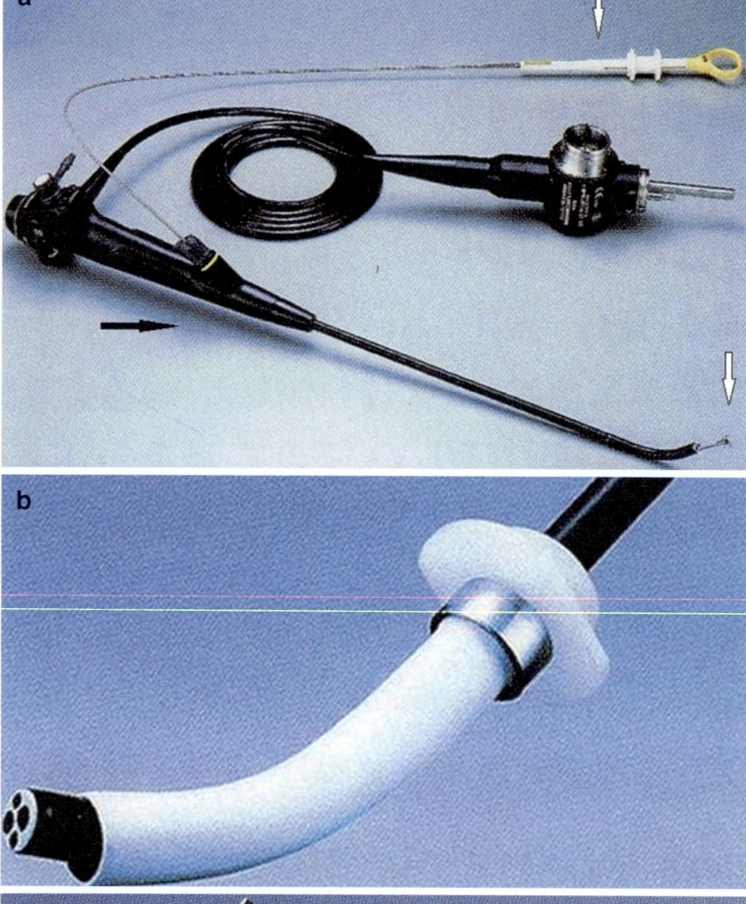
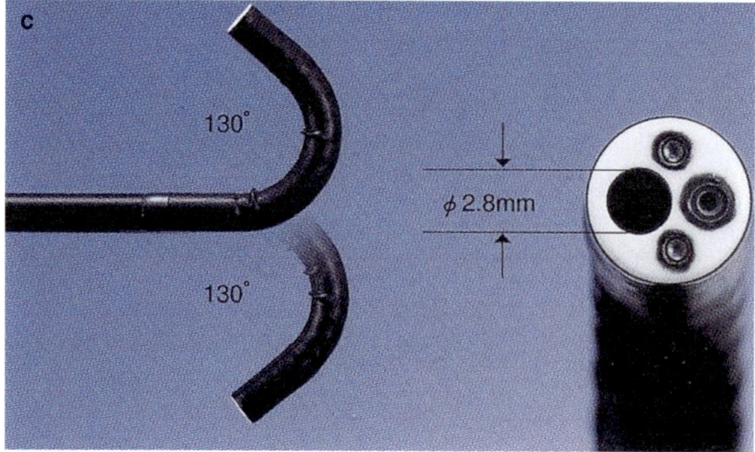

Fig. 27.1 Necessary equipments for the pleura-videoscopy: (**a**) The pleura-videoscope (a rigid thoracoscope with a bidirectional flexible tip – length: 52 cm, caliber: 7.0 mm) (*black arrow*) and alligator jaw-type flexible biopsy forceps through the working channel (*white arrows*). (**b**) The pleura-videoscope inserted through the flexible trocar. (**c**) The tip of the pleura-videoscope (*on the left*) and a view of the working channel (2.8 mm) for biopsy forceps or suction catheter (*on the right*)

(LTF-160). The flexible tip can be controlled by a lever on the handle, which allows for 160° upward and 130° downward movement. The 2.8-mm inner working channel accommodates the biopsy forceps and other instruments including an electrosurgical coagulator and argon plasma coagulation probe. The flexi-rigid thoracoscope model LTF-260 is compatible with the existing video processors CV-200, CV-240, CV-260, and CV-260SL (Olympus), and the model LTF-160 is compatible with the video processors CV-100, CV-140, CV-145, and CV-160 (Olympus). Both models are sterilized by either ethylene oxide gas (EOG) or autoclaving.

The sterile, disposable flexible trocar (MAJ-1058; Olympus) designed for the flexi-rigid thoracoscope is 8 mm in diameter. It is not airtight. There are two types of flexible biopsy forceps available, one without a needle (FB-36C-1; Olympus) and the other with needle between the alligator jaws (FB-55CR-1; Olympus).

27.5 Techniques

27.5.1 Thoracoscopic Procedure

The technique is described in Fig. 27.2. The flexi-rigid thoracoscopy can be performed under general anaesthesia; however, in this chapter we describe our method, the flexi-rigid thoracoscope under local anaesthesia without sedation. The procedure can be performed in the operating room, in the endoscopy suite, or at the bedside in a general ward. Patients are placed in the lateral decubitus position, involved side up. We ask patients to hold a pillow to keep their arms upward and to maintain an adequate intercostal space. The entry point is determined by ultrasonography, usually in the midaxillary line at the fifth to seventh intercostal space. The patients are premedicated with 25 mg hydroxyzine and 15 mg pentazocine given intramuscularly. Supplemental oxygen is administered via a nasal cannula, usually 3–5 l/min. Pulse, blood pressure, and oxygen saturation are continuously monitored. The patient's skin is disinfected, and the physician and assistant clean their hands and put on a sterile gown and gloves. The physician stands on one side of the patient and the assistant is on the other side. The main operator usually faces the patient. Local anaesthesia with 10–15 ml of 1 % lidocaine is instilled to the chest wall at the previously marked site of entry. Entry into the pleural cavity is confirmed by the drawing back of fluid or air into the syringe. A 10-mm incision is made to the skin and subcutaneous tissues with a scalpel, followed by blunt dissection to the pleural space. The 8.0-mm flexible trocar should be held firmly in the palm of the hand and inserted until a release of resistance

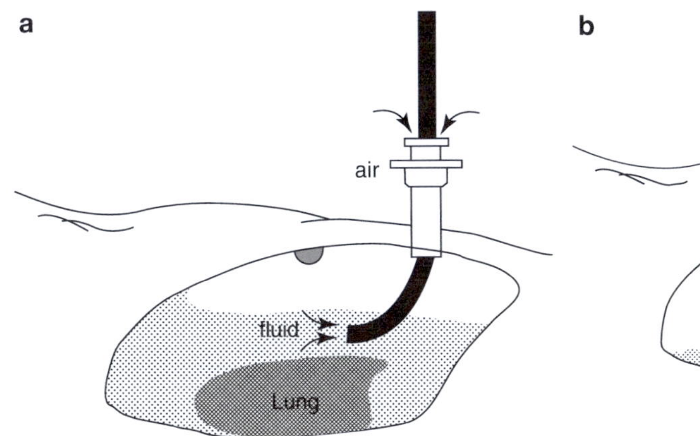

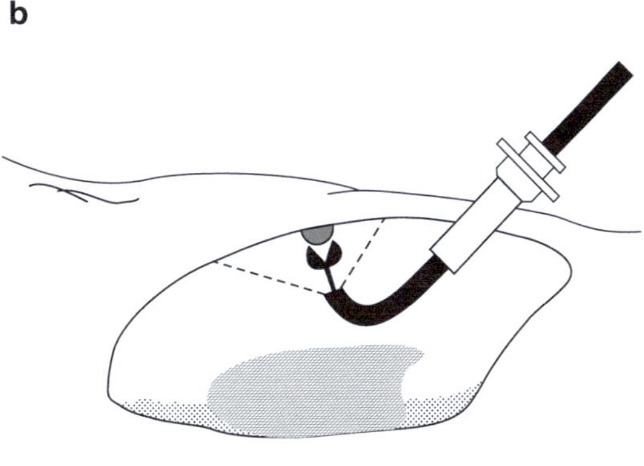

Fig. 27.2 The schema of pleura-videoscopy. (**a**) Pleural fluid is drained through the working channel, and atmospheric air is introduced via a trocar allowing the lung to collapse away from the chest wall. (**b**) Biopsy is performed through the working channel

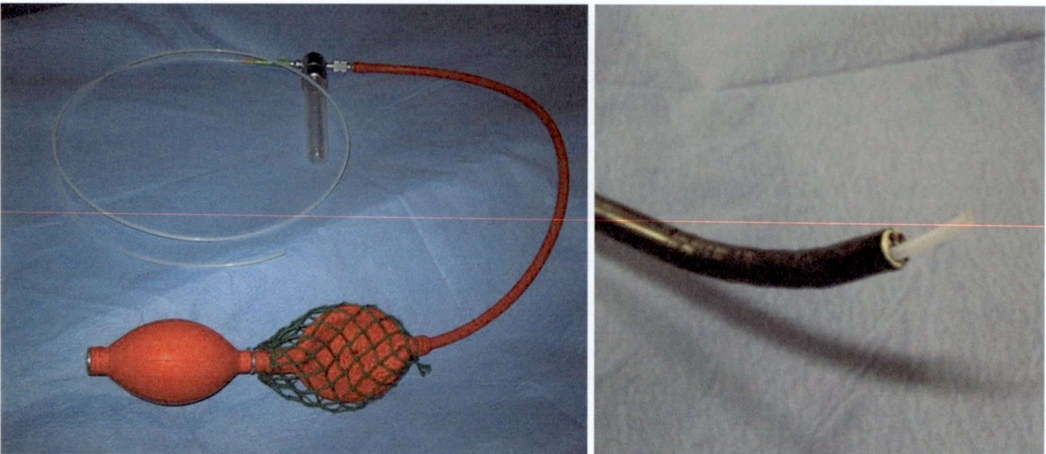

Fig. 27.3 Using a double balloon insufflator, sterile talc (Steritalc®; Novatech; France) is spread into the pleural space through the working channel of the pleura-videoscope

is felt. If the trocar doesn't enter the pleural cavity easily, the physician should perform further blunt dissection. After the flexible trocar is placed, the flexi-rigid thoracoscope is inserted into the pleural cavity. Initially the physician cannot see anything clearly due to the pleural fluid. The fluid is aspirated through the working channel of the scope until the physician obtains sufficient examination space.

27.5.2 Pleural Biopsy Techniques

The parietal and visceral pleura and diaphragm are carefully inspected. Biopsy specimens are obtained from suspicious-looking areas on the parietal pleura or diaphragm using flexible biopsy forceps under direct visual control. Usually 5–10 biopsy specimens are stored in 10 % formalin solution for histologic examination, and 2–4 specimens are stored in normal saline for bacteriological examination.

27.5.3 Talc Pleurodesis

After completely removing the fluid, sterile talc (Steritalc; Novatech; France) is insufflated into the pleural space through the working channel of the pleura-videoscope (Fig. 27.3) or

through the 2-mm Boutin pleural puncture needle (Boutin Trocar; Novatech) placed as the second site of entry. At the end of the procedure, the distribution of the talc on the pleura is confirmed by flexi-rigid thoracoscopy.

27.5.4 Post Procedure

After every procedure, a 20-Fr chest tube is inserted through the same incision used for the flexi-rigid thoracoscope and attached to an aspiration device. A chest roentgenogram is performed following the procedure. For pleural biopsy alone, the chest tube is removed when complete lung reexpansion is confirmed on chest roentgenogram. The chest drain can be removed on the same day. In cases where talc pleurodesis was performed, negative pressure, usually −20-cm H_2O, should commence immediately after the procedure and be maintained for at least 48 h after the procedure until the fluid drainage is less than 200 ml/day.

27.6 Efficacy

The flexi-rigid thoracoscopy has been used for diagnostic purpose (Munavvar et al. 2007; Ishida et al. 2004, 2005) and talc pleurodesis

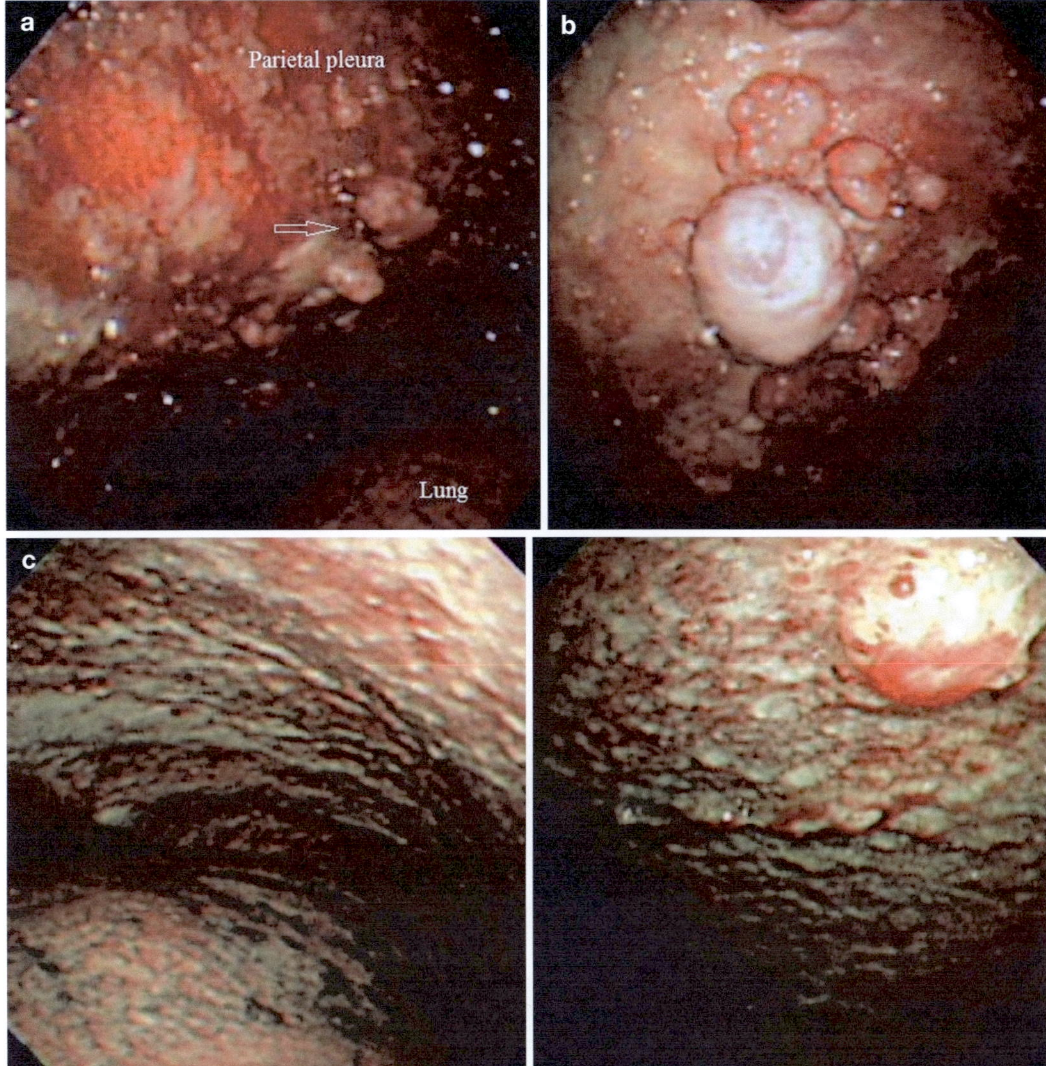

Fig. 27.4 (**a**) A distant view of diffuse malignant mesothelioma inspected by a pleura-videoscope. The *arrow* shows malignant nodules. (**b**) A closeup view of diffuse malignant mesothelioma as inspected by a pleura-videoscope. The uneven pleural thickening and nodules are observed all over the parietal pleura. Biopsy samples obtained from a nodular lesion of the parietal pleura revealed solid and epithelioid form with irregular spaces. (**c**) A distant (*left*) and closer (*right*) view of the pleural cavity in patients with malignant pleural mesothelioma

(Ernst et al. 2002). The diagnostic yield of thoracoscopy using a thoracofiberscope was first reported as 81 % for malignant pleural diseases (McLean et al. 1998). The latest model, the flexi-rigid thoracoscope, provides better diagnostic yields ranging from 89 to 91 % (Munavvar et al. 2007; Ishida et al. 2004, 2005). In addition Ernst (Ernst et al. 2002) and Munavvar (Munavvar et al. 2007) have reported that the flexi-rigid thoracoscope was easy to handle and the image quality was excellent.

Figures 27.4, 27.5, and 27.6 show cases of malignant mesothelioma, dissemination of carcinoma, and tuberculous pleurisy diagnosed by biopsy obtained using a flexi-rigid thoracoscope.

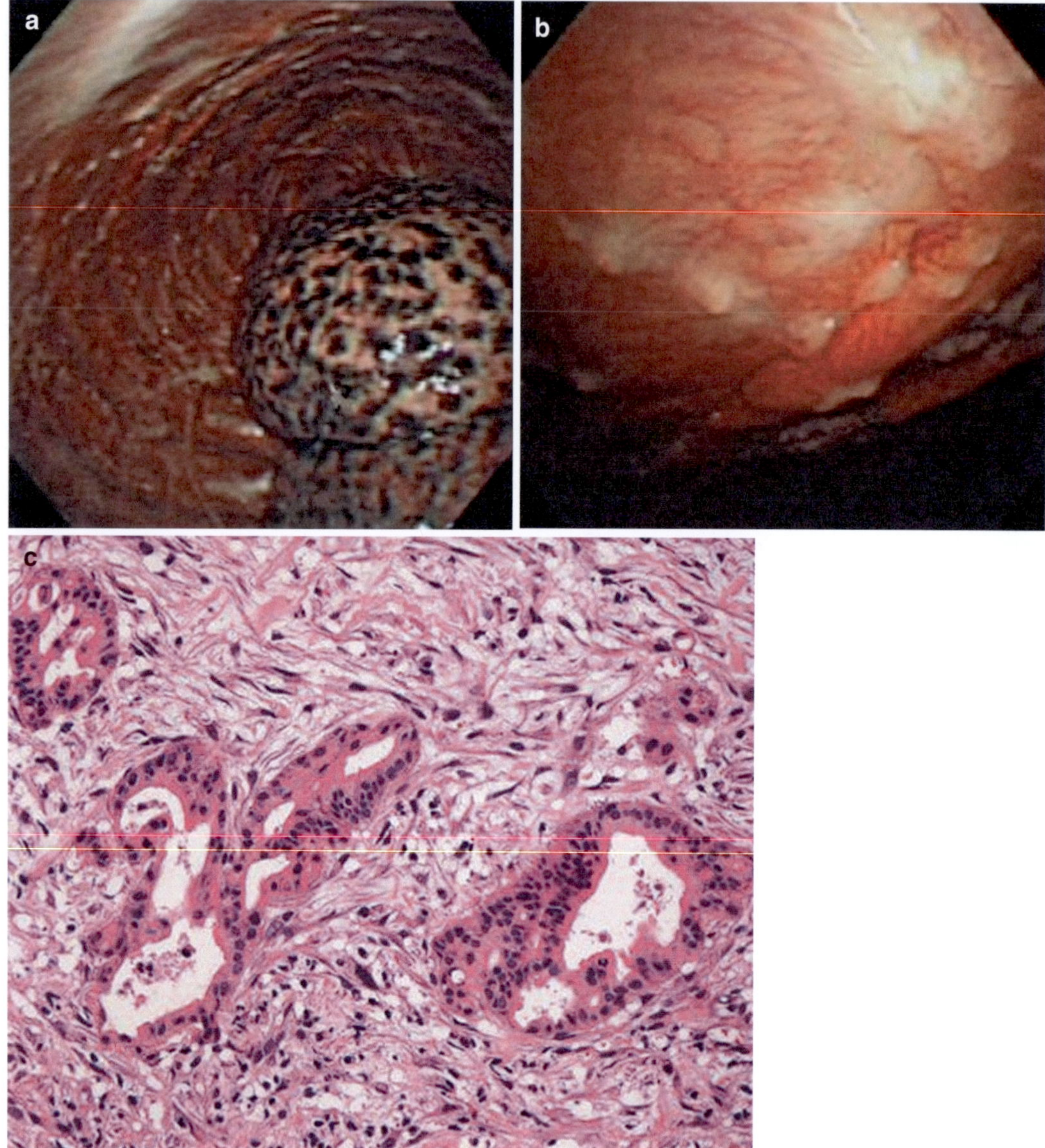

Fig. 27.5 A distant view (**a**) and close view (**b**) of pleural dissemination from a lung cancer inspected by a pleuravideoscope. The small, white nodules are spread over the parietal pleura (**b**). Biopsy samples obtained from the small nodules revealed acinar adenocarcinoma (**c**)

27.7 Complications

McLean (McLean et al. 1998), Ernst (Ernst et al. 2002), and Munavvar (Munavvar et al. 2007) reported that there were no complications for thoracoscopy. However, pulmonologists should be aware of the potential complications associated with thoracoscopy, such as bleeding, hypotension, arrhythmia, desaturation, wound infection, empyema, pneumothorax, reexpansion pulmonary edema, and seeding of the chest wall from mesothelioma.

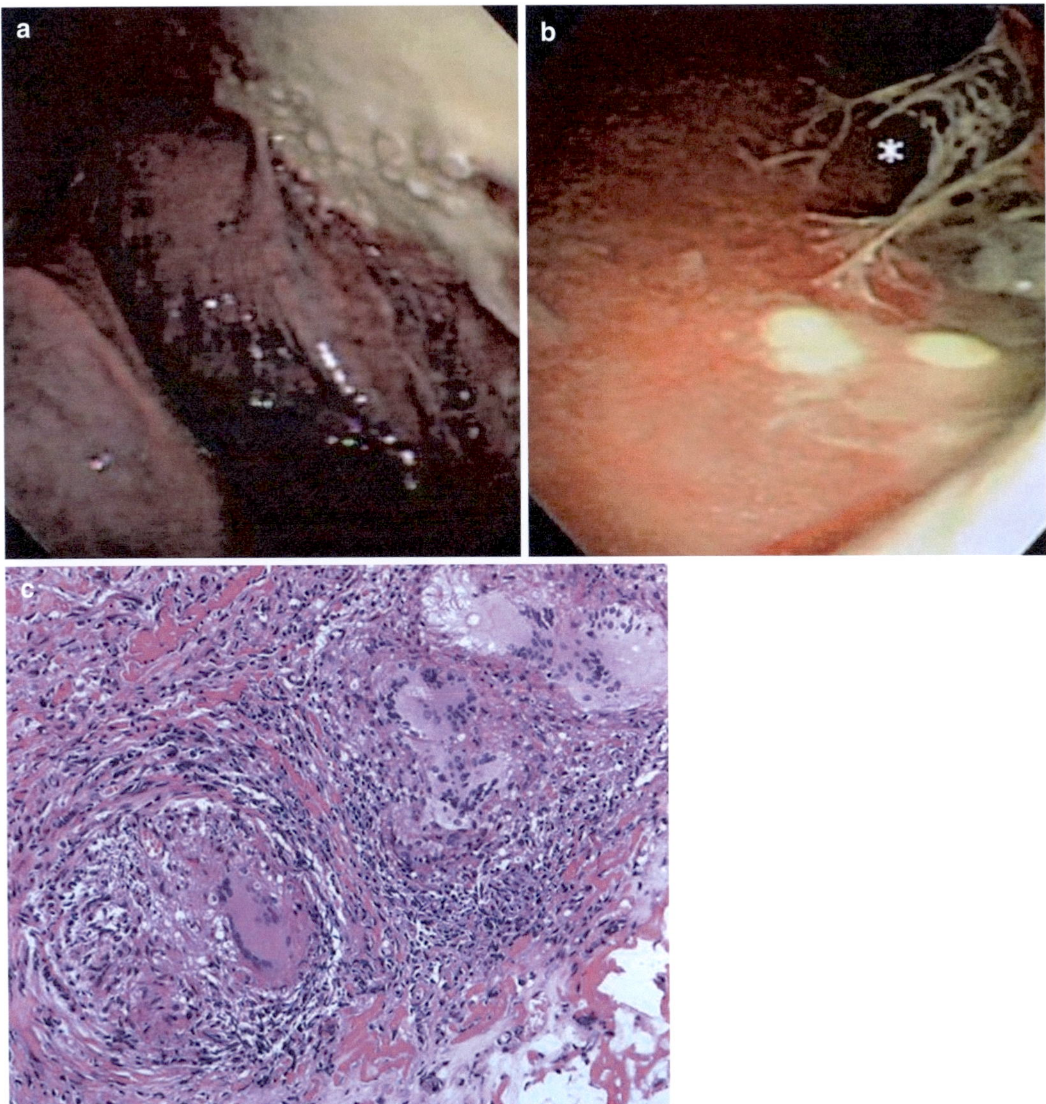

Fig. 27.6 A distant view (**a**) and close view (**b**) of tuberculous pleurisy as inspected by a pleura-videoscope. The close view shows a reddish, rough pleura. Biopsy samples obtained from the pleura revealed granulomatous inflammation with multinuclear giant cells (**c**)

27.8 Limitation

There are some limitations of flexi-rigid thoracoscopy under local anaesthesia. Firstly, the biopsy specimens obtained by the flexi-rigid thoracoscope are smaller compared to samples from rigid thoracoscopy, as they are limited by the size of the flexible forceps, which might result in a lower diagnostic yield. Secondly, since we perform the procedure under local anaesthesia utilizing one port of entry, it may be an inappropriate technique for complicated and/or invasive procedures, such as treatment of empyema and lung biopsy. Although minor adhesions without established blood vessels can be dissected using

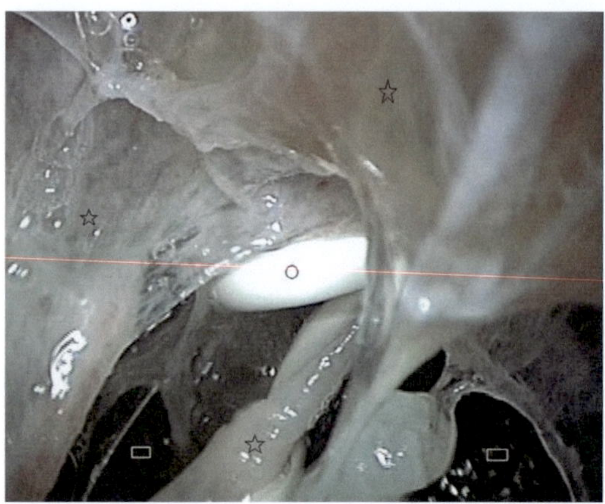

Fig. 27.7 A case of empyema with associated avascular adhesions (☆). The adhesions can be dissected by the pleura-videoscope itself or with flexible biopsy forceps. A pig-tail catheter (O) was previously inserted in the pleural cavity (□) (Courtesy P Astoul – Marseille – France)

the pleura-videoscope and the flexible biopsy forceps (Fig. 27.7), it is our opinion that thick adhesions with blood vessels should not be dissected.

References

Blanc F-X, Atassi K, Bignon J et al (2002) Diagnostic value of medical thoracoscopy in pleural disease. Chest 121:1677–1683

Boutin C, Astoul P (1998) Diagnostic thoracoscopy. Clin Chest Med 19:295–309

Boutin C, Loddenkemper R, Astoul P (1993) Diagnostic and therapeutic thoracoscopy: techniques and indications in pulmonary medicine. Tuber Lung Dis 74:225–239

Colt HG (1995a) Thoracoscopic management of malignant pleural effusions. Clin Chest Med 16:505–518

Colt HG (1995b) Thoracoscopy. A prospective study of safety and outcome. Chest 108:324–329

Davidson AC, George RJ, Sheldon CD et al (1988) Thoracoscopy: assessment of a physician service and comparison of a flexible bronchoscope used as a thoracoscope with a rigid thoracoscope. Thorax 43:327–332

Ernst A, Hersh CP, Herth F et al (2002) A novel instrument for the evaluation of the pleural space: an experience in 34 patients. Chest 122:1530–1534

Ishida Λ, Iwamoto Y, Miyazu Y et al (2004) Diagnosis of tuberculous pleurisy using a flexirigid thoracoscope. J Bronchol 11:29–31

Ishida A, Miyazawa T, Miyazu Y et al (2005) Medical thoracoscopy using a flexirigid thoracoscope in the diagnosis of pleural effusion of unknown cause [abstract]. Chest 128(Suppl):320S

Jacobaeus HC (1910) Über die Möglichkeit, die Zystoskopie bei Untersuchung seröser Höhlungen anzuwenden. Münch Med Wschr 40:2090–2092

Lee P, Colt HG (2005) Rigid and semirigid pleuroscopy: the future is bright. Respirology 10:418–425

Loddenkemper R (1998) Thoracoscopy: state of the art. Eur Respir J 11:213–221

McLean AN, Bicknell SR, McAlpine LG et al (1998) Investigation of pleural effusion: an evaluation of the new Olympus LTF semiflexible thoracofiberscope and comparison with Abram's needle biopsy. Chest 114:150–153

Munavvar M, Khan MA, Edwards J et al (2007) The autoclavable semirigid thoracoscope: the way forward in pleural disease? Eur Respir J 29:571–574

Robinson GR 2nd, Gleeson K (1995) Diagnostic flexible fiberoptic pleuroscopy in suspected malignant pleural effusions. Chest 107:424–429

Tsukamoto T, Nakamura H, Satoh T et al (1991) Comparative studies using a rigid thoracoscope and fiberoptic bronchoscope to treat spontaneous pneumothorax. Chest 100:953–958

P. Astoul et al. (eds.), *Thoracoscopy for Pulmonologists*,
DOI 10.1007/978-3-642-38351-9, © Springer-Verlag Berlin Heidelberg 2014